TRAUMA AMONG OLDER PEOPLE

TRAUMA AMONG OLDER PEOPLE

Issues and Treatment

**Leon Albert Hyer, PhD, and
Steven James Sohnle, PsyD**

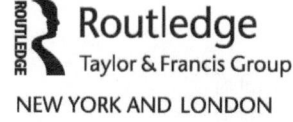

Routledge
Taylor & Francis Group

NEW YORK AND LONDON

First published 2001 by BRUNNER/MAZEL

This edition Published 2014 by Routledge
605 Third Avenue, New York, NY 10017
4 Park Square, Milton Park, Abingdon, Oxon OX14 4RN

First issued in paperback 2014

Routledge is an imprint of the Taylor & Francis Group, an informa business

Copyright © 2001 Taylor & Francis.

TRAUMA AMONG OLDER PEOPLE: Issues and Treatment

Cover design by Robert Williams

A CIP catalog record for this book is available from the British Library.

Library of Congress Cataloging-in-Publication Data
Hyer, Leon Albert.
    Trauma among older people: issues and treatment/ Leon Albert Hyer, Steven Sohnle.
    p.cm.
    Includes index.
    ISBN: 1-58391-081-6 (case: alk.paper)
    1. Post-traumatic stress disorder. 2. Mentally ill-aged--Care. I. Sohnle, Steven.
    II. Title.

RC522.P67 H945 2000
618.97'68521--dc21   00-063057
                                                                CIP

ISBN 13: 978-1-58391-081-8 (hbk)
ISBN 13: 978-0-415-76339-4 (pbk)

To Pete Hyer
and
Ray Saucer,
a couple of WWII vets
who knew trauma

PREFACE

This book is about trauma in a select population, older people. This is important because this group is usually given short shrift because of certain convictions about age, as well as an excessive emphasis on specific trauma-related techniques. In fact, the older group is complex when it comes to trauma. There is much to be exported about older people from knowledge of earlier ages, and there is much that is not. Our basic belief is that the human change process is highly individualized at later life but certainly understandable within an integrated formulation of the person. We address this "formulation."

We have 12 chapters. This is our "Owner's Manual for PTSD at Later Life." In Chapter 1, we are interested in facts on aging as they relate to trauma, a good enough understanding of age. Of course we are interested in trauma, especially post-traumatic stress disorder (PTSD), and we are interested further in the interface of these two: How/where/why do aging and trauma play together. Hopefully this sets the stage for the later chapters on aging, trauma, and its assessment and treatment.

If the first chapter is about aging, Chapter 2 is about PTSD, in general and as it applies to aging. We address all the usual suspects—definitions, changes, types, theories, moderators, trajectory, and comorbidity, among others. We are impressed with the vast array of information available and the almost total lack of discussion of this disorder in both the aging and PTSD literature. Nonetheless, an understanding of the "emotional memory" of the PTSD experience in a chronologically advanced person is important. We provide a primer on this area.

In Chapter 3 we address the self, that strange brew of personhood that organizes life in an interesting way at later life and has some teeth. We also redress what are the needed self-experiences for understanding in a trauma context. Above all, this chapter is about processes of the person, the self components of self-making. Perhaps this is most parsimoniously viewed as modular, but confessing truths from the position of an organized self, sometimes frail, sometimes wise. Of course, in our discussion of self we are considering memory, a series of memories around which the self congeals. Memories are more than a ragbag of events, as the self provides coherence and continuity. At later life, the dream is meaning of a life lived, placing the mystery of life in context and showing the road to humanity through generativity. While there are limits in these strengths, the self through memories does this.

Trauma disrupts this. Chapter 3 morphs to Chapter 4. The narrative is one form of memory, the autobiographical memory. Telling a story about an event is the event in an interesting form, even if negative. Events that play a significant part in one's life become part of the autobiographical memory and may then be used to form part of a life narrative, which is one basis for self-identity. Many things both internal and external to the person influence this process. In Chapter 4 we talk about this—memory as a whole, memory as it is influenced by aging, the autobiographical memory, memory as it relates to trauma, and memory as it relates to PTSD. With trauma, memory processes are uniquely affected at the levels of encoding, storage, retrieval, and recounting.

Over the past two decades we have seen a robust explosion of treatments for trauma. We address many of these but play our cards close to the aging vest. In Chapter 5 we address the treatment of PTSD, overall, as well as provide entrée into the care of older people, older trauma victims. It is the older victim that gives us pause. Again, there is something complex and different about them and their care.

By exposing the field, we attempt to lull the reader into the conviction that treatment can only come in select forms. We give those forms in Chapter 6, the core ingredients of care. These are the sometimes orthogonal, sometimes dependent, and sometimes interdependent curative elements of the treatment process at later life. These are the building blocks on a psychotherapy of older people, especially trauma treatment.

In Chapter 7 we present a model for therapy for older trauma victims. Yes, this is where we have been going and it comes in Chapter 7. In a sense this writing becomes an easy task, as the groundwork is in place. This model of care is intended to provide structure with flexibility: Deal first with perturbation and practical issues, do all the necessary educative and normalizing, coping/social support things, and then attack trauma issues. Above all, we are practical in the treatment of the older victim. In trauma therapy, a balance is always sought between a stable self-capacity and exposure to the traumatic memory, so as not exceed the therapeutic window. That therapeutic window is carefully read at the beginning of therapy with a broad brush. The treatment model has six parts. Here we address the model itself with a special emphasis on the first three components.

We continue with the model of care. Chapter 8 addresses the issue of personality, personality overall, and its problems and use in the context of trauma and aging. Specifically we consider the Millon model and discuss how this interpretation of a person assists in the knowing and caring for clients. Our goal here is not the reconstruction of character, although this is possible, but to provide strategies and tactics for treatment. Knowledge of personality is the best way, we believe, for an understanding and outline of the care of a person victimized by trauma. Because so much of the trauma experience is management, then so much of the treatment is dictated by an understanding of the person(ality).

In Chapter 9 we discuss the treatment of memories. This chapter and the next one are bookends. Here we are interested in core memories that are not trauma-based. Positive core memories (PCMs) are positive and enabling. We just need to understand the way to expose and use these. Use of a client's healthy memories is also helpful. Traditionally, these have not been considered in the treatment of trauma victims to any extent.

In some ways Chapter 10 is the centerpiece of the book. In this chapter we provide techniques for the trauma memory. We include exposure and assimilative techniques, relaxation, and re-narration. The core of our treatment is anxiety management training (AMT) and eye movement desensitization and reprocessing (EMDR). Finally, we highlight issues that are critical for success: booster sessions/relapse prevention, and the broader focus of care, the caretaker/family. These technologies provide the "close-to-critical" material for change. As we have done in many previous chapters, we consider the influence of aging in this mix first.

In Chapter 11 we discuss the importance of grief treatment. Grief is always applicable in trauma. We argue that the traditional approaches to grief are too restrictive. A critical component in the treatment of trauma involves the issues of loss in the trauma re-experience. We outline tenets for the understanding and treatment of PTSD with its grief components. This is highlighted by the hypothesis that the person is best understood in the context of the stored memories that form their identity (as mentioned, a crucial aspect of the self-theory). Treating trauma is insufficient; treating the person and their self-theory is required. We also present a model of the processes and steps involved in grief treatment. In written form this model may seem simplistic and "canned," but it possesses enough abstraction, generality, and flexibility so that respect for the person of the victim can be maintained while still providing a road map for treatment.

Chapter 12 considers assessment, which we save for last. Perhaps our cart is before our horse. We believe that PTSD more than any other disorder requires an understanding of what is going on (i.e., assessment). This provides perspective, flexibility, caring interventions, and monitors for care. We discuss the necessary substratum for an understanding of the trauma victim (i.e., assessment). This begins with assessment, both PTSD and aging. We address each, including their commingling.

☐ Perspective

Our model of trauma includes what other books have—a discussion of pre-individual vulnerability (and resilience) characteristics, the particulars of the stressor, and post-exposure mediating variables. Work on trauma is crowded with "new understandings" on its mechanisms of care. We agree that first (but not foremost), PTSD is a disregulation of biology, in the release of endogenous stress-related neurohormones (e.g., epinephrine and norepinephrine, serotonin, hormones of the HPA access) and endogenous opioids. In fact, PTSD victims often seem to have impaired cortical control over the subcortical areas responsible for learning habituation and stimulus discrimination. Just as important, PTSD consists of painful memories as well as memories of pain. That is to say a memory of the past is essentially painful and the remembering is painful. The content and the experience are in cohoots. Information processing deficits are directly implicated. Trauma-related experiences are stored in memory in a hierarchically organized network (or schema) and are easily triggered by trauma-related clues. The result is greater accessibility of trauma memories and integrated programs of conditioned emotional responses (e.g., physiological reactivity), which leads to an allocation of attention to potentially threatening stimuli in the environment. Trauma-related stimuli are preferentially processed leading to greater interference during normal tasks. Ultimately, individuals respond to trauma events by their own interpretation and by the perceived implications (of the trauma events). Ultimately, core expectations about self (schemas and personality) are disrupted during trauma, resulting in a distortion of cognitive/emotional processing, and not an objective representation of reality.

Then there is PTSD-specific anxiety, the one that gets all the press. This occurs when the individual anticipates future negative events or catastrophic consequences of imagined action but reacts to these in the present as though they were actually occurring now. In this situation, fear is evoked in response to the catastrophic expectation and the appraised threat. Because the person realistically appraises the current situation as safe, however, the fear response is appraised as inappropriate, the action tendency associated with the response (e.g., running away) is prevented, and the person experiences anxiety. The person is mobilized for action but interrupts its expression, often by interfering with breathing, constricting muscles, and not moving.

These core PTSD processes apply to older people. But there is also more. Trauma taps into attachment anxiety and is experienced as a basic ontological insecurity. This is a more global form of anxiety in which the person's sense of coherence and intactness as a functioning self is threatened. Here there is an experience of threat and vulnerability to basic self-organization. When this threat to basic self-organization occurs, the ongoing supportive quality of the therapeutic bond is crucial in helping the person to affirm a sense of self and internalize the therapist's support. The support allows for a calming of the self and the ability to provide support for action from within.

PTSD at later life is not a reaction of a scared person at age 75 with an acute fear. It is a life span reaction of 365 days times 75 on dimensions that we are just beginning to understand. To understand a bone fracture in late life, one must consider inadequate peak bone mass early in life, accelerated bone loss due to menopause at midlife, and physical inactivity in later life. To understand PTSD we also need an archeological telescope, but one that has common sense.

Above all, this book is about treatment. Treatment of the trauma victim requires an integrated approach, a considered attack on the curative elements of exposure and assimilation. For exposure, the process of meaning alteration occurs best in a person that is involved (aroused); for assimilation, renarrative repair and coherence must occur. Yes, these are staples of trauma. At later life, however, the assimilation process seems to be more equal: Trauma beliefs infect the process of living and the balance of the person is realigned. We need to re-realign these beliefs and to address the "living," and we need an understanding of the person. This takes a model.

To belabor this point, psychotherapy for the trauma victim is many things but it is always phenomenological, and psychotherapy for the older victim is always common-sense practical. For discussion, the many variants of therapies can be placed on a gradient ranging from "more core" to "less core." For the former, the emphasis is on cognitive content and specific behavior or cognitive techniques. The emphasis then is accessible thoughts, images, and eventually behavior. The "less core" involves the practicalisms of life, made necessary at later life. Therapists are most often apostles of permissiveness and self-tolerance. They do this well. Treatment of PTSD at later life requires more.

Finally, we bring up one more thing. The trauma victim is potentially transformed in this experience when there is an optimum level of frustration allowing for at least some disintegration, restabilization, and growth. Within this growth-healing we posit that adversity does make a person confront self as in no other way. We believe that this is best done at later life.

☐ Psycho-philosophy

As humans, we have not changed that much in the last 2000 years. But we do get older. Private moments of knowing always matter most. When they happen they become, as Fulgum said, "holy ground." These are the integrating moments that are hard to talk about—like dreams. But we know these and their importance—we are not crazy or superhuman. We are doing what we do. We believe that trauma actually makes this more real. Perhaps people should worry not so much that these events might occur, but that they might not.

In aging there is a distinction between managing the patient and curing the disease. In this book, we are most interested in the former. It has been said that there are four existential crises in life (Plutchick, 1997): (a) hierarchy (Where do I fit in on the salient dimensions of life?), (b) territoriality (What part of the world is mine?), (c) identity (Who am I?), and (d) temporality (How much time do I have left?). Trauma brings problems in all. At later life, however, the chief governor is temporality, the one that pushes issues and ushers in self-reflection. In this book, we dance between aging and trauma and highlight a care model that applies at later life, one based on the science of living.

In fact, treating older folks with trauma problems is not unlike the treatment of a rehabilitation patient with permanent damage. That is, the aim is not cure but the acceptance of a new life. It is an internal process of change and self-transformation so that the world can be accepted on somewhat new terms. Life is not deprived of meaning: It now needs to accommodate to the existential changes that are now a part of life. The battle, if you will, is not between the therapist and patient (resistance), but between the old and new self. This can be quite a battle.

☐ Post Script: A Confession

We started out writing this book with some understanding of trauma from the perspective of that older group in our culture who led the way in PTSD for older people, the combat veteran. Research and clinical experience as well as other studies indicate that veterans from wars experience PTSD symptoms, even decades after the war. Over time, we have expanded this knowledge and have fashioned a much broader book. This is now about trauma at later life.

We also are mini-iconoclasts: We downplay the necessity of the prescriptive role of our diagnostic system and more clearly seek to balance the person in life. This is beyond the treatment tasks of matching client coping strategy with an intervention and more directed to the "righting" of a life style with choice and behavior. The right treatment at the right time in the life of the older person is important. We seek a blended landscape of healing and growth.

We attempt to walk that line between the lighter side—science—and the heavier side—the pulp fiction of the day-to-day response of the trauma victim. We use the words *patient, client,* and *old folks,* among others, liberally and, where appropriate, interchangeably. We do this with an aging population, an area also where information and misinformation vie for conquest. We walk the line then between the bundled, "integrated" packaging of the managed care world and the unbundled and visionary treatment equations of real people with trauma problems. Thomas Moore (1999) says: "Care of the soul observes the paradox whereby a muscled strong-willed pursuit of change can actually stand in the way of substantive transformation" (p. 19).

We also are underrepresented with the use of cases. We do this for reasons of space, as well as the nature of the content that we provide. We invite the reader, therefore, to fill in between the lines. We solicit an active reader.

CONTENTS

CHAPTER 1

Aging and Trauma

"After the first death, there is no other."
Dylan Thomas

Trauma has been labeled as the "soul" of psychiatry (van der Kolk & McFarlane, 1996). During the past decade it has become the most intriguing and studied construct to evolve in mental health. Trauma is ubiquitous. To expect victims of trauma, any trauma, to walk away from the experience as whole people would be unreasonable (Hyer, 1994a). They stand intruded upon with aspects of their personhood eroded. Perhaps the biggest problem of trauma is that it upsets the illusion of a purposeful life. Trauma symptoms are sufficiently prevalent and intrusive as to become a major concern for mental health practitioners, giving rise to myriad pathologies, ranging from subclinical symptoms to full-blown psychiatric disorders.

The study of trauma in older people, especially the diagnostic syndrome post-traumatic stress disorder (PTSD), is fraught with problems related to developmental issues and lifespan patterns, rendering uncontaminated facts hard to come by. Complications are present, related to the nature of trauma and aging decline, to cohort issues, and to the natural transition from an acute to chronic status (of trauma). Often in an almost imperceptible way older people downwardly adapt to meet the needs of life changes. The intimate relationship between symptoms and the unique and complex experience of the individual is lost (van der Kolk, 1996).

There have been major alterations over the 20+ year history of PTSD. In the beginning, for example, the fact of a trauma was considered the principle component in the understanding of psychopathology. Now there is a virtual smorgesboard of elements that cause, moderate, mediate, and influence the experience. The components of the trauma have actually become less important and, in some circles, irrelevant. The fact of trauma has now been found mooring in the role of meaning attached by the person to the traumatic event. It is conventional now to argue (Green, 1991) that the trauma response is a function of: the individual (personality variables), considerations of the trauma itself, and the mediating influences of the recovery process.

In all of this however, the predicament of older people has been wanting or absent altogether. When the aging process is added to the mix, the trauma response is not so easily separated. Where the influence of trauma on aging is concerned, disruptions in lifespan transitions result and alter the acquisition and integration of developmental competencies (Pynoos, Sternberg, & Goenjian, 1996). Like a deathbed confession, trauma needs to be heard and is not very poetic in its expression. If listened to, the voice of trauma can be heard in every part of a person's life and echoes throughout the lifespan. Influencing development, disrupting expectancies and competencies, juggling transition points, and disturbing biological maturation, trauma has much to say in how a life unfolds. The very soul of the person is affected.

It is at the interface of aging and trauma that we seek more clarity. We juggle both issues. If there is simplicity, it is that we believe the operative concerns of trauma are more a function of factors relevant to the variables related to trauma (PTSD) when we consider treatment and more about aging when we consider assessment and the context of care. Regarding treatment, most issues affecting younger trauma groups play similar roles in the experience of the elderly when we address the trauma memory. In this way, we argue then for the "continuity position" as far as the influence of aging is concerned. However, when we address the issues of care in the broader sense, we talk about aging. An understanding of the needs of an older trauma victim rests to some extent then on chronological status and to some extent on a practical knowledge of psychiatric disorders or disordered responses to life (trauma responses). As in any therapy where the more the person knows about the therapy, the better the chances for success, so too the therapist well-versed in the concatenations of aging and trauma is more likely to succeed. It is important to note here too at the outset that this understanding of trauma at older ages is in its infancy (Gurian & Miner, 1991).

This is really a book about therapy that attempts to manage a person of the trauma victim who is older. In this process we attempt to apply what is known about the elderly and trauma. We are interested most in the interface of these two: How/where/why do aging and trauma play together? In this chapter we are interested in aging first, as it relates to trauma, especially PTSD, and the synergistic shadow cast by the interaction of the two. In Chapter 2 we address PTSD first, with aging as the context. Naturally we are carving nature at its joints too finely. The first section isolates key elements of aging, given trauma. Next, we address the key trauma elements of trauma that are intimately related to aging. We then address key moderating variables of trauma and then issues of aging and treatment. Hopefully this will set the stage for later chapters on aging, trauma, and its assessment and treatment.

☐ Good Enough Understanding of Aging

Our culture is reforming by the revolution of the rising demographic tide. The annoying issue, who is old, aside, in due time the crest of the baby boomers will constitute 20% of the population of the United States (Albetes et al. 1997). The fastest growing age group in the United States is the aged, especially those individuals age 85 and older. Neugarten and Neugarten (1994) described the changing age distribution of the population, in which the proportion of old to young is rapidly increasing. At the turn of this century, 1 out of 25 persons in the United States was age 65 or older. Today it is about 1 in every 8. By 2020, when the baby boom will have become the senior boom, it is expected to be 1 in every 6, or even 1 in every 5. By 1985, approximately 70% survived until age 65 and 30% lived to be 80 or more. Now half of all deaths occur after age 80. This trend marks a revolutionary change in human history. There are more older persons and they are older than in previous generations (Siegler, 1994).

Box 1-1 is an effort to downsize "our" components of aging. It is a short summary of relevant facts of aging, loosely related to trauma. Perhaps Einstein's question of life is most relevant to many of the items. He wanted to know the answer to this important question: "Is the universe a friendly place or not?" Most older people have an answer here: It is. Older people are happy, varied, and in possession of considerable experience. They are also not, by and large, passive in the pursuit of tasks. Aging is more an opportunity than a "crisis in slow motion" (Weinberg, 1970).

The developmental process is basically the same in adults as in children: adult development is an ongoing, dynamic process, that there is a continuous and vital interaction between childhood and adulthood; developmental processes are influ-

---

Box 1-1
Age-Related "Facts"

1. Most older people rate life satisfaction high. Even though health-related difficulties increase with advancing age, of persons aged 65 to 74, over 80% report no limitations in carrying out these daily activities; of those 75 to 84, more than 70% report no such limitations; and of those over age 85, half report no limitations.
2. Life-span perspective has multiple interactions (social, biological, and psychological aspects of development). It is frequently pointed out that these issues may have greater interactive consequences with advancing age.
3. In contrast with early development, where knowledge of age provides developmental benchmarks, in later life age itself contains relatively less information. A major difference between theories of child development and adult development is that the former generally try to account for well-known phenomena, and the latter try to point out phenomena to be explained. Whereas childhood development is focused on formation of psychic structure, adult development is concerned with the continuing evolution of existing psychic structure.
4. Interindividual variability is maximal at later life. Pick an attribute (e.g., intelligence, income), the distribution of scores for older adults will overlap to some extent the distribution of scores for younger adults and show more variability.
5. Cohort is as important as age. Cohort refers to the generation into which the person was growing up and growing older in a particular time in history. All we know about stress at later life, we learned from this current older group.
6. The older individual is not simply the passive recipient of events and changes. The individual is an actor in his or her own life, coping and managing.
7. The older the organism, the longer it will take to return to baseline. Not all physiological functions decline with age and not all age related physiological changes result in disease.
8. Disease is most often chronic. The average older person has 3.5 diseases and fills 13 prescriptions annually (Albert, 1989). Common diseases in later life do not start there; thus a life span developmental perspective may be helpful.
9. Chronological age is not the most important factor of adjustment: It may be more important to consider the age of the disease. This applies to chronic diseases as well as psychological stress.

enced by a person's adult past as well as his or her childhood; and physical processes and the awareness of death are central phases that affect psychological expression in adulthood (Colarusso & Nemiroff, 1981; Nemiroff & Colarusso, 1990). In this regard, aging is a highly individualized process. More variability is found at later life on just about every dimension than at other age periods. Because the aged are a heterogeneous group, generalizations should be made cautiously. Along the way people struggle to make sense out of what happens to them, to provide themselves with a sense of continuity and order. People also age at different rates and in various ways. An ipsative lifespan course of unique events and stressors occurs for each person (Lazarus & DeLongis, 1983). Multiple causation—the accumulation of stressors and the concurrent weakening of the person due to age—is considered a basic rule of living. It is also a basic rule in trying to understand the life course.

But older people do poorly relative to younger groups. Three hypotheses have been offered as explanations of aging (Salthouse, 1994). None appear apt. First is the speed. Speed slows with age. This a fact. Peripheral or motor processes decline with age and thereby a decline in cognitive status occurs. However the cause of the decline is not speed by itself as the time on task and signal detection tasks (where central and peripheral tasks are differentiated) show that time required to reach a solution is not just a function of a perceptual motor process deficit. Second, the disuse hypothesis holds that tasks are not exercised enough. If so, then tasks that are continually performed should show small or no declines; however, data show that adults forget meaningful stories systematically with age. In addition, tests high in ecological validity have been found to decrease with age, even when prompted. Additionally, older adults do worse than younger adults remembering familiar sayings, the source of acquired information, and in overlearned actions. In fact, even people in mentally demanding occupations (e.g., faculty professors) perform less well than younger matched participants. Third, the changing environment hypothesis holds that, because with each generation the environment changes, the older cohort is "punished" in tasks because they are less familiar with the tasks or at least its context. This is the cohort effect. These are people with the same environmental and sociocultural influences. But again, data (from the Schaie Seattle Longitudinal Study in 1983) are persuasive. Cohort factors are not responsible for many of the age-related changes on mental abilities tests seen in cross sectional studies because equivalent age-related differences also occur in comparison within the same birth cohort.

The life span implies continuity. On the whole, modifications follow directly from integrating knowledge of life-span development, normative life events, and normal age-related changes with what the astute clinician already knows and practices. To the extent that there are adaptations to be made, they have their basis more in the particular client and the particular attribute inspiring the adaptation (from visual impairment to lack of familiarity with psychotherapy) than in chronological age per se. As implied, discontinuity or a greater respect for issues of aging applies more to assessment than interventions of care (e.g., Knight, 1986; Zarit, Eiler, & Hassinger, 1985).

Of course, the question about aging and health is critical: When a person's age is known, what does one know about that person? Disease exists. Problems at later life are likely to be chronic (rather than acute). This also applies to trauma. Trauma is likely at earlier ages and its residuals are likely to be carried over extended periods of time. Stress is chronic because it represents an accumulation of daily insults (hassles) or negative life events whose effects remain beyond their time (usually one year). Past them is prologue, that is, past psychiatric symptoms are crucial to the understanding of current problems; past problems account for the majority of the variance of a "now understanding."

What we have discovered simplistically is that what distinguishes people who develop trauma problems from people who are acutely stressed and recover is that they start organizing their lives around trauma. A qualitatively different type of reaction ensues in which the primary concern is to survive in order to preserve resources. This is modal "PTSD at later life" and often is a chronic and subclinical form. The variations of a given disorder are very individual and intrinsically idiosyncratic. This is especially true at older ages.

A difficult problem facing advocates of adult development theories is simply defining the field of study. Should we focus on ego styles, interpersonal behaviors, social support, life stories, and so on? What exactly would adult development be? However, psychological development continues throughout life. Hopefully something challenging is implied in an understanding of trauma and later life. At present we know enough about trauma and enough about aging to make both understandable and hopeful.

In light of these factors, we address several issues that are summarized in Box 1-1. This represents our "good enough" understanding of aging as it applies to trauma. We note too that what we know about aging may apply only to the current cohort of older folks. The extent to which age differences also reflect generational differences is not known. So the "individuals now old" may have little to do with the individuals who will be old in 20 years. We know all we know about aging form the current cohort of elders.

The Subjective Nature of Trauma

Trauma is subjective. It is a negotiated product. It is appraised. Whereas other researchers hold that trauma is an objective external condition (Harvey, 1996), Lazarus (1984, 1990) argued that the "stress process" is a transaction between the person and the environment in which the person's psychological resources are taxed or exceeded. Thus, in his model, the source of the stressor is not in the environmental events per se, but in the appraisals made by the person that he or she is being harmed, threatened, or challenged by an event. In fact, the stress response is commonly thought to represent a transaction between the individual and the environment. The most widely cited definition (of stress) is that of Lazarus and Folkman (1984): "Stress is a particular relationship between the person and the environment that is appraised by the person as taxing or exceeding his or her resources and endangering his or her well being" (p. 19).

This definition emphasizes stress (and trauma) as a subjective event. That is, simply knowing an event occurred is not enough to determine what impact it has on an individual; one must also know how it has been appraised. According to Lazarus, once a person has appraised a transaction as stressful, coping processes are used to manage the person–environment relationship.

In fact, as we shall later discuss, both positions and negative events and affects co-occur commonly in people. Folkman (2000) muses that perhaps the more appropriate question is, "How do people keep sane?"

Trauma and "Aging" Filter

Older age implies a filter notably for the better. Elder and Clipp (1989) concluded that compared with younger individuals, the elderly suffer the same, or even lower, rates of PTSD and other psychological symptoms when exposed to severe trauma. He added that premorbid level of psychological functioning and the severity of the trauma are much more important predictors of symptomatology than age. He suggests that "as a group, the elderly (trauma victim) ask less, complain less, and receive less in resources than younger-age ranges of the population" (p. 96). In part, this pattern appears to be due to a reluctance to accept "government handouts." Interestingly, the elderly are more willing to use aid from social agency sources, such as home insurance agencies and the Red Cross or Salvation Army (Green, 1991).

Despite some detractors (e.g., Sandard, 1995), stressful events such as retirement, children leaving the home, death or separation from relatives and friends, physical illness and hospitalization, as well as other precipitating factors, do not seem to potentiate underlying PTSD residual problems that last. But the influence of aging on the effects of a sudden or brief traumatic experience, such as an accident or robbery, has yet to be corroborated.

Despite early reports of increased negative outcomes and consistent findings of increased risk for physical harm among the elderly, the data of the past two decades do not support the hypothesis that older adults are at greater risk than younger adults for negative psychosocial outcome following exposure to natural disasters. Much available data suggest that elderly persons cope as well and at times better than younger adults. If anything, data suggest that age contributes minimally to the prediction of psychosocial outcomes and that variables, such as pre-existing physical and mental health, severity of trauma, and availability of specific resources, are of greater predictive value. There is little empirical evidence that coping mechanisms, cognitive faculties, and affect regulation necessarily deteriorate in later stages of the life. Stressful life events are not sufficient explanations for the re-emergence of PTSD in older trauma survivors. This is not to say that there are no differences in the way in which the elderly experience and respond to a traumatic experience. However, there is insufficient evidence to conclude that disaster causes more negative psychosocial consequences in older adults.

Age and trauma interact. The work of Carolyn Aldwin is most relevant to this issue. Her work upsets the traditional notion that aging causes or results in a diminished capacity to adapt to stress. While several issues related to age and stress are more ambiguous (Aldwin, 1992), Aldwin accepted the idea that changes in sensitivity to stress can occur with advancing age, but she stated that change should not be viewed as a deficit or deterioration. In fact, reactions to stress are indicators of Erikson's notion of generativity. Aldwin adopted a more general view of the generativity trait in considering it as a process whereby an individual becomes more sensitive to events that happen to others in social networks. It is probable that mediating factors are more influential on stress reactions than just age. Older hypertensives, for example, who scored high on measures of neuroticism, endorsed significantly greater somatic complaints than those who scored lower on this index in the presence of stress (Zonderman, Leu, & Costa, 1986).

The question of whether the experience with a previous disaster contributes to a "protective" influence of age (Phifer & Norris, 1989) or not is still in doubt. We know that older age people who successfully adapted to trauma are "predisposed" to do so again (Gibbs, 1989). But we also are told (Lamdou, 2000) that older adults who have survived early trauma retain some long term consequences of early trauma. The overall implication is that older people do well.

The Positive Effects of Trauma

We have intimated then that older people do well with trauma. There is now a growing literature on the positive effects of the perceived benefits of trauma. Simply put, people who have undergone extremely stressful circumstances often report that, in the long run, they have achieved certain benefits, including an increase in mastery, coping skills, and self-knowledge, enhanced social ties, and changes in values and perspectives (for reviews, see Aldwin, 1998, and Tedeschi & Calhoun, 1995). Tedeschi, Park, & Calhoun (1998) coin the phrase post-traumatic growth (PTG) to indicate the increased tendency among researchers to recognize positive change after trauma. Concepts, like resilience, sense of coherence, hardiness, stress innoculation, and toughening populate the landscape of new trauma offerings. This appears to be more than an inoculation to further stress but actually a positive effect of stress. Specific to aging, this was supported by Aldwin, Levenson, and Spiro (1994) who found that the effects of combat exposure during World War II (WWII) and the Korean War on current symptoms of PTSD were attenuated by the perception of benefits from military service. In fact, with older combat veterans Elder and Clipp (1988) found positive outcomes including learning to cope with adversity and self discipline. Of course, negative reactions were also found, especially for older veterans who entered WWII at older ages (Elder, Shanahan, & Clipp, 1994).

In *The Soul's Code*, James Hillman argued that each of us is born with an innate character, a unique way of being and doing. It is the understanding of this character that allows us to become the person we are truly meant to be. In a later book (*The Force of Character*), Hillman argued for the importance of aging. It is in later years that we have the potential to "become more characteristic of who we are." Hillman argued that our culture's tendency to try and deny the sometimes debilitating changes that aging brings is a mistaken impulse. Signs like short-term memory loss and lessening mobility force us to become introspective, to review our lives, and to slow down and take notice of the wonders that surround us every day. These aforementioned signs of weakness allow for the deepening of character. "Aging is no accident. It is necessary to the human condition, intended by the soul." It is, therefore, in the last years that character is confirmed and fulfilled. Perhaps there is a usefulness to suffering in terms of personal development.

Trauma is Hard to Measure

As noted, the experience of stress is a highly individual matter and is thus difficult to measure in a meaningful way. The many complications that accompany aging present myriad stressors (many in the form of loss). As these sources of stress accumulate, the result is a vast array of intertwined issues and it becomes difficult to sort them out.

It is virtually impossible to distinguish between objective and subjective stress indicators on the basis of self-report measures (cf. Aldwin, Levenson, Spiro, & Bosse, 1989). This especially applies to people with personality problems, those "contaminated with neuroticism." Late life is thought to be a time of excess stress, due to bereavement, the loss of social roles, and the advent of chronic illness and subsequent limitations on daily activities, and a time that the elderly report fewer life events on standard inventories.

Box 1-2
Trauma Facts at Later Life

1. Older victims are not worse off as a result of stress.
2. Stress is a subjective experience.
3. Stress at later life has a generativity filter. It is mediated.
4. There are positive effects of stress.
5. Victims at later life react to stress "better" than other age groups.
6. Stress is hard to measure.
7. The best treatment method for older patients with PTSD is unknown.

Inventories that measure loss tend to sample events that are more common to young adults (e.g., divorces, job loss). The earliest approach to measuring stressful life events was the Schedule of Recent Events (SRE) developed by Holmes and Rahe (1967), which contains a list of 43 life change experiences, unrelated to older people. Researchers have criticized the use of these life event scales. Measures that include events that are more common to older adults, such as institutionalization of spouse or divorce of a child, tend to demonstrate little age-related change in the occurrence of life events. This topic is covered in greater depth in Chapter 12.

Best Treatment for PTSD is Unknown

There have been no well-controlled studies of the best methods of treatment for elderly patients who manifest PTSD as a result of trauma suffered years before. Should patients attempt to recapture repressed unpleasant memories after so many years, or is it better for them to try to forget intrusive thoughts? Additionally, the best type of psychotherapeutic treatment—group, individual, or behavioral—has not been determined, nor has the role of psychotropic medication.

In sum, research indicates that older individuals resemble adults of all ages in terms of the impact of stress and preferred ways of coping. If anything, they may be better in the overall reaction to extreme stressors. Older people who do well tend to be average people, those who are healthy enough to cope with disaster, find meaning in trauma, and access inner strength, often for a new beginning (Tedeschi, Park, & Calhoun, 1998) (see Box 1-2).

☐ Moderating Variables of Trauma in the Aging Person

What else do we need to know about the older victims of an excessive stressor? Moderating variables tell us under what circumstances will a stressor lead to, or be associated with, a good or poor outcome. From this knowledge we can direct efforts at treatment. The mixture of the life transition process and the trauma adjustment make for an interesting interaction (Elder & Caspi, 1990; McAdams, 1993). Halligan and Yehuda (2000) suggest that a stress-diathesis model is emerging for PTSD.

Elements of environment, demographics, personality, and psychiatric history as well as genetic and biological influences are cited as risk factors. Even compromised cognitive functioning is seen as a potential contributor.

Characteristics, such as social support, personal resources, and personality traits, become relevant in predicting stress outcomes (Costa & McCrae, 1993). For later life issues, six variables seem especially important: (a) the presence of other stressors, (b) social support, (c) health status, (d) comorbidity, (e) cognitive decline, and (f) personality. To this list, we could add other variables such as age itself as well as gender (Realmuto, Wagner, & Bartholow, 1999), socioeconomic status, and marital status (Bolin & Klenow, 1988). We will consider these important variables in the discussion of the six main variables.

"Hidden and Current" Stressors

Once a stressor has had an impact on the person, the equation alters in terms of adjustment. First, the person may not know that they are experiencing a loss. There are several types of losses, including the many secondary losses that result from a death, for example. These losses can be the role of a partner, a card-playing and paper-reading "buddy," to name a few. Doka (1999) has labeled this phenomenon as "loss without recognition."

Second, older people are vulnerable to the effects of current stressors, many of which may exacerbate latent PTSD symptoms, even after years of being relatively asymptomatic. For most veterans, military trauma remains the most severe stressor throughout the lifetime; for many, however, other recent traumas are rated as more severe (Hyer & Summers, 1995). For those who have experienced a significant trauma and have not placed it into the context of ongoing life, the struggle to contain painful memories can be considerable (Mazor, Gampel, Enright, & Ornstein, 1990) and the likelihood of other stressors (and presumably their influence) is high (Yehuda et al., 1995). So, the identification of the exact loss and the presence of current ones are most important.

We note here that there can be long-term delayed effects of trauma. Clinical studies reveal that survivors of WWII, for example, who were traumatized as children may suffer from a delayed onset or sudden exacerbation of PTSD symptoms during the transition from middle to late life (Bramsen, 1995). These studies are referring to long-lasting severe traumatization.

Social Support

Diagnosis and treatment planning for trauma are inadequate without information on social support. This variable has been implicated in the etiology of PTSD (Barlow, 1988; Flannery, 1990; Lyons, 1991). Arguably, emotional support at the time of the trauma (or shortly after) may be the primary protection against being traumatized (van der Kolk & McFarlane, 1996). In fact, social support probably enhances the emotional processing necessary for integration (Foa & Kozak, 1986). Individuals without extensive social support, then, are at greater risk for disease (e.g., Cohen, 1988).

Interestingly, social support decreases with age, as relatives and friends die, move away, or become seriously ill or incapacitated. Social support also interacts with other variables to either protect or cause problems with adjustment. Kobasa (1979) noted that men who have good social support and internal locus of control did well in regard to suffering from heart attacks than those with neither. Of the two, internal locus of control was more protective. Gatz (1994) also noted that role strains may be as important as the loss itself. Why this is true is unknown, but whatever mechanisms operate they probably do not vary purely as a function of age (Poon & Siegler, 1991). However, social support counts big in the realm of trauma.

Health Status

We are not only dealing with the normal age-associated physical changes. Siegler (1994) noted that theoretical models of aging rarely deal with health and disease. A typical stress model holds that at basal levels, changes in most body systems are slight, and regulatory mechanisms compensate to preserve function. As stress increases, however, the limits of the compensatory processes are reached and breakdown occurs. The most commonly invoked model is the vulnerability model (Dohrenwend & Dohrenwend, 1981). According to this model, exposure to stressors triggers illness onset in already vulnerable individuals.

Regarding just aging, there is considerable biological evidence that suggests that the elderly are less resilient to stresses (Finch & Hayflick, 1977), less physiologically adaptable (Timiras, 1972), have slowed homeostatic-regulatory functions, and are less immunologically competent (Kiecolt-Glaser & Glaser, 1991). There is evidence that health status influences age-related cognitive decline too. The idea that health or disease factors contribute to lower cognitive performance with increased age is plausible, because a variety of diseases have been found to depress the level of cognitive functioning, and the incidence of many diseases tends to increase with age (Salthouse, 1994).

Regarding PTSD, research on the impact of life event stress (more related to PTSD) has also revealed modest, though fairly consistent, relationships between life events and various health indices. Several major models explaining the links between stress and illness have evolved in relation to the study of physical and psychiatric disorders. In regard to PTSD especially, studies have shown that victims reported significantly more illnesses post-assault than non-victims, of females relative to males (Ullman & Siegel, 1996), and male veterans with PTSD compared with matched cohorts without the disorder (e.g., Kulka et al., 1990). In one recent study, Ullman and Siegel examined the relationship of traumatic events to physical health. In a randomized community survey ($N = 2,364$) of Los Angeles residents, they found that 16% had experienced a lifetime traumatic event. Respondents with a traumatic event history indicated poorer perceptions of their physical health, more chronic limitations in physical functioning, and more chronic medical conditions compared with respondents without such a history, while controlling for demographics, psychiatric history, and other stressful life events.

Compromised health status appears to covary with PTSD (Bremner, Southwick, & Charney, 1991). Physical illness and functional impairment increase the degree of stress experienced by these older veterans. There is reasonable evidence for increases in self-reported health, morbidity, and service use following exposure to trauma (Schnurr, 1996). PTSD may even be a mediator affecting health behaviors between trauma and physical health (Schnurr, 1996). This is more obvious for older people as the impact of health status negatively impacts all psychiatric disorders (Gatz, 1994; Haley, 1996).

Finally we note that Row and Kahn (1989) made an important contribution to gerontology in this area. They restated the aging versus disease controversy in terms of risk factor modification. Successful aging in this formulation has different risk factor profiles. Risk factor profiles are related to extrinsic or behavioral aging (rather than intrinsic biological aging) and thus can be modified by changes in behaviors. They call for health promotion and disease prevention interventions, techniques that are central to health psychologists. The research task now is to understand what changes with aging and whether aging is the same in those persons who have specific diseases compared with their peers without disease. Disease-specific data, as with Alzheimer's disease, are important additions to the field. However, it is clear that health status impacts on the trauma experience and vice versa.

Comorbidity

Cormorbidity means two things, the existence of other disorders (traditional comorbidity) and complex PTSD. PTSD is not just a disorder that is comorbid—comorbidity is its natural state (Hyer et al., 1994). In fact, comorbid disorders are probably never truly functionally autonomous with PTSD. Typically around 80% of PTSD sufferers receive an additional diagnosis (Summers & Hyer, 1994). This applies because PTSD cannot be explained by a single pathophysiology. The syndrome of PTSD actually describes abnormalities in a number of clinically distinct domains within the individual, such as memory, mood, bodily experience, interpersonal relatedness, emotion, and behavior.

Depression is a special problem. In later life depression may just be interactive with (Hyer & Stanger, 1997; Lee, Vaillant, Torrey, & Elder, 1995) or significantly related to (Foa & Kozak, 1986) PTSD. Hyer and Stanger tried to argue that, when all is said and done, however, PTSD is an anxiety disorder with depression a necessary part (Hyer & Stanger, 1997). This is what is popularly accepted. However, PTSD and depression do covary, whether as manifestations of the same psychiatric state or distinctive is unfolding. We will address this issue below.

Data on the comorbidity with PTSD apply to other disorders also. This is especially so of substance abuse (Boudewyns, Albrecht, Taylor & Hyer, 1994). In fact, it appears that prior psychiatric symptom level was the stronger predictor of post symptom levels. Smith et al. (1986) found prior psychiatric level to account for 30–40% of the variance of flood victims. In sum, consistent associations have been reported between life events and psychiatric symptomatology, exact prevalence rates (of other disorders) and their influence have yet to be determined.

It is unclear whether comorbidity plays out differently with older folks. It seems not. It is an issue that demands clinical deliberation especially if the effects of trauma have been extended.

Cognitive Decline

Evidence now exists that cognitive decline is present in trauma victims (Bremner et al., 1993; Creamer, Burgess, & Pattison, 1992; Gurvits et al., 1993; Sutker, Bugg, & Allain, 1991; Sutker, Wibstead, Galina, & Allain, 1991; Thygesen, Hermann, & Willnger, 1970; Uddo, Vasterling, Brailey, & Sutker, 1993; Zalewsi, Thompson, & Gottesman, 1994). This is no doubt worse in the older trauma victim. In general, older people experience cognitive decline that influences the processing of information (Salthouse, 1994). Relative to PTSD, Litz and Keane (1989) noted that cognitive processing changes may be found when more sophisticated, higher order neuropsychological instruments were used. Several biologically based studies in both clinical and preclinical populations also suggest that cognitive functions are important in understanding the interaction of psychologic and biologic factors in PTSD (Charney & Heninger, 1986). In addition, memory deficits, amnesia, and concentration problems have been found to load significantly on the construct PTSD (Hyer et al., 1994). That this issue relates to PTSD is evident, but how neuropsychological status affects PTSD is at present unknown. Due to the complexity and confusion of matching cognitive and underlying neurological mechanisms, it is perhaps best to emphasize a distinctive approach to neuropsychological disorders (Stringer, 1996).

Finally, we note that just as in children and adolescents the processing of traumatic memories depends on maturity and understanding, so too it is important to know an aging victim's developmental level. Developmental complexity governs a progressive capacity to integrate sensory information. Different symptoms may represent the reaction to traumatic exposures at different points in development. Many adversities can influence subsequent adjustment. Some examples are caretaking, disturbances in developmental expectations in the acquisition and integration of developmental competencies, the disruption of developmental transitions, disturbances in normal biological maturation and the expression of traumatic expectations and interfering fantasies (Pynoos, Steinberg, & Groetjin, 1996). The cognitive status of the older person, both at the time of the trauma and after, are important and will be addressed again.

Personality

Personality has been implicated in the risk of and expression of PTSD. Hyer and Associates (1994), among many others, discussed the relationship of Axis II disorders to PTSD. People with rigid personality styles or personality disorders (Millon & Davis, 1995) have problems in the negotiation of trauma because of their limited, rigid, defensive organizations. This appears the case with any Axis I disorder. Traits too can have an impact on the expression of related problems such as grief (Lepore, Silver, Cohen, & Wortman, 1995). We believe that, due to trait stability over time, Costa & McCrae (1984) as well as the logical expression of Axis I problems resulting from "trait problems," that personality asserts considerable influence on PTSD. Evidence exists for the influence of more medium or lower level personality variables or stress outcomes. Also, there is evidence that they play a role as potential moderators of stressful events on adaptational outcomes (Solomon, Mikulincer, & Hobfoll, 1987). For example, studies on locus of control (Burgess, Morris, & Pettingale, 1988; Parkes, 1984), self-efficacy (Bandura, 1977), self-confidence (Schaefer & Moos, 1992), optimism (Carver & Gaines, 1987; Scheier & Carver, 1985; Carver, Scheier, & Weintraub, 1989), hardiness (Kobasa, 1979), resilience (McFarlane & Yehuda, 1988), sense of coherence (Antonovsky, 1987), creativity (Strickland, 1989), and intrapsychic strengths (Stutman & Baruch, 1992), Type A personality (see Goleman, 1994; Rhodewalt, Hays, Chemers, & Wysocki, 1984), and neuroticism (McCrae & Costa, 1986; Watson & Clark, 1984) have pointed to the presence of personality factors as modifying the impact of stressors on psychological and physical outcomes. "Person" components influence the stress response.

As in other areas (Rosowsky, Abrams, & Zweig, 1999), the effect of personality on age is now under investigation. On the one hand, there appears to be little or no change in the mean levels of traits in domains of personality in adulthood.

Longitudinal comparisons of personality traits show general stability. On the other, personality disorders moderate and are changed by life changes. Personality "naturally" reformulates to accommodate to the needs of later life. This construct, we believe, is so important that we build it into our trauma model and discuss this in a later chapter.

☐ Older People in Need of Help

Even this late it happens;
The evening of love, the coming of light . . .
Even this late the bones of the body shine
And tomorrows dust flares into breath.
Mark Strand

We wish to make several points about the unique feature of being older and seeking treatment for trauma. First, given problems, older people require considerable effort on the care equation. The biopsychosocial model applies. Age itself presents us with some information on the care equation but often is not the problem (of adjustment). Rather it is the conditions of aging that accompany it. Age may indeed be a "carrier variable" (Leventhal, 1999), as it carries other variables and allows them to be influential at different times. These are the problems of living at later life in our culture. In addition, older people come to therapy because of problems that they have had all their life or current problems of loss or health. Atchley (1991) noted that many older people develop poorer coping strategies that are self-constricting. They just do this as a result of aging. Successful aging is really a full-time job, a life/career choice.

Second, psychotherapy with an older adult is not simply adjustment to current problems of old age (as is often assumed in reviews of therapy with the aged) but is concerned with working through unfinished business from earlier stages of life. Paul Baltes (2000) labels this the aging struggle with incompleteness. People at later life attempt to remedy the defects of aging, physical and psychosocial. Although it is possible for someone to go through all of their life with unresolved identity issues from adolescence, generativity issues from adulthood, or even autonomy issues from childhood, it is not likely. Personal narratives, the stuff of trauma, are not, then, encapsulated intrapsychic constructs, which dwell in splendid isolation within the mind. They are attached to the developmental dialogue of the person and as part of other characters and story-makers (Omer, 1994).

Third, the psychotherapist who treats an older person addresses the fundamental issues of life, assumptions and origins. Carl Jung may be correct in claiming that patients never solve fundamental problems; they outgrow them. But, modern therapists are in the business of facilitating a mellowing process of "life as problem," as well as overcoming the nature of human nature. This is done both with the technology of our therapies and acceptance of the human condition. Unfortunately, there is no easy deliverance from our technologies or easy acceptance of our beings. In psychotherapy with older people the therapist must attend then to the "big" things of living (the essences and meaning of life).

To wax philosophic for a second, at later life one form of anxiety involves existence. To accept life as is, is to transcend loneliness. Aging that is successful entails a series of ego and often practical sacrifices while still saying "yes" to life.

Long have I resisted.
Finally I yielded.
When the old ego disintegrates
the new ego awakens.
Goethe

Done successfully, there is a kind of "egocide" that transforms the person, as one who is on a journey (Boren, 1993). In the context of trauma, good psychotherapy allows the person to appreciate the now by a realization of a life lived.

Fourth, the therapist must also consider the "little" things in life, issues of living in the trenches. We add to this the annoying obsolescence of older ways no longer working. This is the case formulation, the "theory of the client" that can be encompassing. In a consensus statement for the American Psychological Association, Abeles and colleagues (1997) noted that the treatment of choice is a function of the nature of the problem, therapeutic goals, preferences of the adult, and practical considerations. Little things, issues of life, can mean a lot. This is so important that this map of the healing journey must traverse money issues.

Fifth, we argue for an integrated therapy. We are not alone. Regarding older people and therapy, Nordhus, Nielsen, and Kvale (1998) and Bartz and O'Brien (1997), among others, advocate for such a position. Here we highlight the construct personality and petition the therapist to become an integrationist, an orchestra leader who plays every instrument for effect. The therapist does so nomothetically (knowing the science of trauma and aging) and ideopathically (knowing the person). So, the therapist must read interpersonal patterns, as well the symptoms of the patient, and make adjustments, sometimes supportive, sometimes challenging, sometimes directive. The therapist becomes an active caregiver as a well as a psychotherapist. The therapist of the older person indeed is a "new priest."

Sixth, there is no "the elderly." Why are older people even singled out for special consideration? Kastenbaum (1978) has pointed out that a more useful focus might be on specific sub-populations of people, of all ages, with particular types of problems. Therapeutic strategies might be appropriate for depressed persons, widows, people with brain damage, no matter what the age of the individual. In and of themselves the presence of such "negatives" as significant health problems, cognitive slowing, difficulties with memory, or client's place of residence are not reason enough to preclude cognitive therapy, nor to predict treatment failure. As we have intimated, older adults do not show poorer ability than younger adults in semantic processing, strategies for making associations, imagery, or extracting main points from prose material.

As we have argued, for the most part, approaches to psychotherapy and behavior change that were developed for other age groups are also effective with the aged. (The continuity theory of care applies.) Adaptations are made (e.g., psychotherapy is shortened and more focused on immediate reality problems, life review, etc.), but such changes do not represent a fundamental discontinuity of process and technique. Modifications have drawn on what is known about cognition and aging, personality development, and other research literature, as well as the practitioner's direct clinical experience with older adults.

Older folks do not "want" psychotherapy. Problems can be represented in underuse. It is best explained by the concatination of reluctant elders to receive psychiatric care and a reluctant system to provide incentives for such treatment. Take depression as a monitor. As many as 17% to 37% of elderly primary care (PC) patients suffer significant symptoms of depression (Jurte et al., 1999). Up to 70% of patients who meet criteria for depression in PC settings remain unrecognized by generalists (Mulrow et al., 1995). In these clinics it is estimated that $\frac{1}{6}$ patients have depression problems sufficient to result in an altered adjustment and of this number only $\frac{1}{6}$ is diagnosed and treated appropriately.

Why is this so? Perhaps this occurs because primary care physicians don't recognize depression. This may also occur because the older person does not want to admit problems even in this setting. It may be that older people and health care providers "collude" to prevent appropriate psychiatric care in PC settings. Underrecognition is due, then, to the reluctance of the elderly to seek help from the mental health sector (Nadler, Damis, & Richardson, 1997), not being socialized to use psychiatric language (Hasin & Ink, 1988), or, as a group, have a phenomenological experience who appraise self by their physical (and not psychological) health. Negative attitudes for medication as a treatment for depression are also pervasive. Leventhal (1999) found that community-dwelling elders in the Rutgers Aging and Health Study are largely unwilling to seek assistance for depression in geriatric primary care: Elders would not be willing to accept care should they need it. If they did, it would be on a PC setting. However 40% would not speak to anyone about depression if they had problems; only 12% would agree to see a psychiatrist or psychologist. What do you think may happen with PTSD?

Below (Box 1-3) is a "strawman scheme" of therapy positions and probable initial differences as a function of age. Under this schema, older people do not perceive a psychological problem as an opportunity to explore developmental processes. Emotion, for example, is seen as "wrong thinking." Similarly for many younger people resistance and relapse are moments for learning. For many elders these are failures. It is only later in therapy that older people appreciate and can practice the importance

---

Box 1-3
Initial Therapy Positions of the Younger and Older Ages

Issue	Younger	Older
Philosophy	Learning is linear and logical; reality is stable	Learning and development in refinement and transfer of mental processes: existential
Time	Here and now	Here and now and there and then
Control	Demands it	Yields it
Focus	Dynamic	Practical: current problem
Cognition	Prepotent and impulsive	Influential and reflective
Emotion	Information source	Problem
Brain/body	Inseparable	Independent: focus on body
Intervention	Psychological	Medical

of reflection and "knowing about knowing." After socialization the generative and metacognitive issues become important.

One currency of a denial system is somatization. Somatic factors travel with PTSD/depression and vice versa. Older people would rather see psychological problems in the form of physical problems. Avoidance is certainly a part of this. Older people for example can often prevent anxiety attacks by avoidance, often at the cost of greater dependence and disability. In fact, while avoidance is not unique to older folks, a variety of cohort differences that can affect therapy and the client–therapist relationship, including differences in moral values, religious orientations, attitudes toward the family, and tendency to somaticize complaints, does exist.

Being older then is not being particularly psychologically minded. If the chance occurred in life that one were in an idyllic spot and the world was turning slow on that day, the self-actualized person would turn inward. However if you have 70+ years of being practical, of blunting or avoiding, the option to be "inward" is less appealing. For many older people, this is a completely foreign concept. Erikson saw this as foreclosure. It is the weight of many years and considerable learning. Therapy will then require constant vigilance to fight the weight of resistance of therapeutic impact.

☐ Conclusion

The business of trauma is to know: to know how the victim treats his/her inner life, to respect this intrapsychic zone, to reframe this interiority so as to resonate across all levels of the person, and to surface the immense significance of this operation for human choice. These tasks evolve from and are confirmed by the person, not the professional. Mahoney (1991) noted:

> We believe that a current challenge in the field of traumatic stress studies is to avoid the danger of depriving trauma victims of their individuality and uniqueness by focusing exclusively on the commonalities in response patterns among survivors. We must remember that trauma is experienced by persons, not by dehumanized "victims" and their differences, as well as their commonalities, must be respected and understood. (p. 4)

The business of this book is also to know about aging: To know how to balance the person. Wilson and Keane (1997) wrote that recovery from PTSD is a lifelong process. In later life we need to consider the whole life as it is currently and as the past has suggested. We need to respect all parts of the person. And, we have noted, often that older person does not embrace psychotherapy.

PTSD itself is sort of a biopsychosocial happening in which a usual healthful opponent process prevents any exit. It is deviant information processing that involves the overinterpretation of current stimuli as reminders of the trauma, the generalized hyperarousal and difficulty in distinguishing between what is relative and what is not, and a continuation of the use of poor defenses as a way of dealing with related intrusions and other stressors (van der Kolk, 1995). van der Kolk noted that people's life experiences shape the assumptions that determine the perceptions they select in their day-to-day environment. On the basis of severe trauma, the impairment of trust, the lack of a sense of responsibility, negative effects on identity, the impact on play and relationship with others, as well as excessive interpersonal sensitivity along with the compulsion to repeat the trauma, are major problems (van der Kolk, 1995). People cannot go on with their lives. It was Kardiner who noted the deterioration in PTSD, a physioneurosis and a disorder not unlike that of schizophrenia. Not fun!

Regarding older people, there is now an extensive literature that examines the effects of life events, chronic stressors, and daily hassles on older adults' psychological well-being. Older adults experience the full spectrum of stressors; they endure cumulative life crises throughout their personal histories, experience recent life events and losses, and encounter chronic stress brought about by ill health, environmental, and social problems. Tritely we say there are individual differences in this process.

We believe further that trauma forms a context or opportunity for development in adulthood. Trauma may create uncertanties that force individuals to re-examine their assumption system (cf. Epstein, 1991); coping with major stressors may increase an individual's coping repertoire and thus, his or her sense of mastery. It is precisely this increase in knowledge base, coupled with uncertainty, that, Tornstom (1996) argued, was the (dialectical) basis for the development of wisdom in later life. We believe that the older person brings something better to the table of adjustment than those at other ages in this area (of trauma).

In this book we address but do not deliberate on important issues: of how older individuals compare to younger ones; the biology of acute and chronic stress; the neurophysiologic, hormonal, immunologic, sleep, or other changes observed with severe stress; the effect of poor physical health on the manifestation of PTSD symptoms; the influence of developmental issues of late life on the occurrence and nature of PTSD symptoms; how previous life experiences predispose to or protect against the development of PTSD in elderly individuals who are exposed to severe stress; and whether the treatment for PTSD in the elderly differs from the treatment for younger patients.

We do seek the "truth" of PTSD as it applies to the elderly, the older victim. PTSD has several characteristics that "transcend" the Diagnostic and Statistical Manual of Mental Disorders (American Psychiatric Association, 1994) description. We are very interested in these differences. The map is not always the territory: PTSD demands further explanation. Certainty is of course illusory but may actually stifle dialogue. All communication must be placed on a continuum of inferential content. There is some inferential content in all facts, lots on issues of older people.

Finally at later life we know this also: There exists an inexorable gravitational pull of death and dissolution. There is an intrinsic mutagenic process. This is after all the most compelling part of old age.

PTSD in the Context of Aging

*"Style is knowing who you are, what you want to say, and not
giving a damn."*
Gore Vidal

In the last chapter we considered aging with PTSD as a backdrop. This chapter is about PTSD and its legacy, as well as the context and backdrop of aging. If we can say that aging has its own rules, we can surely say that PTSD has its own way in the nosology. At base, PTSD is an anxiety disorder, the most prevalent kind of disorder among the aged. In fact, as much as 20% of older adults have "pathologic levels of anxiety" (Schramke, 1997). Anxiety is pervasive, often comorbid with or masking other disorders, and is actually adaptive for some purposes. But PTSD is also a disorder that leaves the clinician puzzled because a natural (or unnatural) life event causes trouble at the roots of a person. It also appears to hang on over time.

This gives us pause in making any firm statement about PTSD. A position holding that trauma alone is causative of PTSD problems, or that premorbid factors alone dictate symptoms, does not adequately reflect the facts. In a non-definitive study on the effects of war trauma, Grace, Lindy, Gleser, and Leonard (1990) examined the relative contributions of "causative" variables on PTSD: Pre-trauma factors accounted for 9%, trauma for 19%, and post-trauma for 12%. But this study was not performed on older people and the complex contexts of aging were thereby not included. Also, no personality measures were used, again precluding information on the complexities of the person.

In another study, Foa, Steketee, and Rothbaum (1989) discussed the unique features of PTSD: "Three factors appear to be central: the intensity of the responses; the size of the structure, and the ready accessibility of the structure." The distinctive features of an anxiety disorder may not be the unique quality of its principal components (physiologic arousal, cognitive processes, and avoidant coping strategies), as much as its excessiveness (Blazer, 1998). What seems to exist is that, as in other anxiety disorders, a person possesses this ready-state of anxiety, as well as a sense of unpredictable/uncontrollable reactions, to join with the stressor for a chronic victim status to result. Again, PTSD is an anxiety disorder with, at its base, fear stimulus, response, and meaning features, that resist change.

No one-to-one relationship exists between PTSD and the stressor. All 17 of the constituent symptoms of PTSD correlate highly with PTSD as a whole (thereby supporting the construct); however, the actual role of intrusion or avoidance, as well as their actual expression for any one person, is highly variable. At a simple level, acute trauma responses produce intrusions and have little numbing or avoidance. In the chronic form of this disorder, however, victims tend to endorse all criteria but actually develop maladaptive patterns around only selected symptoms, usually avoidance. Information on symptom clusters of PTSD and their relationship to outcome measures is also woefully underrepresented in our research literature. If age at all enters into the picture, the clinician can rightfully ask: Which symptoms are primary and which secondary?

In this chapter we discuss PTSD, its roots and provide background for understanding the older trauma victim. This starts with a discussion on prevalence of PTSD. We then discuss the modal trauma type at later life, combat. This is also relevant because it is the only model for PTSD that we have sufficient cross sectional or any longitudinal data on. We then consider PTSD, its forms, and diagnostic problems. We also consider key theories of PTSD. We then discuss three problems of PTSD as they apply to older victims.

☐ Prevalence of PTSD

Although related, trauma and stress are different: When trauma occurs, its absence does not alleviate symptoms; in stress, it does. Trauma is a major stressor that appears to have a distinct trajectory of decline. Norris (1992) found the lifetime exposure rate to at least one major stressor event 69%. Trauma is common (Kilpatrick & Resnick, 1993). In later life the prevalence of a major stressor appears to be even higher. Most of the elderly are likely to experience psychological consequences, given a stressor (Green, Epstein, Krupnick, & Rowland, 1997; Norris, 1992; Shore, Tatum, & Vollmer, 1986). Ensel (1991) showed that most older community-dwelling adults (74%) had at least one major life event during the past 6 months that produced a negative impact. It is believed that somewhere between 8% and 10% incur PTSD at some time in their life (for all trauma). Given exposure to trauma, the rate is about 25% (more for women). Some trauma as in war and rape are naturally worse.

As with all disorders, the prevalence for lifetime PTSD varies as a function of the sample assessed, methods used, and the definition of trauma. Using just military groups in the United States as a model, prevalence rates are low (at times <2%; Hankin et al., 1996; Schnurr, Aldwin, Spiro, Stukel, & Keane, 1993; Spiro, Aldwin, Levenson, & Schnurr, 1993) when community samples are used. Prevalence rates for community groups in Europe, however, for lifetime PTSD can be high (Op den Velde et al., 1993). Among psychiatric inpatients, rates are high, estimated from 50% to 67% with symptoms enduring over 40 years (Goldstein, van Kammen, Shelly, Miller, & van Kammen, 1987; Hovens et al., 1994; Rosen, Fields, Hand, Falsettie, & van Kammen, 1989; Zeiss & Dickman, 1989). The same applies for prisoners of war (POWs; Tennant, Goulston, & Dent, 1993). Rates of 18% (WWII) and 30% (Korea) has been also been noted for medical inpatients: For veterans who never sought psychiatric treatment, the numbers were 9% (WWII) and 7% (Korea) for PTSD (Blake et al., 1990).

From the PTSD research, we do know that, if the trauma is sufficiently intense, this is correlated with the extent of symptoms in almost all studies. In some epidemiological studies, PTSD is only behind alcohol abuse, depression, and social phobia in its toll on society and problems (Kessler et al., 1995). In others, a brighter picture applies.

With "on time" losses (e.g., death), many older individuals may be able to go through a normal grieving process and even "grow" from the experience. They may even help others (Lyons, 1991; Melick & Logue, 1985–1986). It can also be said that, although stress leaves a negative trail, after six months to a year its effects are modest (Depue & Monroe, 1986).

Finally, the influence of minor stress is a puzzle. Many older people may experience more than their share of minor stress (Ensel, 1991). These can cause problems (Falk, Hersen, & Van Hasselt, 1994; Tait & Silver, 1984), be underrepresented, or altered (e.g., somaticizing; Hankin, Abueg, Gallagher-Thompson, & Laws, 1996). However the opposite may also be true: Older people have reported fewer hassles in part because of the loss of social roles, such as work and parenting (see Aldwin, 1990). Interestingly, Wagner, Compas, and Howell (1988) found that daily stresses play an intermediary role in the process by which major events influence psychological symptoms. This may have a singularly negative impact on older people.

In sum, even when the effects (probably) due to aging are accounted for (e.g., sleep disturbance and memory impairment), rates of PTSD diagnosis and symptoms are still high (Zeiss & Dickman, 1989). Unfortunately the long-term developmental aspects of trauma or stress have been largely ignored because of the absence of longitudinal data (Elder et al., 1994). In one of the few longitudinal studies, Elders and Clipp (1988) presented evidence that, overall, symptoms decrease over time.

☐ PTSD's Historical Roots: Military Combat

This discussion is about what Brokaw (1998) called *The Greatest Generation*. The vast majority of our information on the influence of stress on older people involves war trauma (Ruskin & Talbott, 1996). Over 40% of all PTSD investigations in the last 20 years have involved this stressor (Blake et al., 1992). This heritage includes case studies, WWII veteran studies, POW studies, personality (e.g., MMPI) studies, and a variety of investigations of specific issues of the traumatized combat veteran. In fact, through the years there has been considerable overlap of symptoms between older war-related diagnoses, such as traumatic war neurosis, combat fatigue, and shell shock, and the diagnosis of PTSD as set forth systematically in *DSMs*. Combat or war trauma leaves an "indelible image" on all (Lifton, 1979), and if one knows about war trauma, then one knows about other trauma.

Military Service in the Developmental Context

Most veterans believe that military service affected their personal development (Card, 1983; Elder, 1987; Elder & Clipp, 1989). Negative outcomes are pervasive: disruption of the life course, separation from others, and painful memories. Positive benefits are also noteworthy and include increases in maturity, coping skills, self-discipline, independence, cooperation, and sensitivity to others (Aldwin, 1993; Schnurr & Aldwin, 1993).

Aldwin, Levenson, and Spiro (1994) found both positive and negative outcomes exist and are mediated by the combat experience. These veterans probably addressed life's tasks at earlier ages than their counterparts, thereby developing better lifelong coping strategies. Data also support the view that WWII and Korean War veterans are less likely than civilians to have a psychiatric disorder (Norquist et al., 1990).

However, given a strong stressor, the experience carries to other areas: veterans with PTSD have more marital and family problems and are more isolated. They also have lower educational attainment, both overall and relative to pre-military education, and higher levels of occupational instability and unemployment. In general for most social areas, whatever problems have occurred earlier in life as a result of war trauma, by mid-life these veterans have caught up to their civilian counterparts. Additionally, upward mobility is most evident in minority groups (Schnurr & Aldwin, 1996).

In summary, the residuals of combat stress in the older cohort are experienced commonly (Rosenheck & Fontana, 1994), or in positive and distinctive ways (Elder & Clipp, 1989; Elder, Shanahan, & Clipp, 1994; Lee, Vaillant, Torrey, & Elder, 1995) relative to other wars. Combat seems to mediate life's experiences, especially during early adulthood. In this way military experience can be considered as developmental (Schnurr, 1997). Regarding combat veterans, Schnurr and Aldwin (1996) wrote:

> Military service is a significant developmental experience in the lives of many men and women. Furthermore, the effects of military service, like other developmental experiences, unfold over time. A pattern of outcomes observed 5 years after discharge may differ markedly from the outcomes observed 20 years later (Aldwin & Stokols, 1988). Given these complexities, the best one can do is to delineate general patterns, knowing that they may not hold for all cohorts, social classes, sexes, ethnic groups, or individuals.

Lessons

We have learned some hard lessons from this cohort. Perhaps mostly we know that PTSD symptoms persist. In fact, older people may be vulnerable to the effects of different stressors, many of which may exacerbate latent PTSD symptoms, even after years of being relatively asymptomatic (Falk, Herson, & Van Haslet, 1994). For some veterans, military trauma remains the most severe stressor throughout the lifetime; for many, other traumas are rated as more severe (Hyer & Summers, 1995). You might say that for those who have experienced a significant trauma and have not placed it into the context of ongoing life, the struggle to contain painful memories can be considerable (Mazor, Gampel, Enright, & Orenstein, 1990) and the likelihood of pathological effects from other stressors is high (Yehuda et al., 1995). We will never know, however, the exact prevalence of PTSD of these older men when they were younger because longitudinal data do not exist so we must rely on retrospective accounts of the experiences.

On the other side of the coin, we know that, despite the clinical fact that there is a long history of negative consequences as a result of combat (as we just noted), PTSD prevalence rates are low in the community. Many possible reasons exist, including mortality, cohort differences in war experience and the homecoming, a tendency to deny or minimize psychiatric problems, or generally showing higher levels of adjustment relative to the younger Vietnam veterans. There is also resilience, the "Teflon-shield" coping of many people. This applies for the majority of stressor victims. What are those components of the person most likely to be resilient in the face of trauma? The ways in which an "empowered" self-repair unfolds are unclear.

The mixture of the life transition process and trauma adjustment make for an interesting interaction (Elder & Caspi, 1990; McAdams, 1993). We do not know all the permutations and outcomes. In treatment settings it is common for patients to sense that symptoms have become worse with age. Over time too, trauma-related problems may be reactivated when reminders of the war occur, perhaps also when events associated with aging occur, as in retirement and medical illness. But, neither of these events are stock occurrences or, for most, not even stressful (Schnurr, 1997).

Box 2-1
What the clinician still does not know about PTSD.

1. Why do some and not others develop PTSD?
2. Should the trauma memory be addressed for symptom remission?
3. At what point does the clinician attack the trauma memory?
4. Over time how much does secondary gain influence treatment?
5. Does the clinician deal with the most pernicious stressor, the most current one, and so on?
6. What are the best treatment components and when?
7. What is the role of secondary gains? The longer the trauma response, the stronger the likelihood of this influence.
8. How do symptoms remain quiet over time?
9. What is the cohort influence on denial of problems?
10. What is the relation between the physiological and psychological symptoms?
11. What is the biology of fear and its connection to PTSD?
12. What is the effect of medicalization of problems?
13. What is the place of medication in the long-term care of PTSD?
14. What is the hierarchy of interventions in the care of a trauma victim (safety first but then what ...)?

So, there are things we know about PTSD. We tend to have better information on the questions that apply to PTSD, as well as its very conceptualization. We know more about trauma too. We also know more about those most likely to get PTSD. It is not surprising that, with many older victims, "secondary" issues become important (in therapy) such as a supportive social system, an empowered problem solving focus, and the ability to cope with ongoing (and past) stressful situations. But there is much we do not know. Box 2-1 provides some questions.

☐ What is PTSD?

Acute Trauma and Later Life

Laub and Auerhaun (1993) described different levels of awareness of trauma that can change over time as defenses wane. They are not knowing at all, reliving in fugues or altered states of consciousness, reliving in fragments of the trauma, giving into traits, being influenced by an overpowering narrative, as well as being defined by life themes or eventually using the narrative as metaphor. Whatever happens in the stress reaction, it starts with an acute stress disorder (ASD). This is different from more chronic forms of PTSD. ASD is acute anxiety. In fact, it is a critical variable in the determination of later trauma-related problems (e.g., PTSD and depression) and overall adjustment.

ASD was added to the DSMIV in 1994. It had mixed reception due largely to its lack of empirical justification, its excessive pathologizing of transient stress, its emphasis on post-traumatic dissociation, and its one "skill" of assisting in the prediction of other disorders (largely PTSD) (Bryant, 2000). For ASD, a person should (a) suffer a traumatic experience, (b) display at least three acute dissociative symptoms, (c) have at least one re-experiencing symptom, (d) display marked avoidance, (e) show marked hyperarousal, and (f) have these symptoms between two days and four weeks after trauma.

The acute trauma type that has received the most interest is motor vehicle accidents (MVAs). Limited data show that MVAs can be a significant precipitant of PTSD (Norris, 1992). Estimates range from 10% to 46% (Blanchard, Hicking, Taylor, & Loos, 1995; Blanchard et al., 1996; Mayou, Bryant, & Duthie, 1993), as well as other psychiatric distress at 1-year follow-up (Mayou, Bryant, & Duthie, 1993). Harvey and Bryant (1998) assessed 92 victims for ASD within 1 month of the trauma and reassessed 6 months later for PTSD. ASD was diagnosed for 13% of the sample, with 21% having subclinical levels. At follow-up, 78% of the ASD participants and 60% of the subclinical participants met criteria for PTSD. Similar results were found in one other study by these authors (see Blanchard & Hickling, 1998) and colleagues. None of these studies used an older sample.

In a pivotal study, Blanchard and colleagues (see Blanchard & Hickling, 1998) followed MVA PTSD and subsyndromal victims for 6 months after the accident. Variables that predicted change in status for each, both positive and negative, differed. Frequency and intensity of the accident were the most predictive variables in either case. The intercurrent issues of a new trauma and relative recovery from the injury were also predictive of subsequent trauma response. Additionally, the presence of depression at the time of the initial assessment was a red flag, indicating lack of remission among PTSD. Depression was also significantly related to PTSD and, when PTSD was removed from the equation, it became a significant variable. Treatment itself made little difference in the remission of symptoms. As with other studies, few accident variables (e.g., number of cars in the accident) were significant. Results also showed that degree of initial physical injury and the relative degree of physical recovery at 4 months classified the later clinical status of 84% of the victims with initial PTSD. Older people were not involved.

There appear to be many variables that are potentially of interest in the eventual trauma response among older victims of MVAs. One link between ASD and PTSD, for example, is dissociation, a core element of the trauma response. In general, it is reasonable to speculate that any link between these disorders is multiple, as is the case with PTSD, where the presence of an acute reaction (Bryant & Harvey, 1998), severity of the trauma (Kulka et al., 1990), avoidance (McFarlane, 1992) or intrusions, and arousal (see Hyer, 1994), as well as a host of premorbid factors, such as previous treatment, previous trauma or personality disorder (Hyer et al., 1994), potentiate problems (of PTSD). Social support, physical condition, and severity of or additional trauma also appear important (Hyer et al., 1994).

Another group of studies on acute trauma reactions has involved natural disasters. Several studies have before and after data on older victims of acute natural disasters. Older people do well. Using longitudinal data from 1971 from the Northridge earthquake in California, Gatz (1999) reported that the older groups had lower rates of depression. The older groups required greater amounts of damage to cause problems in adjustment. Using another longitudinal data set, Havens (1999) too reported that in a flood in Manitoba, Canada, older people reacted well to the trauma. In fact, older age seemed to be protective against cognitive decline and served to enhance perceptions of general health status.

On the weight of it, however, there is currently little evidence to support targeting older survivors based solely on their age. Elderly disaster survivors especially appear to be at relatively low risk for developing long-term psychological problems following these events. Their coping strategies, and perhaps their cumulative past experience, allow them to take changes brought on by the disaster events. Additionally, because older people may have reduced burdens in terms of caring for others at this time, they may have fewer worries and more time to devote to dealing with the meaning and the resolution of the event. Finally, older individuals may have a great deal to offer their younger family and friends in terms of positive attitude and calming effect, and this resource should be considered and tapped. As always, those who have the most stressful experiences (e.g., loss or life threat, prolonged exposure) would be at higher risk than those not so exposed (Brewin, Andrews, & Valentine, 2000).

In sum, results of these studies on MVAs suggest that researchers attend to all variables related to ASD, PTSD, and depression, and do so over time. We know further that the role of physical insult and its rehabilitation as a result of trauma are central to adjustment and PTSD. Although there is little data on age as a variable in MVAs and its effects on trauma symptoms, at least one study found such a relationship (Malt, 1988).

DSMs and PTSD

We now take a look at the changes in the diagnosis PTSD and march through the criteria and their measurement. We do this with trepidation. Although the final common pathway that allows for some sanctuary of understanding is PTSD, many subclinical varieties exist and can create confusion. PTSD is a disorder that is imperfectly constructed.

We are faced with a morning goalpost. We have the same key criteria as outlined in the previous DSMs (since 1980) but there are changes from the DSM-III–R to the DSM-IV (American Psychiatric Association, 1994; Box 2-2). The experiences of trauma that may manifest PTSD symptoms possess both objective and subjective elements. Additionally, changes in diagnostic criteria reflect difficulties in identifying and articulating the core symptoms of PTSD. Undoubtedly these criteria will continue to evolve. Overall they reflect the need to objectify the subjective experience of the stressor, to appreciate Criteria C (avoidance) better, and to bring in newer symptoms.

As a general statement, however, only in the last 5–7 years has there been interest regarding the validation of scales on PTSD for later-life sufferers. For the most part, this interest has evolved from the field of trauma in general. We present self-report scales on the symptoms of PTSD in Chapter 12.

Criterion A: The Trauma

Let's look at Criterion A. The only reason that we concern ourselves with the stressor and its quantity and quality is because we must justify the nosological need for a DSM construct. Although this may be a hard, anti-stimulus view, the fact of trauma is but a starting point for a specific inquiry on its potential negative effects. Currently the definition of a traumatic event in the DSM-IV requires that a person has "experienced, witnessed, or was confronted with an event or events that involved actual or threatened death or serious injury, or a threat to physical integrity of self or others" (p. 427).

The nosology follows with two premises: (a) a stressor event outside the normal range of human experience, and (b) one that impacts markedly and negatively on a person, objectively and subjectively. The essential features of a traumatic event are

---

Box 2-2
PTSD Criteria and Changes in DSM-IV

1. Expressed a constructivistic approach in the revised criteria in that stressful stimuli could be unique to the person who experiences them rather than objectively and unequivocally stressful.
2. Adding a distinct hyperarousal symptoms cluster.
3. Combining numbing and avoidance symptoms into the same cluster.
4. Dividing "symptom intensification" into cued physiological arousal and psychological distress.
5. Adding avoidance of thoughts and feelings.
6. Dropping guilt and non-specific memory impairment by adding memory impairment related to the trauma.
7. Having "sense of a foreshortened future."
8. Adding the requirement that the syndrome will cause significant distress or impairment in social or occupational functioning.

---

that they represent a threat and that there is a response. This definition also requires that the person's response involve intense fear, helplessness, or horror.

We see good news and bad news here for older people. Life-threatening illness is explicitly named in the DSM-IV. The good news then is that diseases, such as cancer and myocardial infarction, qualify. All of these diseases increase with age. The bad news involves the meaning of these events. With many of these diseases the immediate "death encounter" is not experienced in the initial episode but rather looms ahead. This type of threat is vague and has been labeled as an "information stressor" (Green, Lindy, & Groce, 1994). The threat in many cases, therefore, is in the future. As aging and medical illness often co-occur in later life, what is trauma in this context?

How do you decide the difference between symptoms characteristic of the stress response and those typically produced by the illness and threat itself? Use of radiotherapy and chemotherapy is especially a problem. What does intrusive thinking mean in this context? For some, the contents of the images and thoughts might be hypochondriasis and even a future orientation; for others there may be a recollection of past events. What does numbing and denial mean in these contexts? How does one's "foreshortened future" play out in this context? What is hyperarousal? These might simply be hyperalert focus to bodily changes.

While these concerns might be symptoms of hypochondriasis, they also might be appropriate cueing for trauma problems (Green, Epstein, Krupnick, & Rowland, 1997). Additionally, somatic reactions are not only common at later life but they require unique assessment as their place in the context of emotional experience is unclear.

Now the DSM-IV emphasizes the subjective side of the stressor. It now can include death, physical illness, and injury. Of course Criterion E demands that this event "causes clinically significant distress or impairment in social, occupational, or other important areas of functioning" (p. 429).

To evaluate the importance of Criterion A, Kilpatrick et al. (1994) conducted a multisite study to assess the associations between a variety of stressors and PTSD symptoms. High-magnitude events (typical Criterion A events) and low-magnitude events (those not included) were in the mix for over 500 treatment-seeking and community-dwelling participants. These were lifetime events. Most participants (71%) had a combination of events and most had experienced more than one high-magnitude event. Predictably, PTSD rates were highest with physical and sexual assault and combat. In this culture we seem to incur stressors.

Kessler and colleagues (1995) performed a state of the art large-scale epidemiological study of PTSD prevalence and comorbidity. Although there were gender differences, PTSD was alarmingly associated with all other anxiety disorders, including Generalized Anxiety Disorder (GAD), panic disorder, simple phobia, and agoraphobia. Depression and its variants as well as conduct disorder, and drug and alcohol abuse were also highly represented. Approximately 88% of men and 79% of women had a comorbid diagnosis.

☐ Oh, Well, What's in a Diagnosis?

At the risk of iconoclasty, PTSD is not the only disorder to emerge specifically from a compromised trauma response. The conventional categorization of trauma, the criteria for PTSD (American Psychiatric Association, 1994), may not serve the study of trauma (Green, 1991) or older people (Summers & Hyer, 1994) well. With the aged, this formulation does not adequately represent the influence of fear memories that depict erroneous messages that generalize to behavior in life (Hyer & Summers, 1995). Trauma's position as a risk factor for future psychopathology is well established. Trauma's role as an etiological factor, however, is not yet corroborated (Maughan & Rutter, 1997). In fact, factors that initiate psychopathology are generally not the same as those that maintain its persistence into older age (Rutter & Maughan, 1997). Myriad factors related to abuse (nature of the trauma), the balancing of risk and resilient components, extant cognitive schemata, the social network, and predisposing factors interact to "produce" a response to trauma, most often one that results in adequate adjustment (Paris, 1997). In effect, the trauma response is both more and less than PTSD, and at later life PTSD is more than a trauma reaction.

The panorama of trauma models is broad. The creation of diagnostic systems, such as the DSMs creates order but does not provide the clinician with specific and individual realities of the pained person. Their ratio of speculation to data is high: A virtual reality of hunches surrounds possible truth. The search for truth in a scientific sense often comes up short.

In the strict diagnostic sense there can be confusion about the presence of PTSD. We do not just refer to the psychological space where PTSD symptoms coagulate. We mean the logic of the disorder and the disorder of the disorder. In the early phases of PTSD, for example, the presentation of symptoms seems normal. Symptoms may not be symptoms in the psychiatric sense. The opposite can also occur: some symptoms are worse (than "typical" PTSD), especially the presence of dissociation or depression. Unlike other anxiety disorders, then, PTSD symptoms can be both natural and unnatural, thereby confusing symptom relevance.

In this process, PTSD can be bigger than life. The prototype appears "real." It has become a type of Platonic form. The connection of symptoms to the particular and complex experience of an individual is in danger of being lost. In effect, the concept of PTSD becomes reified (Pynoos, Steinberg, & Goenjion, 1996). We count intensity and frequency of intrusive images, making clinical and antiseptic these reproductions of the original scene. We often miss the experiential and clinical significance. Intrusive images are memory markers that represent moments of traumatic helplessness, horror, and loss.

What is PTSD in later life? This is a question that is often asked of depression. In later life the effects of trauma are encoded in the heart of an aging process, suffused with the meaning and context of being older. As a consequence, PTSD in later life is both similar to and different from other ages. It is made so because the older person is "different," and because PTSD has been filtered by time.

PTSD and Anxiety

Anxiety disorders are the most prevalent disorders in later life (Schramke, 1997). It can be argued that anxiety among the elderly is viewed as similar to other ages (Salzman & Lebowitz, 1991). The expression of anxiety at later life, then, is straightforward, expressing itself without the intricate conversion mechanisms frequently seen among the young (Blazer, 1998). Similarities are far more striking than the differences.

It can also be said that anxiety among the aging is different from other ages. Johnson (1991) noted that he found "not one case of uncomplicated acute or chronic anxiety syndrome" (p. 213) in the past 21 years of practice, as all cases were contaminated by many other symptoms. Moreover, virtually all of his patients revealed some form of anxiety. Salzman and Lebowitz (1991) wrote, "Anxiety may be experienced as cognitive apprehension, behavioral agitation, or somatic symptoms with hypochondriacal components." Pfeiffer and Busse (1973) underscored the somatic presentation: "Anxiety in the elderly may be displaced into high bodily concern and expressed as hypochondriacal symptoms." Among older persons, the expression of anxiety is more direct, appearing as overt fear, panic, worry of bewilderment, and without the intricate conversation mechanisms. McCarthy, Katz, and Foa (1991) suggested that significant anxiety disorders among the elderly are likely to be phobias, with components that represent exaggerations of rational concerns, as well as generalized anxiety and mixed anxious-depressive states.

Most anxiety disorders in the elderly are continuations of life-long illnesses rather than the sudden, late-life development of panic-agoraphobia, generalized anxiety, or social phobia in previously healthy individuals. Additionally, patients who are over 85 may be substantially different from patients who are between 65 and 75. As is the case with other areas of aging, we need to consider sub-populations, young old, middle old, and very old.

What about PTSD? In two published reviews of geriatric psychiatry (Busse & Blazer, 1989; Nussbaum, 1997), no reference to PTSD appears despite the fact that these volumes contain chapters on anxiety disorders, sleep disorders, and the epidemiology of psychiatric disorders in the elderly. Just as surprising is the omission of any discussion of PTSD in a work devoted entirely to anxiety in the elderly (Salzman & Lebowitz, 1991). Summers and Hyer (1994) noted that older people who have PTSD or PTSD symptoms are likely to be of two types based on onset. Early onset is characterized by a PTSD pattern of both intrusions and avoidance, that is similar to that of younger groups, whereas late onset probably is more characterized by avoidant symptoms.

Anxiety appears to be a very common symptom but an uncommon syndrome. It seems reasonable to question whether the elderly manifest anxiety in the same way and with the same frequency as do younger patients. Should the criteria be the same across all ages? Is the DSM classification of anxiety disorders appropriate for older persons (Box 2-3)? It is appropriate to question also how PTSD, an anxiety disorder, falls in the constellation of symptoms of the DSM categories. Regardless of the background consideration on this important issue, the presence of anxiety is pervasive in this population and has many starting points, causes, contributants, or maintaining factors.

PTSD and Depression

Are anxiety and depression separate entities or are they aspects of the same disease? Many believe that clinical criteria used to determine when an older person is anxious are outmoded or unhelpful (Gurian & Miner, 1991). Studies have shown that approximately 80% of patients with a primary diagnosis of depression have a high degree of anxiety and that about 50% of patients with a primary diagnosis of GAD have symptoms of depression (Zung, 1971). In the often recognized national study on community-dwelling Vietnam veterans (Kulka et al., 1990), major depression was reported in 26%. Similar findings were also reported for a non-veteran community sample of crime victims with PTSD in which approximately one-third had a diagnosis of major depression (Kilpatrick, Saunders, Veronen, Best, & Von, 1987).

In samples of older trauma victims, contradictory results are present. In a WWII and Korean Conflict POW sample, for example, Sutker and Allain (1996) reported a lifetime prevalence of major depression ranging from 42% to 13%; however, it was not clear how depression influenced PTSD. To the contrary, Lee, Vaillant, Torrey, and Elder (1995) studied predictors and correlates of PTSD in a community sample of WWII combat veterans and concluded that symptoms of PTSD and major depressive disorder were not significantly correlated.

Interestingly, several researchers point to an overlap in the symptom criteria between PTSD and major affective disorder (MAD; e.g., Brewin, Joseph, & Kuyken, 1993). In fact, seven PTSD symptoms are related to depression. Criterion features of PTSD, such as emotional numbing, avoidance, and decreased activity are character-

---

Box 2-3
Common Causes of Anxiety in Late Life

1. Major depressive episode
2. Environmental stressors
3. Medical illness (known or occult)
4. True late onset neurotic disorder
5. Life long recurrent anxiety
6. Late onset acute phobic anxiety (in response to acute severe illness)
7. Hypochondriasis
8. Early dementia
9. Episodic and self-limiting anxiety due to bereavement or anniversary reaction
10. Paranoid psychotic state
11. Obsessional states
12. Withdrawal reactions
13. Medications and caffeine

istic benchmarks of depressive disorders (Brewin, Joseph, & Kuyken, 1993; Joseph, Williams, & Yule, 1995). In addition, depressed people often experience intrusions (negative automatic thoughts) and avoidance of specific instances of adversity and have abuse or trauma backgrounds (Brewin et al., 1993). Brewin even noted that "it may be worthwhile considering adding a trauma processing component to the standard cognitive therapy of depression" (p. 338). This appears to also be the case with bereavement (Parkes, 1971).

It has also been argued that depressive symptoms of PTSD are not simply manifestations of a concurrent major depressive disorder (MAD) but are distinctive (Marin, 1997). They may be atypical depressions, characterological depression, or something else (Southwick, Yehuda, & Giller, 1991). Southwick et al. used the Depressive Experiences Questionnaire (DEQ), a depression scale that assesses self-critical and dependent depressive styles, and the Hamilton Rating Scale for Depression with veterans. Results showed that, although participants with both PTSD and MAD were similar on both DEQ scales, those with PTSD were worse off than the MAD participants on all Hamilton-Depression symptoms, especially somatic ones. In other words, if you had PTSD, the tendency was to be similar to MAD participants on both scales, even worse on a traditional scale for depression. In this study too, depression co-occurring with PTSD among war veterans was more resistant to conventional antidepressants and biologically and psychologically different from major depression in the absence of PTSD.

Implied is that several cognitive/affective mechanisms are involved in the understanding of PTSD and depression. First, both PTSD and depression result in an increased access to negative memories and decreased access to positive ones (McNally, Kaspi, Reimann, & Zeitler, 1990). Second, both diagnoses represent "poorer" emotional processing, perhaps in similar ways. Rachman (1980) noted that factors that impede cognitive, behavioral, and emotional processing lead to both PTSD and depression. Intrusions, perhaps the core symptoms of PTSD, are similar to automatic negative thoughts as noted in depression (Joseph, Williams, & Yule, 1995). Avoidance also is a problem with both conditions: Is avoidance a symptom of PTSD or a mediator of the trauma and subsequent emotional state of depression? In this regard too the Foa group (Foa & Kozak, 1989) noted that trauma victims experience emotions as secondary reactions to avoidance. These affective responses can be fear-related (PTSD) or loss-related (depression). Each appear to have their own place in the symptom picture and timing of trauma responses.

Third, attributional styles appear similar. The attribution of positive events to more external and uncontrollable causes and the attribution of negative events to internal and stable and uncontrollable causes results in psychological distress that has been applied to both PTSD and depression (McCormick, Taber, & Kruedelbach, 1989; Mikulincer & Solomon, 1988). Self-blaming attributional styles and a negative self-focus predisposing one to stress are additional commonalties. It is unclear, however, how these features interrelate, present independently for each disorder, and vary as a function of increasing age or changes in health status.

Fourth, depression has also been viewed as a feature in the symptom pattern of PTSD such that an affective disorder represents a phase in the manifestation of PTSD (Wang, Wilson, & Mason, 1996). According to these authors, depression should not be diagnosed as a comorbid diagnosis as it represents only a stage of decompensation. Over time the symptom constellations may change. Mellman, Randolph, Brawman-Mintzer, Flores, and Milanes (1992) investigated the primary and secondary diagnostic relationships associated with PTSD comorbidity, suggesting that these co-existing syndromes may be manifestations of a response to trauma as well as to the chronicity of PTSD.

Depression and PTSD are kindred spirits. Hyer and Stanger (1997) found that 90% of PTSD combat victims had significant depression problems. This is not good news as the two separate diagnoses co-mingle and affect quality of life and outcomes in various noxious ways. So, the treatment of PTSD in later life necessitates consideration of the treatment of depression.

PTSD and Grief

The core of PTSD is that the person's assumptive world is altered. This involves issues that are relevant to the world and to the self. This is also true of grief. In fact, there are several arguments for acute grief being "PTSD-ish." Both involve a loss and an association with anxiety. There is similar manifest symptomatology and the alternating modes of regulation that accompanies both. Grief is then part of and complicates the trauma. Care involves a mixture of PTSD treatments and grief treatments (loss). We will address this in a later chapter.

Partial PTSD

There has been a robust debate among researchers regarding the categorical or dimensional nature of psychiatric disorders in just about every area of psychopathology. The critical issues of PTSD in the nosology, including the best exemplars of the disorder, continue to change. Although this debate is likely to continue without conclusions for some period, several studies have made the point that the disorder PTSD may be a special problem. Data from the National Vietnam Veteran Readjustment Study (NVVRS; Kulka et al., 1990) and one study on premorbid PTSD characteristics (Schnun & Aldwin, 1993) addressed various decision rules (of PTSD), and expressed concern about the limits of the DSM decision rules.

In reference to just older veterans, a number of studies have discussed the notion of a below threshold (PTSD) disorder that is representative of older groups (e.g., Hyer, 1994). Various authors have speculated on the causes for this "partial problem": PTSD as a "delayed recognition"; as a disorder that is "fluid in nature"; as a syndrome that at later life is characterized by "underreporting"; and when measured as "Partial PTSD" as a disorder with a high "lifetime" prevalence (47%) (Hyer, 1994). Green (1991) and Norris (1990) lamented that the diagnosis PTSD requires six symptoms and that, if the right symptom configuration is not present, a diagnosis is not forthcoming. Green (1990) even noted that the diagnostic label PTSD may not have facilitated our understanding of PTSD as it applies to older people.

Partial PTSD was used in the NVVRS (Weiss et al., 1992) on Vietnam veterans and was considered as important as full PTSD (with about an equal prevalence). As there is no set way to define the "middle-range" partial group, Summers and Hyer (1994) evaluated this PTSD group in two ways—according to NVVRS criteria (Criteria A and B plus C or D) as well as a stricter criteria of one symptom in each category (plus Criterion A, the presence of an extreme stressor). In this study regardless of strictness of criteria, the prevalence rates were generally the same and the pattern was the same—partial PTSD victims possessed problems at a level slightly less than full PTSD, but greater than no PTSD. These data were based on standardized interviewer rated measures of PTSD. Highly significant differences were found also on several symptom and adjustment variables among full and no-PTSD groups, with full-PTSD veterans scoring significantly higher than the no-PTSD group. The middle group, veterans with partial-PTSD, was always in the center of the groupings. Results suggested then that the construct partial may be an important subclinical variety, with a high degree of potential for suffering and problems. As the nosological construct PTSD is rationally derived, its expression may involve lowered thresholds of its criteria. Even the criteria may be altered as the monitors of this problem undergo revision outwardly.

At later life, however, this may be a special problem. When an older victim refers to a previous trauma that may be activated by current circumstances, the possible PTSD problems should be considered. Interestingly, partial PTSD data follow depression research findings in older people. Symptoms of depression are highly prevalent and cause problems.

PTSD and the Person

We end this section with a discussion on PTSD and the person. The occurrence of extreme stressors or traumatic events are not sufficient for the diagnosis of PTSD or its short term counterpart, Acute Stress Disorder. Rather, one also must experience anxiety (emotional distress), which serves as a stimulant to subsequent problems. The trauma that leads to problems starts then with a platform of anxiety and multiple associations that are deeply stored in the form of stimulus, response, and meaning propositions (Foa, Bothbour, & Riggs, 1993). Other anxiety features, like a chronic readiness for action, lack of control, self-focused attention, and presence of "hot" survival-based cognitions probably contribute. Perhaps the reason that the severity of the trauma is so highly related to PTSD is that stress potentiates this "ready" state as an illicit substance would do for an addict.

We know that the presence of trauma problems is related to the intensity and severity of the person's experience with the trauma. But, despite the fact that the stressor can precipitate the trauma reaction, the person of the victim largely dictates the type and quality of the disorder. Each person creates his/her own representational models of the world, and the individual is the one who ultimately determines whether the experience is traumatic and, if so, how this is to be played out. We develop a ready-made early warning system and one that both shapes the form of anxiety and seeks to adapt to it.

☐ Theories of PTSD

Trauma is learned, perhaps by imprinting or by sensitization. In the former, the influence of later problems has occurred as a result of the learning during the trauma (probably because of the biological functions of noradrenergic activation and Hypothalamic Pituitary Axis) or after the trauma (kindling or memory consolidation). The former model over-emphasizes the trauma and the latter one under-emphasizes it.

In the last two decades, several theories have tried to explain the components of PTSD and their ascent in the person, including behavioral (Keane & Kolb, 1988; Kilpatrick & Veronen, 1983), learned helplessness (Seligman, 1975), biological (e.g., Friedman, 2000; van der Kolk, 1988), intrapsychic (e.g., Horowitz, 1986; Krystal, 1978), psychosocial (e.g., Lifton, 1993), self (e.g., McCann & Pearlman, 1990; Mahoney, 1991), psychodynamic (e.g., McCann & Pearlman, 1990), and information processing (e.g., Litz & Keane, 1989). PTSD is the unsuccessful balancing of one's style for controlling the flow of ideas in order to avoid entering painful states. There is no "right balance" of the problem maintenance structures of PTSD—behavioral, biological, and interpersonal or some combination. Any good explanation of who gets this pain and how it leaks over time is not present. Theories of "mind," espoused by Horowitz, McCann, Pearlman, Epstein, and Herman (see Hyer & Associates, 1994) expand on this. Theories of the life span also expand on this. There are the life history and the life cycle speculations on trauma, chiefly those espoused by Erickson, Levinson, and Lifton. They discuss adult life structures and frozen souls.

Despite shortcomings, however, Mowrer's two-factor theory has been proffered as a stable model of PTSD: Trauma symptoms develop because of the dominance of both classical and instrumental conditioning. For the former, new stimuli associated with the original trauma become like henchmen and elicit the same response over time. Anxiety associated with original stimuli do not extinguish because of avoidance. For the latter, avoidance behaviors continue because they are negatively reinforcing, thereby reducing anxiety. In time, responses become highly idiosyncratic, indeed psychoanalytically rich, as they beccome derivatives and apply to a large number of situations (Horowitz et al., 1984). So, the processing of information can indeed be complex for the person and befuddling for the therapist. Is it real or is it Memorex?

It is information processing that best addresses faulty "thinking" as a result of trauma. Sufferers do not accommodate well to new information. Lang (1979) proposed that emotional memories are stored as associative networks consisting of sensory elements of the experience. They are activated when a person is confronted with situations that stimulate a sufficient number of elements making up these networks. This occurs with excessive frequency with unaccommodated trauma. Reducing these is a goal in treatment. Regarding PTSD as seen by the DSM, van der Kolk and McFarlane (1996) noted that intrusions prevent the person from attending to incoming information as the individual eventually bails out of such a situation. At some point the avoidance tendency becomes excessive and eventually gives way to generalized numbing of responsiveness. Over time too, victims are often unable to modulate their physiological responses to stress in general, leading to an inability to deal with life and utilize signs as guides for actions.

Results of several studies using a Modified Stroop Color-Word Test indicate that in explicit memory testing PTSD participants exhibit a greater bias than control participants in relative recall of combat words. This also applies for PTSD participants for implicit memory tests where bias is also shown. McNally, Kaspi, Beumann, and Zeitlini (1990) argued that only information that is personally threatening is preferentially processed. Only disorder-specific threat information, therefore, is associated with bias and physiological activation. This is distinct from the work of the Litz group (Litz et al., 1996) where information processing biases appear to be both trauma-specific and dependent on other factors in the cognitive processing.

Interestingly, the Litz group (Litz et al., 1996) showed that the failure to process emotional events fully leads to physiological and psychosomatic problems. The latter are related to emotional numbing—you might say an advanced stage of avoidance. Information or experiences of trauma that are too discrepant cannot be understood. Over time PTSD does not subside and a "psychic surrender," a freezing of affect, results (Krystal, 1968). Dissociation (Spiegel et al., 1988), alexithymia (Steinberg, 1978), and disorganization (Hyer et al., 1994) are other words used to describe this state. The information is not moving in the system (Shapiro, 1995).

Because at later life older people suffer from generalized problems of attention, distractibility, and often cognitive decline, needs for the processing of information regarding the trauma are not all met. The processing of information is already compromised; the mechanisms become "comfortable" with patterns of approach/avoidance that reinforce the status quo (Litz & Keane, 1989). Given this problem, older people also have an advantage—they can rework earlier stories, now as meta-historians, in a natural way. Later life is the time to renegotiate these choices. History and identity are both made and discovered. Whether older people can overcome the problem of the conditioning and the faulty processing is unclear.

PTSD plays out on the stage of the mind and body. We separate these only in our professional texts. Traumatic stressors cause distinct biological, psychological, and social responses in life. Alterations in one of these will intimately affect the other two. In fact, it is not the direct experience of the trauma itself that marks PTSD. It is the persistence of the intrusive and distressing recollections, the psychological dimensions of PTSD that are its hallmark. Although a poor reaction to trauma has sediment in reality—the concrete facts of the traumatic experience—PTSD victims are bothered by their memories and, as a consequence, a host of other situations become problems themselves.

☐ Other Influences of Trauma

It is only in retrospect that the person of the trauma victim is assessed. Different symptoms of PTSD often represent the outcome of specific features of traumatic exposures at varying points in development, secondary adversities that develop along the line (including adverse caretaking), disturbances in the acquisition and integration of developmental competencies, the disruption of developmental transitions, and disturbances in normal biological maturation. We consider then several other PTSD and aging-related issues and discuss their impact and interaction.

Biology

We start with the biology of PTSD. PTSD is biological. With few exceptions (Freidman & Southwick, 1995), PTSD does not conform to the classic biological or neurological lesion analysis. There are few or no corresponding neuroanatomical correlates that are pathognomonic and identifiable via autopsy, computed topography (CT) scan or magnetic resonance imaging (MRI) scan. There is a biological smorgasbord of reactions: a probable kindling where trauma leads to hypersensitivity and vulnerability, a perverted display of sympathetic nervous system arousal (increase startle response), hyperfunction of the hypothalamus-pituitary-adrenocortical axis, dysregulation of the endogenous opioid system, and changes in the physiology of sleep and dreaming (insomnia). These changes combine with psychoendocrine disorientation of cardiac reactivity, elevations in blood pressure, and elevations in urinary catecholamine levels, at least (see Foa, Davidson, & Francis, 1999; Friedman, 2000). In addition, van der Kolk (1999) outlined the significant immunological abnormalities in women with histories of chronic sexual abuse.

Other biological data collude also. Perhaps the most important is that provided by LeDoux and colleagues. They have shown that, once formed, the subcortical traces of the conditioned fear response are indelible and that an "emotional memory may be forever" (LeDoux et al., 1991, p. 24). At a neural level PTSD can be a strange brew. Biologically, if one is traumatized by a dramatic event, the emotional component of the experience is coded in the limbic system. Circuitry of the brain's fear centers is activated more intensely in PTSD than normal participants. In fact, we process fear at two levels: one is processed through the higher brain (cortical level) and the other occurs in lightning speed just below the radar (subcortical level). LeDoux believed that it is the amygdala, in the center of the lymbic system, that causes the problem at the subcortical level. It only takes one event for the amygdala to process incoming data in milliseconds. Later fears do not travel to the thinking part of the brain, implying that we become afraid and never have an awareness of that state. We have a separate memory of the feared stimulus informed by the terror of the event, not consciously experienced.

van der Kolk (1999) believed that memories of intense events become engrafted into the mature brain. Repetitive presentations are usually at the core of learning and memory. Frequent exposure leads to sensitization and kindling. Once sensitized, only mild external stimuli are required for a response. As the individual moves along the threat continuum (calm arousal to terror), different areas of the brain control and organize the response. The more threatened the person, the more primitive the area of the brain.

So some trauma occurs, a neural circuit develops, and the future is acted as if the event were occurring again. The shear act of imagination powered by the human cognitive machine (or a simple stimulus) now creates havoc in day-to-day acts. This seems to be what PTSD is about: An endless debate between fear and reason played out over time, often in imaging form. There is, therefore, a complex relationship between brain and body, mediated through a disregulated hypothalamus pituitary adrenal axis, and resulting in what we know as PTSD.

Lest anyone be ambivalent about a dysregulated biology, recall the study by Shalev et al. (1992). They found that both the central and autonomic nervous systems that mediate the conditioned response failed to habituate in over 90% of the PTSD group compared with 22% in the controlled participants. People with PTSD and those exposed to trauma without PTSD continue to show failure of habituation. Something is wrong in the hard wiring.

McFarland and van der Kolk (1995) believed that biological data have prominence and tend to dominate the study of PTSD just as in other psychiatric disorders. But, in a simple way of looking at this condition, practically everybody who is exposed to extreme stress develops intrusive symptoms. Only some, however, develop avoidance and hyperarousal. For them, it is thought the persistence of intrusive and repetitious thoughts, perhaps by means of kindling, sets up a chronic pattern of arousal. In addition, after being chronically aroused without being able to do much about this, people with PTSD experience feelings of being in a dangerous situation. Because of these difficulties of using emotions to help them think through situations and come up with adequate schemas to help them deal with things, these emotions themselves become dangerous. While it may be easy to make biological findings the metaphors for psychosocial models and thus to disuse what we do not know, something in the biology is amiss, and this may have special applicability at later life where an intrinsic mutagenesis is taking place.

Heterogeniety

Heterogeneity is maximal at later life. There is considerable diversity among normal older adults in the general population. Although no one has looked particularly at the variance of older PTSD victims relative to younger ones, it is probable that this disorder has more varieties at older ages, even subclinical. A number of factors define subtypes of PTSD, such as chronicity of illness, severity and type of trauma, developmental phase when the trauma occurred, comorbid symptoms, and prior psychiatric illness. This explains in part why no single medication or modality has emerged to date as the treatment of choice. Perhaps generalizations are achieved by replication of a case by case basis only.

Valent (1999) reminded us of the "normal" unfolding of the trauma. The person transits through given trauma: impact phase (saving life and property), post-impact phase (insuring vital resources and preparing for recurrence), taking stock and re-building, and healing and building up reserves. Each phase has its own stresses and problems. Valent (1999) also discussed survival strategies, biopsychosocial tactics that develop to enhance maximum survival within social limits. Their understanding is necessary to specify and make sense of acute traumatic stress responses and their developments. They include both successful or unsuccessful responses to a trauma.

Complex PTSD

PTSD is best viewed, not as a continuation of the acute response, but rather a distinct state that develops from the acute stress response based on a host of factors in addition to trauma severity, such as genetic liability and family history, psychiatric history, trauma history, current and past familial relationships, current social support, and the pre-trauma personality. As the distinction between the acute traumatic response and PTSD is clarified, the etiologic model (which elevates trauma as the primary causal factor) appears increasingly inadequate.

A number of authors have suggested alternative classification schemes to better describe the range of difficulties found among survivors of chronic trauma (Herman, 1992; Pelcovitz et al., 1997; Terr, 1991; World Health Organization, 1994). Complex PTSD has been noted. This has been referred to in the literature under a number of names, including disorders of extreme stress not otherwise specified (DESNOS) and complicated PTSD (Hiley-Young, 1992; Herman, 1992; Pelcovitz et al., 1997; van der Kolk, et al., 1999).

Complex PTSD is associated with PTSD as it requires a trauma but is also different as it possesses unique symptoms. Empirically it is independent (Ford, 1999). It has several features. They include (a) impairment of affect regulation; (b) chronic self-destructive behavior, amnesia, or dissociation; (c) somatization; (d) alterations in relationship to self; (e) distorted relationship with perpetrator; (f) distorted relations with others; and (g) loss of sustaining beliefs. van der Kolk (1999) believed that these conditions are prevalent among most outpatient populations, and that the elements of care that are optimal for this type of trauma are different than those for PTSD. They include symptom management, the realization of repetitive patterns, the connection of internal states and actions (aggression, sex, eating, gambling, and cutting), and then the identification of traumatic memory nodes.

Interaction

PTSD of course cannot be explained entirely by the emergence of traumatic memories and their associated cognitive and biological processes. People bring to the table their own baggage. Schnurr, Friedman, and Rosenberg (1993), Kessler et al. (1995), McCranie, Boudewyns, Hyer, and Woods (1991), and Breslau and Davis (1992) have shown the role of prior disorders and family history make a difference. Resnick et al. (1993a) noted that women who had been raped tended to have lower acute cortisol response to a subsequent rape than women who had been raped for the first time. Clearly they are at an increased risk for PTSD. And, one must be aware of prior symptoms in the constellation of PTSD. In the Times Beach situation when symptoms existing prior to the event were taken into account, only those problems related to depression and PTSD remained as being significant in the prediction of later adjustment (Hyer et al., 1994).

The response to trauma is determined by many factors including individual vulnerability or resiliency at the time of the trauma, as well as being appropriately supported and not "abused" by rescue efforts. Adaptations to chronic trauma are also important as many of the problems in people who suffer from PTSD are actually consequences of the secondary effects of the disorder that include the appraisal of the experience as it unfolds. However, with older people, the idea that PTSD exists as it was or de novo does not serve anyone well.

Shalev, Peri, Caneti, and Schreiber (1996) summarized 38 studies on the predictors of PTSD. The existence of PTSD is no accident but can be complicated to predict. These predictors relate to pre-trauma vulnerability, magnitude of the stressor, preparedness for the event, quality of the immediate and short-term responses, and post-event recovery factors. Although the predictors of PTSD present a complex picture in the development of the disorder, there is a "bad" combination of the variables and these appear to lead to a genuine traumatic stress response. Prior experience in the resolution of a trauma assists in the next trauma; the obverse is true also. Often PTSD does not emerge immediately after a trauma. It is probable that a delayed response emerges out of the pattern of the acute distress caused by the trauma. What this means is that a delayed response to trauma occurs and is even predictable to many, especially if the response is disallowed in the immediate aftermath. This latency of response is especially fascinating at later life as the press of living seems to potentiate earlier problems.

It is true that there is a general decline characteristic of PTSD. For those who decline over time there is usually a reduction in intrusive symptoms despite the potential ongoing expression of arousal (McFarlane & Yehuda, 1996). You might say there is an acute and chronic reaction, the latter being a reaction to the initial symptoms of the disorder: The longer PTSD lasts, the less important is the role of the initial trauma exposure.

Trajectory

The relationship between symptoms and adjustment alters over time, suggesting that the relationship between these is fluid. It is probable, too, that the constellation of symptoms changes with the march of time. The neurobiology seems to alter over time even as the importance of the trauma itself wanes. An understanding of the longitudinal course of PTSD is important, as it will assist in the caretaking at later life.

A poor trauma reaction begins of course with an acute reaction. Acute reactions are highly variable and change rapidly in their presentation. Beardslee (1986) also noted that individuals rework the original trauma at each subsequent developmental stage, as new cues become salient. Therefore, relapses over the course of the lifetime can and should be expected. As trauma survivors get older, they may become increasingly likely to experience severe symptoms of PTSD, and even formerly asymptomatic individuals may develop problems.

It is no surprise that the rates of PTSD go down over time. Foa, Routhbaum, Riggs, and Murdoc (1991) showed that PTSD symptoms existed in 94% of rape victims 1 week after the event, 52.4% in 2 months, and 47.1% 9 months later. McFarlane and Papay (1992) assessed 469 fire fighters: 15% had PTSD. After 42 months, 56% of the PTSD group had PTSD again. Years later only 4% had PTSD but 62% had significant intrusive symptoms and arousal (avoidance criterion was not reached). Intensity went down also and the generalizability of the symptoms were greater.

Weisaeth (1984) noted that the initial reaction makes a difference. He noted that sleeplessness and agitation, along with anxiety, are special predictors of PTSD. In one interesting study, Shalev et al. (1996) evaluated 51 civilian trauma survivors, 13 of whom had PTSD. Of the PTSD participants, the symptoms of avoidance increased between 1 and 6 months; of the non-PTSD participants, avoidance decreased. The intrusion scores on the Impact of Events Scale (IES) went down for both groups. Avoidance may then be a defensive strategy to handle intrusion. Intrusive symptoms may not be specific to PTSD, however the combination of intrusion and avoidance are. In fact, evidence exists that the immediate reaction to a trauma influences the eventual reaction to the trauma. The Foa group (Foa et al., 1991) showed that, if arousal symptoms are evident early, this is a good sign; avoidant symptoms later in the course of a trauma reaction are usually negative. Intrusive symptoms have a low diagnostic specificity but the combination of intrusions and avoidance does.

We are of course talking in generalities as the variables that influence the trauma response differ over time, those directly influential after the trauma differing from those 30 or 50 years later (Schnurr & Aldwin, 1993). We know that the consequences of PTSD persist. Knowledge of a trajectory of the (mental) health problems of trauma victims can provide important information on prognosis and care (Mellman, Randolph, Brawman-Mintzer, Flores, & Milanes, 1992). In regards to combat trauma, roughly 20% are continuously troubled, 20% are symptom free totally, and the remainder experience intermittent symptoms (Hyer & Summers, 1995). The typical pattern of decline involves a continuation of lifelong problems, not a sudden development of a new disorder. Delayed PTSD happens but is less usual. A tardive reaction to trauma happens, but it is really a different reading of the trauma that was always there. A subclinical state may have been present (Summers & Hyer, 1994). Perhaps too, at remitted periods the older victim practices "escapist" coping (Aldwin, 1995), or "downward adjusts," (Suls, Marco, & Tobin, 1991) to cope in the real world. Often too, the symptom expression of trauma alters and mellows at later life, as aging-related variables assert a greater influence.

☐ Special Problems

We end by identifying three issues that are special problems for the safe and appropriate processing of trauma. They are not typical in the prevention of trauma problems at later life. Nonetheless they do occur. We have not considered these separately before.

Past Sexual Trauma

In the PTSD literature the phenomenon of delayed memory due to child sexual abuse has been instructive. It occurs, even for older adults. A substantial percentage of adults with child sexual abuse histories report that there was a point in their lives when they were not aware of their abuse history. There is some indication that the likelihood of forgetting this abuse may be associated with more violent abuse, ongoing abuse that occurs earlier in life and that ends before adolescence, and more extended abuse. The age of the abuse, the severity of the abuse, and the type of abuse often prevent meaningful storage of the event and subsequent cognitive processing. This especially applies to abuse that occurs in childhood before the age of 6. Little or no recall of the experience occur in children before ages 7 and older (Yule & Williams, 1990).

Whereas the presence of an early trauma, such as sex abuse, is not modal in older victims, the presence of trauma in other forms may be (Hyer and Summers, 1994). For research purposes the active suppression of the memory may be a black hole, the subject for investigation of amnesia, the typical mechanisms of forgetting and current needs/mood states are more familiar to clinicians. In later life the developmental milestones and losses are at the ready to unleash the occult suppression of trauma. Over time also, the active suppression of thoughts about trauma predispose individuals to stress-related illnesses (Pennebacker, 1985). It is the gift that keeps on giving.

Dissociation

Dissociation occurs with PTSD. Clinicians do not need this headache. This is described by DSM-IV as "a disruption in the usually integrated functions of consciousness, memory, identity, or perception of the environment" (p. 477). Braun (1988) postulated that consciousness consists of the four domains of behavior, affect, sensation, and knowledge, and that dissociation involves the splitting off of any one of these experiences from others. Cues or triggers associated with any one of these four domains can also lead to the retrieval of memories or the reconnection of memory fragments (Courtois, 1992; Olio & Cornell, 1993). van der Kolk, van der Hart, and Marmar (1996) believe that trauma victims hold trauma in mostly primary (fragmentation of the experience) or secondary (out of body experiences) dissociation. The net effect here is the creation of "states of mind."

A wide body of research documents the presence of dissociative disorders and experiences in both child and adult sexual abuse survivors, as well as war trauma victims (Hyer et al., 1994). Nonetheless, "pure" dissociation is relatively uncommon in older victims (Summers & Hyer, 1994). The Dissociative Experiences Scale (Bernstein & Putnam, 1986), a self-report questionnaire, can be used to document dissociative experiences and phenomenology in older PTSD victims.

Type II Trauma

Type II trauma refers to the extent to which the trauma is severe or continuous. This can make a difference in memory. Terr (1983, 1994) noted that the post-traumatic reactions of some individuals are associated with clear, detailed recall of events, whereas others are associated with loss of memory. She proposed that Type I trauma involves single-blow traumatic events of a circumscribed nature and is associated with relatively complete memory. Type II trauma, on the other hand, is related to repeated and prolonged trauma. Herman (1992, 1993) proposed that trauma reactions can be best understood as a continuum of disorders ranging from PTSD associated with circumscribed trauma to complex PTSD (her term for DESNOS), which are associated with chronic and prolonged trauma.

In both Terr and Herman's formulations, more memory problems result from multiple or complex forms of PTSD. In fact, current formulations of PTSD do not adequately attend to many of the long-term symptoms of PTSD and associated problems, including somatization, dissociation, affective changes, identity alterations, revictimization, and characterlogical changes that mimic personality disorders (Herman, 1993). Older people who have PTSD as a result of Type II trauma are difficult to treat, often frozen in time.

☐ Conclusion

In this chapter we saw the essential tension of precision in science. On the one hand, we require exactness. Kasniack and Christenson (1994) hold that "the risks of misdiagnosis, and the potential benefits of accurate diagnosis, make strong arguments for the importance of careful diagnostic evaluation." In fact, this is one of the first rules of medicine, diagnosis then treatment. On the other hand, a precise theory of care with older people does not exist. At later life there may be little specificity in the form of the disorder. PTSD and depression may, for example, both be served by negative thinking with PTSD patients represented with more danger and safety schemas. They may have developed a learned helplessness. Very old people (>85) may be different still: Evidence exists that the very old may long for death, making therapy different to say the least. The DSMs and our working rules of care may not apply.

Regrettably, we have ignored many "critical" questions. Research on the organization, decision rules, and best exemplars of PTSD at later life have been left behind. What really is PTSD at later life? We do not know what potentiates problems for the most common variety of the aging person, the appearance of PTSD symptoms after remitted periods: Do trauma symptoms occur as a result of age-related coping decline, recent stressful events, or is it just the nature of the disorder? With regret, we simply assume that the DSM is the best model for the categorization of a person who experiences trauma.

Finally, we note that no other disorder in the DSM appears to share more symptoms with other disorders or is as conceptually related to other disorders as PTSD. Conceptually, we can examine this "system" from a logical perspective and playfully challenge: Does not PTSD constitute an expected response or is it rightly a non-normative response? Or more aptly, what is normal for one who is violently abused? Although the DSM is an important element in the understanding of PTSD, it is not the only resource. In 1994, Hyer wrote:

> While consensus exists on the symptom clusters of intrusion, numbing, and increased arousal, confusion prevails around the makeup of each. Symptoms can be so bizarre (e.g., illusions or hallucinations, flashbacks), so distancing (e.g., emotional deadness), so embedded (e.g., hyperarousal even to stimuli remotely connected to the trauma), or so pervasive and recalcitrant to change (e.g., intrusion or sleeplessness), that the diagnosis of PTSD easily extends to other disorders and its treatment is an imposing task. Nonetheless one feature of PTSD seems firm: as the psychiatric community "traveled through" the DSMs since 1952 (DSM-I), the idea of a stress reaction changed from one emphasizing its transient nature to the current view that extreme events have long and lasting sequelae.

This still applies.

Life Story of the Aging Person

Tell me the story now
Now that it's over
Wrap it in glory
For one Irish rover
van Morrison

The archtypical story of the archer holds that the minute the archer focuses on the target, he becomes nervous and misses; when he lives in the whole experience, he is successful. This chapter is about how the whole person, the multiple levels of the person, especially the storied self, and the processes of aging, both faces of age, apply in a trauma context. We have argued that knowing the person and the self well requires an exploration of those aspects of living that are less amenable to just one analysis. We need to know the personhood and have some understanding of the self.

Memory is most parsimoniously viewed as modular. A memory is but one story that represents only a selection of events about a life. It is the person's own view or story of self. No single truth exists, only different perspectives, each one a perspective of the world from different vantage points. Through the mechanisms of therapy and the gradual discovery process with other stories, the original story can have a new voice. This after all is what is occurring in the reintegration of the trauma memory. The existence of other stories can also emerge through the gentle massage of the schema that lies beneath memories. These will be rendered more understandable if we know the person (the levels noted above and the transiting process—the life cycle).

Most elders will experience the full normative life course, and think of themselves as growing, changing, moving through passages. The self assists in the formation of a trajectory of life development from the remembered past to the anticipated future. This is a comfortable conceptual environment for notions of progress and self-improvement over time.

To more fully appreciate this, we look again at the aging process. Aging has some benefits, not the least of which is that it is a time for life review. This allows for order and meaning to life, and an ability to defend the dignity of one's own lifestyle. We really become "inward" creatures for meaning-making. At later life we have privileged access to ourselves through inner reflection.

In this chapter we address the face of aging, the good and the bad. We then explore what we mean when we say we "know" a person, at any given time or across the life-span. This is a conceptual view of a practical clinical issue: people grow with some consistency across time and the life story serves as a needed guide. Next we discuss the life-story as the means by which people understand and define themselves—the culmination of (selected) events in an autobiography that explains the self that one knows. Finally we consider language and the part it plays in the unfolding of the life story.

☐ Two Faces of Aging

The Tension

Perhaps the experience of aging is best viewed as a series of confrontations with self (Whitbourne, 1985). People punctuate aging by noticing the body (physical appearance, physical competence, and health), cognition (intellectual self-efficacy, memory self-efficacy, and wisdom), and personality (sense of self and traits, emotions, and coping/defenses). In this way people come to some understanding of the aging process. It is not hard to see how, given varied circumstances, age can be either a risk or a protective factor in the development of psychiatric symptoms (Lyons, 1991; Realmuto, Wagner, & Bartholow, 1991). Cath (1963) eloquently identified a key struggle at later life: growth versus depletion. The older person establishes a balance between factors that promote self-esteem and sense of self (e.g., past accomplishments, wisdom from experiences, past philosophical world view, etc.) versus factors related to depletion (e.g., failing health, cognitive impairment, etc.). Through the balance between these two sets of forces, the person adapts, often in one of two forms, well-being or depletion/depression.

If stress is too intense or if internal changes are major, the adaptive process may go awry and becomes increasingly maladaptive. This has been labeled a "social breakdown syndrome," a vicious cycle of increasing incompetence (Bengston, Beedy, & Gordon, 1985). This is of course the negative side. Kuypers (1974) described another aspect of aging, "social reconstruction syndrome." This construct (from social psychology) emphasizes a benign cycle of increasing competence through internal and external social system inputs, such as positive self-labeling, development of coping skills, positive self image, and environmental support. Paul Balter (2000) views people and the aging process as compromising, "selective organization with compensation." Through these, ultimately the aging person can reduce his/her dependence on the environment or at least reach a better acceptance of his/her limitations. This represents the positive side.

Below we discuss how this process, along with the nature of the life review process, assists in the integration of trauma. Here we view these two faces of aging.

Debilitation

Kipling noted that a look at the best deserves a look at the worst. Older people respond to social changes as a function of the interaction between personality style, the subjective meaning of aging, and the context in which aging occurs. All three are important. Older people experience both minor (Ensel, 1991) and major (Hyer & Summers, 1994) negative life events, often are bothered by these (Falk, Hersen, &

Van Hasselt, 1994; Tait & Silver, 1984), and underrepresent or alter (e.g., somaticizing) problems (Hankin, Abueg, Gallagher-Thompson, & Laws, 1996), or have a more closed view of mental problems (Logsdon, 1995). When an elder becomes frail, as in a nursing home setting, a different set of rules applies regarding psychopathology. In fact, we would argue that, if debilitated and no current control of the situation or ability to reconstruct memories exist, symptoms naturally result.

A list of the issues related to frail elders is given in Box 3-1. Frail older people show some common characteristics. There is a remarkable stability of the self across time. When the process is moving along as it should, this person adapts to the situation. Older people in a frail situation, however, become less aggressive, rely on the past, and cope in more religious ways. Many give up the fight, become less introspective and less troubled by minor issues. Older people who are debilitated also handle distortions better and allow unacceptable motives into consciousness with greater ease. They accept more dissonance and ambiguity than at other ages. This occurs with relative ease compared with other ages. As we will see, older more debilitated people have an autobiographical impulse, probably as a way to keep self constancy and esteem.

There are many negative features also. Mild ones are almost romantic. Older frail people also show a tendency to mythologize the past. Past and present become interchangeable. The frail older person will often note that they are in charge now, when in fact they are reflecting past times. Older people will say that the family is the best ever, when in fact this was never the case. Nothing terribly wrong here.

Box 3-1
Characteristics of Frail Older People

Positive/interesting issues:
    Interchange of past and present
    Distortions
    Lessened introspection
    Reliance on the past
    Aggressiveness
    Magical coping
    Religious coping
    Transference (needy)
Minor problems:
    Poor health
    Say "no" (expectations)
    Say "yes but"
Worse problems:
    Social support poor
    Poor cognitive strength
    Cognitive decline
    Hopelessness
    Personality disorder
    Depression (endogeniety)

But there may be other problems. The person who was in control earlier in life now has little control. If trauma has been dragged into later life and debilitation exists, the residual effects of trauma at later life can have all the problems of other ages *plus*. As a result of poor health, poor social support, or cognitive problems, the frail elder withdraws or becomes agitated. Often the person will show delusional confusion, have nightmares, and experience severe intrusions. Often depression or rigid personality patterns surface. PTSD now is most severe as it is fanned with disinhibition or general debilitation. This is beyond "complicated PTSD" in which characteristics of the person maintain and direct the expression of PTSD. Here the process of aging, the disease process, drives the PTSD (Box 3-1).

As the battle with the normal and not-so-normal slights of age unfolds, the issue of narcissism peaks (Joubowty & Newton, 1999). Along with childhood, adulthood brings on new narcissistic challenges. Forces that modify the adult self are fueled by narcissistic gratifications and disappointments in adulthood. In the integrated person this is closely related to reality and leads to healthy action (healthy self-aggrandizement). This involves normal mourning as well as a constant restructuring of self with age-appropriate mechanisms of obtaining gratification. Pathological forms of incomplete grief or depression do not surface. In a sense the self is respected, reality is preserved, and growth is possible.

In sum, the combination of frailty in aging and trauma can be its own undoing. Plasticity is out, decline is in. Psychopathology often drowns in the sea of debilitation. Here, the clinical focus is management.

Wisdom of Age

For years growth across the life cycle has been discussed. Developmentalists too, like Maslow, Allport, Rogers, Jung, and Erikson especially, argued for a continuing process of self-discovery and self-development. Jung let the uninformed public know about the sources of "other" growth that occurs at later life. Among others, these involved the spiritual sense of self and the individual's relationship to self. This included individuation, the continuing process of self-discovery and self-development. This was the time too when the individual resolved the internal and external realities and integrated opposing functions that would mark the culmination of development (thought and feeling, sensation and intuition). Similarly, for Erikson the last tasks of life—love, care, and wisdom—are different in kind (Erikson, 1975), and present themselves with the hope that a sense of integrity can be achieved.

When patients make progress after a siege of medical problems, we say that they have spirit and a will to live. In fact, there is a long tradition of systematically attending to assets and strengths of older people (Neugarten & Neugarten, 1994; Kivnick, 1996). Kivnick and Murray (1997) noted that the older person has a vital involvement, an innate and vigorous engagement with the elements of the environment. This is an active state that presents a readiness to act on inclinations that have not been activated yet. It is the "thing" in the person that does not allow for distractions—it is the "who am I" part of the person. This is really a reflector of the person's lifelong purpose and meaning that reflects identity. It is the self of the person.

The process of aging can be highly functional (Box 3-2). With aging, an eventual "adaptation to lessened resources" (Dibner, 1978) occurs that helps to compensate for the intrinsic mutagenesis that leads to senescence. This selective optimization with compensation (Baltes, 1987) allows older people to use energy more efficiently. Kastenbaum (1985) noted that older people essentially adapt to stress as well as novel

---

Box 3-2
Aspects of the Wisdom of Age

1. Individual differences
    Interiority
    Hyperhabituation
    Autobiographical impulse
    Mellowing
    Integrity-seeking (loss of egocentrism)
    Well-being factors (Ryff, 1984)
    Passive mastery
    Reminiscence
    Stability of the self
    Adapt to lessened resources
    Seek teachable moments
2. Cognitive
    Wisdom (descriptive and interpretative knowledge)
    Cognitive complexity
    Postformal reasoning
3. Transpersonal
    Gerotranscendence
    Cosmic, cohesive, and solitude

---

stimuli. He labeled this "hyperhabituation, the well-entrenched tendency to assimilate the novel to the familiar, to devour the stimulus" (p. 111). This is the way it is supposed to be.

Still others see the aging process in even more optimistic ways. It is the time to see life as it is (Baltes & Staudinger, 1993), and to appreciate universal and cosmic properties (Chinen, 1986). Van den Dale (1975) and Chinen (1984) have suggested that cognitive behavior in later life is characterized by a "swing back from the highly relativistic, contextual thinking of middle-aged postformal thought to a renewed appreciation of the universal, perhaps in the form of aesthetic or affective properties" (Stevens-Long, 1990, p. 135). Several writers borrowed Piaget's emergent and invariant sequences of cognitive development as a basis for proposing changes beyond the endpoint of formal operations. This is a stage present by young adulthood and characterized by the ability to formulate and test hypotheses and thus deal with variability (Stevens-Long, 1990). Commons and Richards's (1982) notion of structural analytic thought, and Basseches's (1984) stage of dialectical thinking, are both proposed as postformal stages in which an individual develops the ability to understand and compare competing sets of relationships or systems. Over time, adults begin to think more relatively and less universally, appreciating the tension between their own perspective and those of other systems. Labouvie-Vief (1982a, 1982b) labels this autonomous or intersystemic thought, in which older thinkers can "integrate logic and the irrational aspect of experience ... [they] see not only how truth can be a product of a particular system, but also how the thinker participates in creating the truth" (Stevens-Long, 1990, p. 133).

Just when we thought that we had run out of terms for successful aging, a new one appeared, *gerotranscendence*. This represents a "developmental process" in which the individual gradually experiences a new understanding of fundamental questions of life (Tornstam, 1994). Tornstam conducted an empirical study on gerotranscendence, assessing 912 Danish men and women between the ages of 74 and 100 years of age. Participants were measured by a series of statements in which the respondents had to agree or disagree on a 5-point scale. The overall impression was that a large proportion of responders recognized in themselves the content of various statements. Those high in gerotranscendence tended to have a higher degree of self-control and social activity, a high degree of life satisfaction, greater satisfaction with social activities, and less dependence on social activities for well-being. Even individuals who had negative changes in life satisfaction tended to be aided by the development of gerotranscendence and its more active and complex coping patterns.

Tornstam (1996; 1997) followed up his initial gerotranscendent study by conducting a mail survey of 2002 Swedish men and women between the ages of 20 and 85. This was a cross sectional design that was intended to determine if different age groups would be in line with the theory of gerotranscendence. He identified three levels: (a) cosmic applies to the transcendence of space, time, and objects, the connection of earlier generations, a rejoicing in life; (b) coherence involves an increased ego integrity; and (c) solitude involves a changed meaning and importance in relationships. Results suggest that cosmic and coherence levels are continuous processes that begin during the first half of adult life and gradually develop to the maximum in the later half. The need for solitude also reaches a maximum at late life but develops more rapidly during the first half of adult life. Of importance, crises do have an impact on this phenomenon.

Sherman (1981) outlined several aging-related components for integration in relation to stress. These included increased interiority, internal locus of control, passive mastery, reminiscence, and a self-orientation that seeks to set the past right (life review). Perhaps the most important of these is a natural retrospective focus that seeks to meld present (and future) concerns to allow for self changes. Although resistance or closure (moratorium) can and does occur at later life, it is less virulent than at other ages (Sherman, 1991).

Additionally, the idea of wisdom has surfaced in the last decade. Measures of wisdom assess three areas: cognitive (is able to see to the heart of important problems); affective (is giving, behaves empathically, is likable, is compassionate, and has integrity); and reflective (is tolerant of ambiguity, is introspective, has insight, and does not project). Stretching data somewhat, what appears to be at the core is that there may be a state of chronological giftedness in many older people. They possess an expert knowledge system on the pragmatics of life. It is a pursuit of truth and the ability to see life as it is. It represents a true dialectic on life issues with less emotionality and more understanding and acceptance.

Older age then may not be just a continuation of earlier ages, not just mature resilience of coping or improved stress inoculation. It may be the time, the only time, to see life as it is (Baltes & Staudinger, 1993) and to appreciate universal and cosmic properties (Chinen, 1986). It is now clear that objective life conditions (socioeconomic status, physical environment, financial status, social relationships, and social supports) are not sufficient alone to account for life satisfaction. Personality (Costa & McRae, 1990) and developmental influences across the life span (Elder & Caspi, 1990) as well as wisdom (Baltes, 2000) contribute measurably. As argued, the element of maturity provides its own expertise.

Finally, we note that most older people are happy. Life satisfaction according to Neugarten has been frequently used as a measuring gauge. Although there are objections to life satisfaction as a measure, perhaps the best way to find out whether people are healthy or happy is simply to ask them. In one highly relevant study by Dorfman and Walsh (1996), 28 community-dwelling participants were selected and assessed. Focus groups at two senior activity sites were used to obtain data. Successful aging consisted of a complex pattern of interrelated constructs, including mental activity as the dominant aspect. Included in this were components relating to memory, flexibility, challenge, curiosity, alertness, busyness, and a sense of humor.

Most people desire to age successfully although they have no conception of what this means and little agreement exists in the scientific community on what constitutes successful aging (Ryff, 1984). According to Havighurst and Albrecht (1953), high levels of involvement and activity define successful aging. Ryff suggested that such involvement is the means by which older people meet the unique challenges of later life and enhance their personal growth. She identified six factors in this effort: (a) a positive evaluation of one's self and one's past (self-acceptance), (b) a sense of continued growth and development as a person (personal growth), (c) the belief that one's life is purposeful and meaningful (purpose in life), (d) possession of quality relations with people (positive relations with others), (e) the capacity to manage effectively one's life and surrounding world (environmental mastery), and (f) a sense of self determination (autonomy). Despite criticism of what these mean, they represent common sense standards of growth.

Clearly the therapeutic design for this emphasis of the straw man (of debility and wisdom) is one of optimism. The elements of resilience and psychological well-being are operable here, through the power of the life story.

☐ A Developmental Synthesis

There is an order to the conversations, memories, and personal theories of older people. It exists somewhere on the continuum of health and frailty. People do seem to want to fill the incomplete mind, more so at later life. This may only depend on locating oneself in relation to goods and commitments (Taylor, 1998). Whenever we act as an interpreting human being, we construe ourselves and our lives in terms of inescapable person (moral) questions. If we fail to find application for these questions, then we fail to find application for the notions of self and person (Taylor, 1989). Kivnick and Murray (1997) labelled this vital involvement, the necessity for each individual to enact his/her personal strengths and commitments on life at each moment. As trite as it sounds, the "whole" person acts and the "whole" person suffers.

We argue that the examined life is important; it is also natural. The person crosses life with both personal and sociocultural engrams. The marker, age, allows us to visit this in selected ways. For many older people, the past comes into the present and the two commingle until the strength of the past (or present) provides necessary support for the faltering present (or past). Neither self-validation nor contentment care if the operative time was then or is now.

Nicely, many clinicians have now moved beyond psychopathology to focus their investigations on constructs of invulnerability, growth, competence, meaning-making or cognitive adaptation, coping, and resiliency, to name a few. As social scientists, we are looking in other places for answers to problem states. Perhaps this is not new, but it is not just postmodernism either. It is the language of forming answers, of healthy uncertainty, of better valuations.

One Point in Time: What Do We Know About a Person?

A tale is woven here, a model of a person. We start with an overarching model given by McAdams. It is a model for understanding the process of the person at a point in time. Later we will address the person across time. Again, we borrow from McAdams. Then we discuss the importance of the story or narrative and place the autobiographical memory at its center. Consider the following example.

Case X

Ralph, a 74-year-old, retired mechanic and combat veteran (Korea) had lost interest in the things he used to deeply enjoy. Not least of which was his family. His children told of how he "began to change" after retiring in 1990. He had to give up running his garage when his doctor told him he had to take it easy. A heart attack had done extensive damage and he would never have the physical capacity he enjoyed until recently. In 1995, Ralph lost his wife, Rosa, with whom he'd spent 47 years and raised four children. He took the loss very hard and went into a depression. His children noted that he'd lost what used to be a powerful interest in his grandchildren. Concerned for his emotional well-being and pained by seeing him suffer, they persuaded him to see a therapist.

Ralph was by all accounts stubborn. Previous psychological testing confirmed Ralph's strong tendency toward independence and not wanting anything from anyone. He managed his life his way. He could assist others but only through a barrage of later "comments." At times he could be gruff, even hurtful. Ralph was the type of person who knew how to actively engage his environment and create what he wanted. He knew how to "get the job done" in order to get his needs met and had done so many times. On one occasion he borrowed money from a friend of his father's who'd seen his passion, appreciated his talent, and taken a chance on him. This was the only time he had asked for anything. It was easy to see how it would be so very difficult for this self-made man to "take it easy" and passively experience life rather than shape it as he always had.

Ralph never thought that he would be the one to be alive after so many years. After all no one really understood him except Rosa. He related to her that he was the "tough seed" and that he took care of others. No one trampled on him when he was growing up unless they paid a price. He liked to tell the story of the early winters and how he would challenge the coal man after he refused to give his mother coal. Even at age 5 he had to be restrained as he threatened this man. Now he felt vulnerable, perhaps for the first time.

How does one make sense of this? How can the therapist really understand this person in such a way as to be in a position to open him up to a new way of being? Do we know Ralph through the clinician's eyes of independence and perhaps avoidant traits, his place in the family, his symptoms, his story? How could the health care provider understand Ralph's pain surrounding the loss of his wife without knowing the context of his life? Are these the "right" fibers a therapist must be familiar with to work effectively not to change them but reweave them. Without the story, there could be no meaningful therapy.

McAdams (1995) raised the issue of what do we know when we know someone? He envisions a scaffold that consists of three parts. Each describes a way of understanding individuality: How a person is similar to and different from other persons. The first of these consists of dispositional factors that are relatively unconditional and decontextualized, generally linear. They are noted by traits, such as independence or dominance. Perhaps traits are seen to be more than linguistic conveniences, remarkable for longitudinal consistency (McCrae & Costa, 1990) and, when aggregated across time, seem to predict a substantial amount of variance in behaviors and to be reducible to three to five factors. Traits have been studied extensively from the personality theory (Millon & Davis, 1995), as well as the organization of the traits themselves.

Although traits are important, as they are not mere labels, they do have problems. They lack precision, disregard the environment, and they don't explain anything in any important psychological sense. They apply mostly to distributions in groups and not to individuals. Traits are comparative. In effect, traits represent the "psychology of a stranger." They offer us information, but information from a distance.

Going beyond traits to specific times, places, and roles are more personal issues. McAdams calls these personal concerns. Compared with dispositional traits, personal concerns are motivational and developmental. They address what people are after, what they want and the methods, strategies and plans that people use to obtain or avoid important issues in their life. Personal concerns have a long tradition in personality, being associated with personal strivings (Emmons, 1986), life tasks (Cantor & Kihlstrm 1987), attachment styles (Hazin & Shaver 1990), and core conflictual relationship themes (Luborsky & Crits-Christoph, 1991; Luborsky et al., 1995), among others.

Perhaps personal concerns are derivatives of traits that provide form. In a sense, personal concerns represent the contextualization of behavior in a place. They give life to the situations that the person is in this as a part of this social world. To know a person well, then, it is wise to know most of the scripts or conditional patterns that prevail in the key settings the person is in.

Conceptual efforts integrating this level and that of traits have been described. Kaisor and Ozer (1996), for example, found that personal goals, or what they term *motivational units*, do not map onto traits, the five-factor structure. Their study suggests that the structure of personal goals may be more appropriately conceptualized in terms of various content domains (e.g., work, social). Olgilvie and Rose (1995) proposed that certain motivational constructs within personal concerns may be organized into four categories; acquire (obtain a positive state), keep (maintain a positive state), cure (make a negative state positive), and prevent (avoid a negative state).

Something is missing from this picture of the person. McAdams (1993) noted that we move from the psychology of the stranger to a more detailed description of the flesh and blood person, situated in place and role expressing him or herself in and through strategies, tactics, plans, and goals. What is missing is a purposeful telling of life, the story of the person.

One other level, therefore, is the level of the story. This is the central narrative of the person, the one that finds unity, purpose, and meaning in life. This is the personal story of a person. It is inside the person in perhaps the same way that a motive is. It is the autobiographical story. Person and psychological constructs are best told through story telling anyway. It may be seen as the central quality of the person but it is not the person. It is a good deal of what this book is about.

A number of theorists believe that the only conceivable form for a unified and purposeful telling of an individual life is a story (Bruner, 1987, 1990; Charme, 1984;

Cohler, 1982; Hermans & Kempen, 1993; Howard, 1991; Kotre, 1995; MacIntrye, 1984; Polkinghorne, 1988). The "story is the person's identity" (Erikson, 1975). The story provides the person with a sense of purpose in life. The person is both a historian and history—a story teller who creates the self in the telling (McAdams, 1985, 1987). We are born to become tellers of stories. The story is the answer to the question Who am I? and How do I fit into the adult world? The life story of course is a joint product of the person and the environment.

Information, then, is organized in stories. This is a characteristic way of forming stories. For now, we might say that the self or identity is the core story, one that makes optimal sense of life for the person. It is a root metaphor. The self story can be seen as the most vivifying life story(s), the best and most accurate meaning that is purposeful and meaningful. Through the story I confer meaning on me, specific events to the general themes that are unfolding. As powerful negative events are not integrated into the person's life stories, the task of the clinician is to rescript these stories so that adapted scripts can evolve.

There is of course one other level. This is the Axis I Disorder or clinical symptoms. It is the squeaky wheel. The requisite "clinical formulation" is the DSM. Its strength is that most everyone knows this model; symptoms can be treated according to reasonably standard procedures; and actuarially it is a reasonable grouping of symptom states.

A full knowledge of any one of these levels does not provide sufficient information in any psychological sense for an understanding of the person. All levels need to be considered. Additionally, the levels do not "integrate" with each other in obvious, ready-made ways. The boundaries among these are fuzzy. Indeed, they may not integrate at all. Personality psychologists have become more interested in personal accounts and stories as methods for collecting data on the social-cognitive-motivational aspects of the person. Newer models explicitly mimicking story terms are present, as witnessed in Tompkin's (1987) script theory, and theories offered by Hermans and Kempen (1993). How traits fit in here is unclear: Are they prepotent (McCrae, 1987), can they be considered the narrative ("voiced characters"; Hermans & Kemper, 1993), or do they just have a "privileged status" (Polkingham, 1988)? Nevertheless, the best handle for understanding the person (the organizing construct) will involve all levels.

Across Time: What Do We Know About a Person?

The most influential figure in the past 50 years regarding the aging process is Erik Erikson. Adult development is an ongoing, dynamic process. Erikson proposed an epigenetic or invariant sequence of eight stages of development with approximate age ranges, driven and shaped by biological, psychological, and social forces. Within each stage is a tension between ego syntonic and ego dystonic forces that each individual must navigate through. At any given age one becomes prepotent and forms the developmental crisis of the moment; the others percolate in the background or await their turn in the future. Erikson identified four integrating statuses: integrity achieving, foreclosed, dissonant, and despairing. Only in integrity does the person's examined life result in an acceptance of one's life-span. This of course is never total. Although Erikson (1950) does specify in somewhat vague terms the resolution of developmental crises, a limitation of theories of adult development is that they tend not to specify how it is that development occurs.

McAdams (1993) provided a model adding the importance of the life story and identity: the life story is a model of identity and is the most natural vehicle for transporting one's identity. People are reasonably consistent in their life stories. A central dimension of this dynamic is power versus intimacy. The relative influence of each of these has a significant impact on how one's life is lived.

Throughout the life-span the person allows consistency and change to unfold. From infancy or early childhood up through middle and late adolescence the person develops first a tone, later an image, and eventually a theme of either agency (power) or communion (intimacy). A story begins to form using this motivation system. It is the bedrock for the origins of the later stories that will be enriched. Eventually in adolescence the person has the potential to become a historian and can reflect on self. The typical 6-year-old does not have the capacity of self-awareness. He/she cannot see self as others do (the I-cannot-see-Me in a mental sense). In adolescence, however, the self-as-subject starts to see the self-as-object. The autobiographical memory, impossible in youth, marches through the Piagetian conservation tasks, and builds to a point where it (they) can write its own story. At some point in adolescence a change occurs: There is a view of depth from the outside. Kotre (1995) said:

> You now have a vantage point that allows you to see how discrete episodes of your life interconnect, how stories from a life become stories of a life. You can also think about your own thinking. You can say: "That's not the way things are; it's only the way that I have been looking at them." With the new thinking cap of adolescence we all become biographers of the self—a self with a beginning, middle and end. (p. 145)

In adulthood nuclear episodes are added—the most significant single episodes in the person's life. Persons might be high in intimacy motivation or high in power motivation and the nature of the nuclear episode will form accordingly. Often these are meaningful, continuous, or changing events in the person's life, such as Martin Luther's fit in the choir or revelation in a thunderstorm. Eventually in later adulthood, the individual comes to develop images which are dominant characters in the story. They tend to re-arrange themselves often in dialectical fashion but represent characters that the individual becomes modeled after. In a sense the individual asks how they are the same person, as an idealized image of self that is evolving. These are personal and ideal agentic and communal views of self.

Enter the generativity script. Perhaps this is always there in the person throughout life (Whitbourne, 1995). The generativity script is one that specifies what one wants to put into life and what one hopes to get out of life before one dies. This occurs through midlife areas and on into later life. It represents both a legacy and the gift to be given. It represents how one's life story is to end.

Unfortunately, the generativity script is not always positive and not always easy to reach. It is true that prototypical stories of commitment identified in the accounts of highly generative adults occur. But, intimacy and generativity must be contextualized in the temporal life span if these are to be properly understood. In fact, both high and low generative adults present with life stories showing a mixture of positive and negative affect (McAdams, 1993). What distinguishes the accounts of the highly generative adults from those of the contrasting sample is the sequencing of affective scenes. Bad scenes tend to precede and eventually give birth to good ones. Put another way, good scenes often have their origin in bad scenes. This may have something to say about trauma—generative adults prepare the way for the emergence of good scenes by accentuating the good scenes through narrative contrast.

Regardless of the content of this script, age is on the therapist's side here. McAdams (1990) noted that older people (as do younger ones) rework earlier stories but now as meta-historians. At later life, the life-span developmental tendency to integrate, to review, to be interior, and to create meaning exists. The past, then, is a malleable, changing, and resynthesized series of previous life choices. Later life is a time to renegotiate these choices. History and identity are both made and discovered. Even to a troubled person, this is good news. McAdams (1990) wrote:

> Up until old age, the adult operates both as historian and history, the agent and the object of his or her own story making. In the later years of adulthood, however, he or she may step away from the history and the process of becoming a historian. The history that has been made and the process that has made it become the objects of conscious reflection and review. (p. 189)

As we have intimated above also, a life story need not make everything fit together in a person's life. That occurs in a good movie, perhaps. Modern adults do not need perfect consistency to find unity and purpose in life. Indeed, a good life story is one that shows considerable openness to change and tolerance for ambiguity. From the standpoint of postmodernity, it may be that we are influenced by temporal coherence of our lives more than we like. We suppose this is a period effect. The stories are then not really "inside" the person, subject to the person's revision, waiting to be told, continuing to be enacted. Instead, the older person seems to reside amid the stories. The self is as much "out there," in the swirl and confusion of the postmodern world, as it is "in the mind" of "the person" (Giddens, 1991). Both the person and the context matter.

As we noted above, memory is the content that forms the stories carried into later life and stories take on varying levels of complexity, ego complexity or narrative complexity to be exact. These are the plots and subplots that provide the rich texture or absence thereof of the life story. They represent, as Levinson (1978) noted, ego development and can be rather simple to complex. Through the emotional power of the memory, the narrator tells the story, controls the story, masters and reconfirms the life as well as if times change this. McAdams (1993) said: "We cannot just live but we must step back and see the meaning, the value of our lives" (p. 119).

☐ Life Story

Personality/Schema

In 1994, Hyer and associates wrote that the person could be best understood by the concept of schema. People order their lives according to higher order constructs such as order, perfection, safety, esteem, etc. Mahoney (1991) labeled these as tacit, core ordering processes. We argue that personality is the method of operation, the enforcer of this process. Personality also provides the mechanisms for transition. This book retains these constructs, but specifically attends to the life story.

We know that schemas of self and others develop over the lifetime (Beck & Freeman, 1990). Ultimately they are reasonably consistent and they form the person. Given trauma, the maintenance or re-establishment of a sense of self-coherence and feeling of continuity becomes an important goal. For change then, acceptance of one's past *and* present is a necessary condition. Both issues of aging and trauma must be respected.

Personal stories play a critical role in the way that people live (Omer, 1997). Perhaps the story is most essential because it allows one to organize human life into temporary human episodes. If so, psychological change would involve "something deep," an alteration in personal meanings regardless of how these are brought about. This is why trauma is so noxious and (you would think) especially so at later life. Survivors of trauma have to deal not only with the losses accompanying older age, but the losses at the time of the traumatization and the changed self at the time of the traumatization. A working knowledge of personality, the schema as well as the life story, assists in care giving.

Therapy of course utilizes knowledge of personality/schema to assist in this process. With a vision of care, therapy uncovers unique and hidden truths of the past, a growing belief that one's thinking construes the perceived world, and a rising interest in the philosophy of language, imagination, and hermeneutics. Now we know that the life story provides the understanding of the person's aptitude for change. Age, in terms of time, necessity for completion, core learning, memories, and the life story intermingle to allow for this.

Life Story/Narrative and Memory

William James (1963) claimed that a person has as many selves as there are people who recognize him or her. So, does the person have a self or multiple selves? The self is complex. Even though narratives or stories have the capacity to integrate the individual's reconstructed past, perceived present, and anticipated future, rendering a life-in-time sensible in terms of beginnings, middles, and endings (see McAdams, 1985; Polkinghorne, 1988), modular selves reflect the person better and represent core aspects of the narrative. In effect, the self can be better seen as a modular synthesis by interdependent organized schematic processors that can be synthesized into awareness. The person then is an active agent in a dialectical synthesis creating meaning from immediate experience.

How does the life story fit here? We believe that the story is best viewed as an internalized and evolving narrative of the self that incorporates the reconstructed past, perceived present, and anticipated future (McAdams, 1990, 1993, 1996). It is the core self, if you will. Where the self-concept is the day-to-day organizer of the person, the life story is the narrated product of the characteristic way in which the person arranges and reacts to life and creates themes. The idea of a story is one that suggests that the self through the story evolves and is "sayable": The person can tell you about themselves. It confers unity and purpose by constructing more or less coherent, readable, and vivifying stories that integrate the person into society in a productive and generative way. The person then has a purposeful self-history that explains how time connects within the person, yesterday, today, and tomorrow.

The narrative is the word, then, given to the core set of memories that tell the person's story. This can be considered the storied self. In this way the narrative is an accumulative structure of meaning making that unfolds across the life span. The fact that storied accounts are embedded in the discourse of everyday life does not mean then that these stories are ephemeral. They do not transform themselves with every move in discourse, as some postmodernists seem to suggest. A "real," inner, essential self lies behind the public presentation of the self in everyday life (Jung, 1959).

More important then, the core story has enough solidity that it does not typically change from day to day, but it is supple enough to undergo remarkable transformation over time. The self also is broad enough to include both those private narrative musings about "who I really am" and those public narrative maneuverings that are strongly driven by role and situational demands.

The narrative or core story really represents a special selection of memories. If the memory is core to the person, self-representational or self-defining, then it is part of the narrative or story. Some theorists argue that all thought is narrative (Howard, 1991), whereas others describe narrative as a distinctive form for the expression of meaningful human events (Bruner, 1986). Regardless, narrative/story is the best mode for the contents of the autobiographical memory to be recounted. It is the telling of a sequence of events that are important to the person.

The narrative/story in a sense is meaning making of a higher order. It integrates and it organizes information. It is a journey; it is the shaping of selves into a coherent life. It of course takes the form of memories, events told to a listener when asked. And as noted above, we believe that the self's core is translated best from the stories that are told, even though different in content. Again, it takes form from schemas of vulnerability, order, safety, esteem, agency, communion, etc. These schemas and the consequent protector, personality, provide a way to reformulate and measure the core life stories. They form the themes and the protective processes of the stories.

I and Me: Me and the World

This section is provided to delve into the core memory. It is a more microscopic view of the core memory process. William James (1961) and later Sherman (1991) and Chaudhury (1999), among others, discussed how this might play out. William James distinguished between the self-as-subject (the "I") and the self-as-object (the "Me"). It seems that there are two dialectics that occur in people. It is based on the "I" and the "Me". The Me signifies "yesterday." The I has more to do with the ongoing reflective process. The dialogue between the I and the Me has much to do with reminiscence. In reality, there are two dialogues. One is the dialect between the self and the world. It is an outward look at the world. This is between the Me and the World. The other one involves the I and the Me. This concerns the process of experiencing throughout the life cycle and ultimately with the integrity of experience from a life-span prospective.

Therefore, the Me—World is social and cultural in its manifestations. It is stable with time. In later life there is likely to be a decreased dialectic interaction between the Me—World due to loss, retirement, and such. Not so the I—Me dialectic. Here an increased interaction occurs. This has been noted as the increased interiority (Sherman, 1991). As one ages, it can be seen that the "dialect" between the I—Me reflects generativity. Perhaps too this can be labeled wisdom as information that is interior enhances the tacit knowing of data of the life-span and culture.

Guidano (1991), among others, articulated the interplay between the experiencing "I" and the explaining Me. If you ask a person to step out of the story and talk to you, what happens? You get information about self: You get a reflection on what was happening. You see a reflexive stance on self actions, a reaction on the just completed experiencing. Freud made this distinction in referring to the experiencing ego versus the observing ego.

This process is very relevant for treatment. The I is *selfing* (narrating experiences to create a self) and the Me is the self that the I narrates. The I is a process and the Me is the product: The I is a verb and the Me is a noun. With age, the I—Me becomes more active and "interior"; the Me—World, more stable (personality). Over time, the Me develops a sedimentation, a tacit knowing noted above. This is knowing that is a "felt sense," prior, or more fundamental than explicit knowing. In fact, it can be argued that, just as the I narrates and produces the Me, personality characteristics reside in the Me. It is probable too that the process of selfing is part of personality itself, although traits, concerns, and stories are not "parts" or "components" of the I. Everything, however, is recursive.

Therapeutically at later life, the dialectic between experiencing and explaining, the I and the Me, is the process of self-understanding. Self-knowledge entails an endless circularity between the immediate experience of oneself (the acting and experiencing I) and the sense of self that emerges as a result of abstractly self-referring the ongoing experience (the observing and evaluating Me). Listen to what Kotre (1995) said:

> If you look at a video of yourself, you may say "This is me and this is the way that I got to be the way that I am." The remembering self, both the keeper of the archives and as maker of the myth, fashions a remembered self. "I establishes me." (p. 118)

It is this inner dialectic that exists throughout the life cycle. It becomes amplified in later life with this increasing interiority. In this way the integration between the Me and the World and the I and the Me dialectics is an ongoing, emergent process into very old age. Jung (1959) believed that individualization at later life resulted from the integration of thinking and feeling, as well as sensations and intuition. These components become integrated and synthesized in a more balanced way as a result of this process. Gutman (1966) referred to this as a shift from active mastery to passive mastery. Neugarten and Neugarten (1994) found that in older individuals (generally over 60) the environment could no longer be reformed in line with their wishes, so they tended to see themselves as accommodating more to the demands of the outer world and they become in effect interior. More recently, Susan Whitbourne (1985) used the concepts, accommodation (the process that accounts for change in adulthood), and assimilation (the process responsible for stability), as a similar dialectic at later life.

The person or self is the superordinate category under which one may subsume the I-process and the Me-product. The I is not a thing but rather a process. By selfing, the person implicitly knows that he or she exists as a source, an agent, a locus of causality in the world—distinguished from other sources, agents, and loci of causality. Selfing also brings with it reflexively—the sense in which the I looks on the Me, as an observer (as well as a creator and critic) of that which is "mine," a human experience developed very early in life, probably in the second year (Harter, 1983; Kagen, 1989).

This is the playground of the inner dialogues. It allows for a sense of self to be maintained, and those with greater self-complexity (inner dialogues) have more self-aspects and probably can reduce the harmful effects of stress to degrees greater than others. In a sense, individuals with greater self-complexity are less subject to "spill over" effects of only one self (Linville, 1985). Markus and Nurius (1986) believed that these people have more possible selves and can master problems better.

Age and the Story

The narrative or core story consists of knowledge structures of one's own person, stored in memory, and similar to other knowledge structures. It reflects an ongoing behavior and mediates and regulates behavior. Once it was thought that these were a stable and generalized average view of the self, but they are now considered dynamic and multifaceted phenomena comprised of sets of images, conceptions, theories, goals, and tasks. If so, altering these is critical in the change process of therapy.

Age plays a role. It is not until late adolescence and adulthood that the person is "rich enough" for the life story, even though it has been in progress. A 5-year-old is too young to have an identity in this sense because he/she is generally not able to experience unity and purpose as problematic in their life. He/she may know that he/she is a very good ice skater (domain-specific skill), loves baseball, and hates school; however, this list of attributions does not an identity make. As we have intimated we need the story level, and this applies richly to older folks.

Our focus on life shifts over time. Self-integration becomes transformational as the life course transits (at later life) to generativity. Like the law, it changes ever so slightly over time to meet the needs of the situation. Being a self, then, is not prepackaged. It is not passed down from one generation to the next. This is why the story is so important. It is by the story, the storied self, that the clinician can understand what the individual is like, who they are as people. The person eventually arrives at a self, more or less in final shape through the synthesis of contradictory identifications and greater individualization, and through the turbulence of adolescence, through the transition periods of adulthood, through middle-life, and eventually into older age. A cohesive identity often involves such constructs of the person as a realistic body image, as a subjective self-sameness, consistent self-attitudes, a sense of temporality, and gender.

We do not know answers to the critical questions: How does the narrative influence the coding, storage, and retrieval of data, at any moment in time but also across the life-span? How does the aging process influence self and vice versa? Results of research have yet to show whether the victim's developmental stage at the time of abuse contributes to specific types of problems, such as memory loss or damage to the self-concept. But we do have information on the best practice guides and on clinical experience to allow for good care.

Power of Language

About trauma, Janet (1911) noted: "Unable to integrate traumatic memories ... as if the personality has definitely stopped at a certain point, and cannot enlarge any more by the addition or assimilation of new elements" (p. 532). This formulation of the effects of trauma is based on the notion that extreme emotional arousal resulted from a failure to integrate traumatic memories. The 1990s saw a resurgence of trauma from the perspective of failed meaning integration. Janet proposed that people experience "vehement emotions" and a "phobia of memory," the mind being incapable of matching their frightened experiences with existing cognitive schemes. The result of this is that the memories of the experiences cannot be integrated into personal awareness. They are split off from consciousness and from voluntary control. It is as if the personality rigidifies so that further integration by assimilation of new elements becomes impossible. In this sense, dissociation became a core pathogenic process that gives rise to posttraumatic stress. People are "unable to make the recital which we call narrative memory, and yet they remain confronted by (the) difficult situation" (Janet, 1909; see van de Kolk, Weisaeth, & van de Hart, 1996).

The exploration of personal meaning of the trauma is critical: The pursuit of the meaning of the trauma is the central goal of therapy (van der Kolk, 1988). van der Kolk outlined problems with specific limbic system abnormalities in PTSD particularly the connection between the amygdala and the thalamus. He held that people experience sensory elements of a traumatic experience and may be physiologically prevented from translating this experience into communicable language. They are in the limbic system. When PTSD victims are having a traumatic recall, they suffer from the speechless terror in which they are literally out of touch with their feelings. In effect, they are not able to narrate their experience.

If the narrative is what makes sense of life, then it is this that must be addressed. "Storytelling is an excellent way of caring for the soul" (Moore, 1994). As we noted, somewhere in adolescence we become our own biographers. We create a narrative whole and put unity and purpose around it. We continue to evolve into life. At each stage we have something to add and something to integrate—past, present, and future. But there is a sense of inner sameness. What this means is that people make sense of their lives by their narratives. It can be good or bad. We continue to construct life stories that reflect our identities (personalities). "We tell ourselves stories in order to live" (Didion, 1979).

In the chapter on treatment we will see the importance of language altering the trauma memory. The renarration of the trauma story provides the assimilation and integration of the experience. It is the meaning-making; language allows the person (and therapist) to hover over the experience. Over time it dilutes. Vaillant, Torrey, and Elder (1995) found that, of the 200 undergraduates who were in WWII interviewed 45 years later, those who did not have PTSD consistently altered their original accounts to more diluted levels. They also could dialogue these. This group also was more likely to be in *Who's Who in America*. Those who kept the PTSD did not modify memories. We think this modification occurs at later life.

☐ Conclusion

Narrative is a paradox construct: It has been seen as central to mental health (as in identity) or the cornerstone of psychopathology (as in trauma narratives). We know now that the life story is a developmental construct that builds (probably on a theme of autonomy or belonging) and forms a core of narratives that provides consistency and understanding of the person. Age seems to make them obvious, as generativity, in all its forms, seeks expression. Perhaps an elegant solution to the issues of later life involves a discovery of the connection between the normal vexatious needs of the life lived and the issues of being. This is probably not done without considerable effort. But, as one gets older, the use of one's memory, the unearthing of previous life events, approximates such a task.

Memory is always present consciousness: It becomes alive as a "new then." So, although memories of the past may be flawed, it is the experiential context of the present that gives the memory its meaning. The "late organizes the early" or the new organizes the old. In a sense, the person's inner dialogue and identity organize this past process. We will address this in later chapters.

4
CHAPTER

Person and Memory

"... the act of imagination is bound up with memory. You know, they straight-ened out the Mississippi River in places, to make room for houses and livable acreage. Occasionally the river floods these places. "Floods" is the word they use, but in fact it is not flooding; it is remembering. Remembering where it used to be. All water has perfect memory and is forever trying to get back to where it was ... remembering where we were, what valley we ran through, what the banks were like, the light that was there and the route back to our original place. It is emotional memory—what the nerves and the skin remem-ber as well as how it appeared. And a rush of imagination is our "flooding."
Toni Morrison (1990, p. 305)

Generally, researchers do not study the autobiographical memory. They deal in the "less important" issues of the information processing (Hyer et al., 1994) that are accounted for by memory. Memory is usually studied then from the perspective of ability and decline. But there is also this other memory, the autobiographical memory, of which the narrative is one form. Telling a story about an event is retrieving information in memory. It is organized data: Events that play a significant part in one's life. This is a life narrative instantiated in the storied words of the time and context.

Unfortunately and naturally, this process is influenced by many things both internal and external to the person. One is aging. And, one of those things is trauma. Given trauma, memory processes are uniquely affected at the level of encoding, storage, retrieval, and recounting. In this chapter we talk about this—memory as a whole, memory as it is influenced by aging, the autobiographical memory, memory as it relates to trauma. We also consider the systems of the core memory, its traditions and context. In so doing, we attempt to build a case for our conceptual model, the psychotherapy sections.

☐ Memory Overall

"Everything should be made as simple as possible, but not simpler."
Albert Einstein

A memory is a kind of chaotic attractor. Systems models can be described as chaotic, nonlinear dynamics, and self-organization. Complex systems are often best represented by nonlinear dynamics. Over time these tend to settle down. They are attractors. Neuropatterns or electroencephalogram (EEG) patterns of an odor, for example, are not the same each time, not like a fixed photo. So too memories are not the same each time. The change in the EEG structure is dependent on the meaning of the stimulus at the time and not only on its presence. In a sense the structure of the old learnings reform in the context of new ones. The nervous system is dynamic, a chaotic attractor. So too, the memory system is such a dynamic, a chaotic attractor that is both unpredictable and somewhat irregular.

Your memories are your poetry. They are "the thick autonomy of memory," "not easily penetrable by the direct light of consciousness; resistant to conceptual understanding; sedimented in layers; and having 'historical depth'" (Casey, 1999). This is an immersion in the temporal, meaningful environment. Memory is not confinement of information within the person. For Casey, memory is already everywhere: "Memory is ... more porous than enframing." We know, for example, that the mind does not capture memories by internalizing exact replicas of experienced events. Rather, people find themselves surrounded by layers of meaning, awareness, and reinterpretation that are affected by social and cultural constructions. Individuals are not in command of memory as an internal store of facts.

Casey used one more term that applies: He spoke of memory as commemoration, the act of intensified remembering. Commemoration signifies solemnity and seriousness, the importance and centrality of certain memories. It is a purposeful, transformative process. It is more than "doing again": It is "remembering through." Memory is a process. It is best thought of in this sense as a verb not a noun, reconstructive, not reproductive. Various stages of processing are influenced by active meta-models or schemas that link together associated memories and emotions, and prior learnings. At a higher level, memory is a symphony of meaning seeking. Robert Kegan (1983) in *The Evolving Self* writes: "The activity of being a human being is the activity of meaning making. This lasts until death."

The brain is no single memory system. Memory is not a closet in the brain in which things are stored. It is not a unitary thing. There are several forms. There exist several types of memory agencies that work in somewhat different ways. Some memory mechanisms retain records of sensations for only seconds. Other types form habits, goals, and styles that we hold only for days: Others are used for personal attachments that endure. We also modify memories that seem quite permanent. In fact, it may be argued that we remember little of any particular experience. At some point we transfer information to the long-term memory. There we classify as controlling, dangerous, important, and so on.

Simply to maintain vast stores of unclassified memories is not efficient. We do not need to search through all data to recover what is relevant. We have ways to organize our memories. This process is largely inaccessible to consciousness. In this process, however, we are democratic. We have other agencies (of mind) that give voice and make input. Minsky (1985/1986) noted that, as human beings, we use machinery evolved from fish, amphibians, reptiles, and earlier mammals to use different kinds of organizations for achieving many kinds of goals. We do not need perfect methods because we remember how perfect methods fail (Minsky, 1985/1986). He wrote:

> Each of these dimensions ... offer(s) alternative ways to proceed when any system fails. If part of your society of mind proposes to do what other parts find unacceptable, your agencies can usually find another way. Sometimes you merely need to

turn to another branch of the same accumulation. When that fails, you can ascend to a higher level and engage a larger change in strategy. Then, even if an entire agency should fail, your brain retains earlier versions of it. . . . Finally, when even that won't work, you can usually switch to an entirely different family of agencies. Whenever anything goes wrong, there are always other realms of thought. (p. 210)

Again, we simplify to argue issues. Memories are complex. The relationship between memory and just about anything else cannot be captured simply: A complex interaction between the type of the event (emotional and neutral), type of detail (central or peripheral), information preceding or succeeding an event, time of test (immediate vs. delayed), length of retention interval, and retrieval conditions (retrieval cues, mood and other contextual clues, single or repeated testing) make a difference (Christianson, 1992). Subcortical (limbic) and cortical memories coexist—the amygdala, the thalamus, as well as parts of the cerebral cortex, interact in the formation of new memories. There is a complex rail system between the two that has yet to be mapped. Subcortical and hypothalmic pathways are most apt for immediate reaction, enabling a quick response before the organism fully realizes what it is reacting to (Cristianson, 1992). These are the "limbic memories," which often assert a strong influence over the person causing nightmares, flashbacks, and repetitive perception of threat triggered by associated stimuli. There are, of course, cortical memories, where meaning making occurs.

Processing of trauma information is supposed to work in a straightforward way: The survivor of trauma reconnects the self and the past by capturing with each retelling new meanings and greater insights about the impact of traumatic events. The non-processing of trauma also works in a straightforward way: Because the future is inextricably linked to the past and because many trauma survivors cannot recall much of their past, there is often a corresponding inability to anticipate or plan for the time ahead. Information is not moved. No new learning occurs. Locked in the present, survivors may be unable to dream of a future for themselves because of its inescapable contiguousness with an "unspeakable" past.

We do not enter the debate on the believability of trauma reports. On the one side stands a group of cognitive and social psychologists who advocate for the fallibility of memory, the ready availability of suggestability, and the flimziness of research on recovered memories; on the other are therapists who contend that child (sex) abuse is common, that forgetting does occur, and that recovery of the memory is necessary for cure. We are most interested in a reasonable rendition of the event. There is evidence that this occurs with regularity showing neither exaggeration nor underreporting of such events (Brewin, Andrews, & Gotlib, 1993). This assumes that the person is old enough and well-placed to see and experience the event.

☐ Autobiographical Memory and Decline

The most usual way of "carving nature by its joints," in terms of memory, is by differentiating the procedural and declarative memory. Procedural memory refers to the procedures and rules that are necessary for an understanding of storage and retrieval of events. This memory is what psychologists study, involving abilities to recall and to use the rules of learning. Declarative memory, on the other hand, is what we have been discussing. It involves both factual and episodic memory. Facts are just facts, no context. So, the episodic or the autobiographical memory is what we are most interested in.

Remembering is best viewed as encompassing three steps—acquisition/encoding, retention/storage, and retrieval. Problems can occur at any of these phases (Loftus & Davies, 1984; Perry, 1992). Additionally, three types of memory evaluation—recognition, reconstruction, and free recall—are impacted differently by the complexities of retrieval and remembering. Patients with dementia, for example, evidence a severe impairment of episodic memory (i.e., memory information that depends on temporal and/or spatial contextual cues for its retrieval), which is thought to be mediated by damage to the hippocampus, as well as to the cholingeric neurotransmitter system. This deficit is characterized by ineffective consolidation or storage of new information, a rapid rate of forgetting, and an increased susceptibility to proactive interference.

There is then bad news and good news about aging (and perhaps PTSD). Deptula, Singh, and Pomara (1993) noted age-related decline is fact, attributable to many factors, including cognitive loss, insufficient use of cognitive strategies, lack of practice in performing cognitive tasks, and decreased emotion. In addition, older participants are more vulnerable than younger ones to the adverse effects of negative emotional states. Even among the normal elderly individuals without a diagnosable psychopathology, negative states, such as anxiety or depression, interfere with memory functioning. Interestingly, these authors note also that introversion is associated with poor recall memory and higher levels of physiological arousal (Deptula, Singh, & Pomara, 1993). Introversion may increase with age (Gutman, 1966).

As if to rub in the many forms of problems with older folks, Schacter (1998) described seven sins of memory (while not directing his thoughts to elders or trauma). Three of the sins included different types of forgetting: (a) transience, which involves decreasing accessibility of information over time; (b) absent-mindedness, which includes inattention and shallow processing (contributes to poor future recall); and (c) blocking, which refers to the temporary inaccessibility of information that is stored in memory. The next three involve inaccuracy: misattribution involving the attribution of a memory to an incorrect source; suggestibility, referring to the implanting of memories as a result of leading questions or a poor context; and bias, which refers to retrospective distortions and unconscious influences that are related mostly to current knowledge. Last there is persistence. These are events that we cannot forget. This relates to PTSD. Evidence for persistence comes from several sources including studies on directed forgetting (trauma participants cannot forget even when instructed to, relative to normals), excessive rumination over depressive or PTSD symptoms, as well as neuroimaging on increased activity of the amygdala weeks after the viewing of emotional films.

Memory can always, of course, be influenced by one's current state. Learning is state dependent as mood associated with events can influence one's ability to recall events (Bower, 1981). The accuracy of recall is not uniform, generally worse over longer intervals and generally better when events are salient (unique or important). Recall content is also relative. Recall of dates is quite poor, but objective facts are recalled better than subjective ones (Rockey, 1997).

Memory is a process; it is reconstructive and not reproductive. Research on autobiographical memories especially suggests that recall is highly prone to both error or bias. Despite the fact that the autobiographical memory by itself is not well-studied (Brewer, 1986), we know that recollections are not simply a direct retrieval of information from a decaying archive. In fact, this form of memory degrades with time. Memory relies on heuristic strategies to reconstruct recalled events. Recall for particular episodes can be disrupted by interference from other similar events that occur perhaps before or after the episode and by important schemata that may describe a protypical class for the event (e.g., medical event). Memories also are distorted by post-event information and by the extent to which events are rehearsed (Loftus & Davies, 1984; Wells & Loftus, 1984). Additionally, memories are also altered by the respondent's preconceived notions about the event or by their attempts to salvage self-esteem by creating a similarly coherent and consistent narrative.

Now the good news—most autobiographical memories for major life events are relatively accurate. Among the elderly, events such as marriages, deaths, births, holidays, injury and illness, education, family, war, love, love affairs, and recreational sports are remembered just fine (Cohen & Faulkner, 1989). Current findings suggest that highly salient or stressful events may be recalled more accurately than information associated with laboratory studies of memory (Goodman, Hirschman, Hepps, & Rudy, 1991; Yullie, 1993). False memories occur more for peripheral details and not for central features of events (Terr, 1994). We know also that reconstructions of major personal events represent "relatively minor editorial revisions that bring the past more in line with a person's current self-image" (Ross & Conway, 1986, p. 139). A "fundamental integrity" of most major autobiographical recollections is the rule (Barclay, 1986). It may be that what a person remembers depends on existing mental schema. Once a particular event is integrated under the existing mental schemes, some distortion occurs as the schema alters the memory to fit its needs.

Degradation occurs only to a small extent with normal aging. Memory at later life for normal aging is often seen as impoverishment, beset with an overgeneralized coding proclivity, sometimes lack of effort or distraction. Problems, however, involve the working memory and the problems in retrieval, other memory tasks, or storage problems. When forced to engage in elaboration or semantic processing of information during the study phase of the free-recall task, the performance of normal elderly adults, but not that of dementia patients, is even enhanced (Reese & Rodeheaver, 1985). This finding suggests that the severe episodic memory impairment of dementia is not primarily due to difficulties in retrieving information but rather reflects a deficit in consolidation or storage.

In addition, there is little evidence that people with diagnosable psychological disorders are more likely to experience memory distortions than other people. It appears that confidence in one's memories is moderately related to demonstrated accuracy of recall. This is, of course, related to health problems—associated with higher levels of memory complaints and problems (Siegler, 1994). Interestingly, older adults appraise their ability to remember in ways that are at least as accurate as those of younger adults (Herzog, 1997). Overall a partial reconstructive perspective of autobiographical memory is more accurate than the espousal of either literal reproduction or substantial alterations in adult memories of childhood events. Research ("fuzzy trace theory") too, which has demonstrated that "gist" memories and "verbatim" memories are functionally independent and have different properties, may ultimately have an impact on how autobiographical memory is conceptualized (Reyna, 1995; Reyna & Brainerd, 1995). We must never forget that the unburdening of a memory is always a function of the psychosocial and cultural influences as much or more than of storage and retrieval systems.

There are lots of facts here (Box 4-1). However, such musings are absent critical evaluation about changes in linguistic and syntactic characteristics of memory. Little

Box 4-1
Facts of the Aging Memory

Core Autobiographical Memory Processes
  Encoding
    Salience—the more salient the experience, the more likely that it is to be remembered. This refers to the emotional arousal of the event (positive or negative). This may not apply to extreme events such as a rape.
    Frequency—this component determines that the details will be forgotten but the memory of the class of the event will be excellent.
  Storage
    Rehearsal—this positively influences memory. The developmental level of the person is critical: up to age 5, children depend on cues and prompts to form organized memories.
    Intentional forgetting—this can result in a diminished capacity to recall events. The to-be-remembered items are elaborated relative to the re-pressed items.
  Retrieval
    Reinterpretation—changes in the subjective interpretation of events can re-sult in recalling inaccessible information.
    Hyperamnesia—repeated retrieval of the information improves the likelihood of accurately retrieving the information. This can also enhance the possi-bility of false recall. Suggestive procedures may result in an exaggeration of the memory.
    Encoding specificity—when the conditions of retrieval match those of en-coding, chances are best for recall. State specific conditions (emotions) enhance the recall of the event.
    Implicit memory—the nonconscious part of the memory seems to encode data that is different from the explicit memory and can be recalled at a later time to degrees over those of the central memory.
Aging Memory Problems
  Acquisition: What is learned? The working memory is a problem. Memory is a process, is reconstructive, not reproductive. The problem may be in attention flexibility. When induced to encode effectively, the older learner does well.
  Storage and retrieval: In normal aging problems of retrieval are evident. Ac-curacy is not uniform because of time; interference for similar events after the target event; unique events are recalled better; schemas, as in proto-typical class, preconceived ideas/models, a need to salvage self-esteem, or create a coherent narrative, play a role; objective facts are stored better than subjective ones. Recollection is not simply decaying material.
  Overall: Episodic memory degrades with age. Memory is not entirely accurate or inaccurate. Although not precisely accurate, once formed, memories are hard to eliminate. It is prone to error or bias. Inaccuracy is both random and systematic (as in a systematic bias with depressed people).

(continued)

Box 4-1
(Continued)

Reasonable Facts of the Autobiographical Memory
Most autobiographical memories for major life events are relatively accurate. After a period, they tend to remain.
Metacognition, the awareness of cognitive functioning, is accurate at older ages.
There is little evidence that even people with diagnosable psychological disorders are more likely to experience memory distortions than other people.
Age of trauma, intensity/complexity of stressor, and dissociation influence memory.
Emotion appears to facilitate the accuracy of recall of central details. High emotion appears to slow forgetting.

---

attention has been devoted to studying the dissociation between affect and declarative knowledge in emotional memory, to describing the content and characteristics of intrusive memories (fragments, entire episodic memories, emotions, sensations, self-talk, etc.), to determine what it means in operational terms to have control over remembering processes, or to identify linguist and semantic cognitive strengths that are predictive of recovery. Additionally, the combination of the degradation of the autobiographical memory as well as the psychological trauma itself (including dissociation) is likely to make individuals vulnerable to suggestion or construction of explanations for their trauma-related affects that may be of little relationship to the actual realities of their lives. This can be rather confusing to the clinician over time. Increasingly, however, clients discuss aspects of the trauma in a repetitive fashion with which there is no change, often over many years. This, of course, is a treatment focus.

Our best summation is that the autobiographical memory then is imperfect and involves a "constant process of selection, revision, and reinterpretation" (Brewin, Andrews, & Gotlib, 1993, p. 85). Recall processes may introduce systematic bias also as evidenced by depressed patients who consistently over-estimate the occurrence of negative events, often in a summary fashion. Difficulties in retrieving specific autobiographical memories also may contribute to emotional disturbance in several ways (Williams, 1994, 1995). Depressed patients cannot retrieve specific memories about themselves and often experience difficulty benefiting from cognitive therapy because of the emotional quality of these autobiographical memories. An inability to retrieve specific positive memories may even blunt positive affect (Rubin, 1986). Interestingly, it has been reported (Schachter, Kihlstrom, Kihlstrom, & Beran, 1989) that autobiographical memories are difficult to retrieve only in depressed patients with histories of abuse and not in those without history of abuse.

Perhaps, as McNally, Lasko, Macklin, and Pitman (1995) suggested, preoccupation with intrusive memories of trauma may consume cognitive resources rendering it difficult for traumatized persons to use memory in a specific adaptive fashion. As if by backlash, PTSD researchers have noted that cognitive representations of the self are often distorted, giving rise to problems. People who later develop PTSD see themselves as weak, vulnerable, and untrustworthy (Janoff-Bulman, 1989). Such conjectures indicate that disturbances in self-representation in PTSD imply that negative attributes or traits dominate the schemata relative to positive ones. Autobiographical episodes exemplifying positive traits, therefore, are more difficult to access (McNally, Lakso, Macklin, & Pittman, 1995).

In sum, memory and age are natural brothers. Memory does degrade with age. Older people base their identity on a core but changing life story or personal narrative (McAdams, 1985). As we age, many pick their favorite decade and replay the memories. Often the older the person, the more the decade sneaks into the past. Things that occurred dramatically or are novel are recalled with more frequency and with more vibrancy than others. Contrast effects too predominate especially if there are problems in life (as in PTSD). Memories too are many-formed: they are instrumental. They underwrite lessons learned in the past, such as in the Depression. They are transmissive, that is, they pass on to others messages of one's heritage or wisdom. They also seek inner changes; life reviews put life in order. Often we change memories for the better simply because we have aged ("we should be mature"), and when memory results in positive reactions for older people, generativity is involved. Typically, this occurs in predictable ways: biological (offspring), parental (nurturing children), technical (teaching), and cultural (leaving something for culture, art, business, etc.). These issues are summarized in Box 4-1.

☐ Core Memory

We borrow from five "models" of psychotherapy and aging/trauma to build a case for our psychotherapy model. We discuss each and draw conclusions about later life and therapy. We pick this up once again in Chapter 9 and make a case for the application of the core memory in therapy.

Reminiscence

"In reminiscence my experiences do not fade, they grow more vivid."
Marcel Proust

In 1911 Sir Francis Galton studied autobiographical memories. He requested that people associate to words like *book* or *machine* and provide an early memory. Alfred Adler picked up the issue and proposed a complete theory and psychotherapy around this construct. However mostly the theories that provide understanding for the use of reminiscence as a therapeutic technique have evolved from people who wrote about the elderly, Erikson (1963) or Butler (1963). Butler extended Erikson's views by postulating that reminiscing is a way of achieving ego integrity. Coleman (1986) is not alone in noting that close similarities can be detected between the concept of a normative life-review and Erikson's notion of the developmental task of achieving integrity. These techniques have also been used in many venues, including educators and community education workers (Duffin, 1992; Lawrence & Mace, 1992) and oral history (Samuel, 1975; Thompson, 1988; White, 1980), to name two. Regardless, reminiscence has been used almost exclusively with older people (Butler, 1963). Butler (1995) noted:

> Only in old age within the proximity of death can one truly experience a personal sense of the entire life cycle. That makes old age a unique stage of life and makes the review of life at that time equaly unique. (p. 17)

Older people use reminiscence more than other age groups. DeVries, Blando, and Walker (1995) showed that older adults do review a greater number of events than younger people. It appears too that negative events are processed in a more complex way than positive ones. Reminiscence also allows for an achievement of self-cohesion (Kohut, 1984), for an improved connection between interpersonal relations (Klerman & Weissman, 1993), for mourning (Molinari & Reichlin, 1984–1985), as well as for the integration of the life story (Shafer, 1992). It assists in depression, in stress reduction, and even in dementia. Evidence exists too that integrative reminiscing increases during transitions, bereavement, and medical setbacks (e.g., hospitalization; Rybarzyck, 1995). This is as it should be. This is where the action is in a person's life. Still, integrative reminiscence most often requires encouragement. "Narration confers spellbinding power on older people" (Garland, 1994, p. 23). About this "good" reminiscence, David Gutmann (1990) said:

> Through reminiscence, older persons may creatively revisit their past to conform to some sustaining personal myth; by finding or constructing the threads that connect the current self with some past, idealized self, they can overcome the devastating experience of discontinuity and self, they can overcome the devastating experience of discontinuity and self-alienation. (p. 43)

Wong and Watt (1991) provided a taxonomy for reminiscence: integrative, instrumental, narrative, transmissive, escapist, and obsessive. Greater amounts of integrative and instrumental reminiscence characterized the better adjusted people in their study. The former conveys a sense of meaning and coherence to the life-story. The latter recalls past attempts to cope with difficult situations and thus may contribute to an enhanced subjective perception of control. The less well-adjusted people were characterized by greater amounts of obsessive reminiscence. Molinari and Reichlin (1984–1985) saw life-review in terms of mourning with stages encompassing reorganization of relationship to lost others; obsessive recounting and reiteration; reflection on self-absorption; and the end result—learning to relinquish what has been lost.

Life-review is often seen as an active grappling with the past. It is a healthy activity that depathologizes older stereotypes of remembering. This is an intrapersonal and interpersonal procedure that involves both personal integrative and interpersonal transmissive functions. Viney (1995) noted that older people lose many of the sources of confirmation for positive stories that are necessary for good mental health. Reminiscence possesses many instrumental and integrative aspects that act as coping strategies to stave off depression. In effect, this strategy accesses prior problem-solving strategies and positive self-attributions. Coleman (1994) noted too that reminiscence teaches important shared moral values and links the person to society.

In an effort to better understand reminiscence, Webster (1997) developed the Reminiscence Functions Scale (RFS). It consists of seven factors: boredom reduction, death preparation, identity/problem solving, conservation, intimacy maintenance, bitterness revival, and teach/inform. Reminiscence is a process that begins early and ends late. In fact, there is a stability of reminiscence across the life-span but the functions change with age. Older people use death preparation and intimacy maintenance more than do other groups. From the typology of Watt and Wong (1991), the healthier forms of reminiscence are integrative and instrumental with obsessive the least adaptive.

One example of the use of life review (our reminiscence) is in a nursing home. Molinari (2000) used a group format with only motivated, verbal, introspective, and non-crisis patients. It lasted from 60–90 minutes and was closed (involved the same group of people from beginning to end with no newcommers). It was also social in nature. The therapy was structured and had a topic for each session, as well as an overall syllabus. It started with an education on the value of life-review, its differences from reminiscence. Members were encouraged to prepare for each week's theme. Some of the topics included relationships with parents, regrets, unfulfilled desires, and major transitions. The task of the group leader was to keep people on target and to focus on content and not process. The end was used to tie up loose ends, to summarize content, and to affirm the self. This was found to be an overall positive experience.

Finally, we note similarities/differences between reminiscence and life-review pointed out in the literature. Similarities between the two are that both involve memory and recall, have a structure of free-flowing process, access happy or sad memories, are implemented predominantly with the elderly, and serve as a therapeutic function. Differences, on the other hand, are highlighted in that life-review is a more integrity-seeking process that is more intense, focuses on issues across the life-span, is a more psychoanalytically based theory, involves a more active role on the part of the clinician, and often targets painful memories and issues. The process is usually structured with the work being internal and directed toward integrity. We will develop our view of these two in later chapters, but stress now the importance of the integrity-seeking process noted above.

In addition, we note this: Research conducted on the efficacy of reminiscing as a therapy have yielded conflicting results—some positive (e.g., Fry, 1983), some negative, and some mixed (Frey, 1983; Molinari, 1999). Methodology has been predictably shoddy in this area (measures, definition of population, and methods), but there is a certain consensus. In general, the application of memory work in reminiscence has been criticized for (a) a lack of clarity on how to apply procedures; (b) overreliance on clinical judgment of how to use it; (c) little scientific validity; (d) limited use in handling specific problems (such as adapting to organic dysfunction); and (e) a lack of clarity about how this therapy might benefit persons with reactive depression or conflict with other therapies. Additionally, several writers have recently suggested that men and women communicate and tell stories differently (Gray, 1992).

The researcher's task is represented in the question provided by Kastenbaum (1987) over 10 years ago: "Under what circumstances ... is life review a valuable form of prevention, and under what circumstances is it useless or potentially harmful?" (p. 325). Molinari and Reichlin's (1985) questions have not yet been answered also. What is the optimal time, ideal frequency of sessions, type of content? What processes lead to what kind of positive (or negative) outcome? What older people can benefit? Does the nature of life-review vary according to age? How is life-review experienced from the client's perspective? How does life-review affect reactions to ongoing problems? Is reminiscence important in the process of aging?

In sum, life review has now progressed to the state where the theoretical and practical aspects of the process can be researched and applied for meaningful treatment. Reminiscence too is satisfying in itself without necessarily leading to psychological insight. Recall that stories help everyone to develop and maintain a sense of identity, provide everyone with guidance by which to live, enable everyone to place order on the sometimes chaotic events, and gives everyone more power than they might otherwise have. Additionally as we noted above, the very processes, which Butler (1963) viewed as characteristic of life-review, are found in psychotherapy. But in the end, it is the person who influences the memory. Nietzsche reminds us, when memory and pride debate an event in a person's life-story, pride usually wins.

Older folks appear to be primed for a life review. This includes three core functions: to integrate the disparate aspects of self, to assist in current problem solving, and to bequeath a legacy. The overarching goal of memory therapy is to deconstruct an individual's perspective on his or her life history into a more positive and coherent life history emphasizing strengths, successes, and lessons learned (Molinari, 1999). Some of the functions of life review are given in Box 4-2.

Life Experience Interview

"It is a luxury to be understood"
Emerson

There is tradition in psychotherapy that addresses narrative issues and reminiscence. Where the narrative approaches are used almost exclusively by psychotherapists, primarily allied health professionals working with older adults use reminiscence. Reminiscence therapists work within an existing life story, to help the client get new perspectives on current issues or to facilitate the integration of unresolved past events and choices. Narrative therapists focus on changing or "rewriting" dysfunctional stories about the self. Narrative therapists often focus on parts of the life story that deal with those aspects of the self. Reminiscence workers address positive aspects of the individual's life story, focusing on the past exclusively.

Box 4-2
Functions of Life Review

Provides coping mechanism for management of grief, loss, and stress.
Lends consistency to self-concept.
Links present to past and past to present.
Provides reminder of past mastery.
Reinforces sense of identity/roots.
Lends meaning to one's existence.
Reconciles what might have been.
Gives perspective on survivor guilt.
Provides access to repressed material.
Helps address fear of death.
Helps identify past strengths.
Yields written family legacy.
Creates opportunity for socialization (in groups).
Enhances long-term memory.
Can be a recreational function.
Systematically identifies accomplishments.
Provides intergenerational benefit to others.
Fosters transition to other forms of psychotherapy.

Rybarzcyk and Bellg (1997) improved on the use of the narrative and operationalized their methods. They advocated two approaches with memories. In one, the "counselor" takes on a primarily supportive role, approaching the older adult as a "wise teacher" (Biner & Deutchman, 1991) and focusing mainly on rose-colored memories. Choosing what to emphasize is the point at which narrative therapists attempt to intervene. This life-experience interview (LEI) is based on the premise that the positive feelings elicited by simple reminiscing will effectively counteract anxiety triggered by a stressful situation. The LEI covers topics that frequently evoke positive emotions, such as childhood activities, family traditions, adventures in adolescence, and early dating experiences. No direct effort is made to guide the interviewee toward remembering events that relate to successful coping. The goal of reminiscence interviewing is not to gather information but to create a positive psychological experience for the storyteller. To put this more succinctly, "The process is more important than the product" (Rybarchyk & Bellg, 1997).

The other approach is more active and involves more challenging memories. Rybarchyk and Bellg (1997) endorsed such an approach at least 25% of the time. The therapist plays a more active role in trying to help the client integrate memories into a cohesive and positive life story. Reminiscence is stretched, focusing on challenges successfully met, underscoring the strengths and resources used to meet those challenges, and summarizing key lifelong attributes at the close of the interview. The overall goal is to increase interviewees' awareness of their coping strengths and resources by directing them to recall past successes in meeting life's challenges.

Regardless of the approach, results were very encouraging for patients on medical units (Rybarchyk & Bellg, 1997). Participants in either of the two reminiscence interviews experienced a decrease in anxiety after the interview, compared with an increase in anxiety among the participants who received the present-focus interview or no interview. Life-narrative interviews led to substantial reductions in the anxiety that patients commonly experience when facing an invasive medical procedure and were as effective as the relaxation techniques and interventions widely used in health care settings to alleviate stress. Finally, when an interview focuses on past experiences of successful coping, it leads to a positive change in the patient's appraisal of his or her coping abilities and resources. While these approaches await support, they apply considerable common sense to understanding memories in a clinical setting. The enigma of the person unfolds naturally.

Self-Defining Memory

Self-defining memories (SDMs; Singer & Salovey, 1993) are not the structural factors of memory but are key episodes in the person's life, the declarative and episodic memories of the self. They are central to one's past, interpretation of the present, and possible predictions of the future. They represent two ends of the narrative continuance, that part that preserves the affective immediacy of the moment and the one that subserves the power of the summarized account.

Singer and Solovey (1993) believed that each person carries around a unique collection of autobiographical memories, a sort of carousel of slides of the most important personal memories of life, witnessed by their vividness and intense affect. These memories are snapshots that represent core slides to which people return to repeatedly. In a moment they convey representation and instantiation. These images crystallize characteristic interests, motives, and concerns of the individual into a short hand moment. These memories contain many false recollections and embellishments, thereby not having to pass the test of historical truth.

SDMs then are prototypical and exemplify the person. These memories are a blend of summary/single event memory, a blend of abstraction and immediacy, a blend of reason and emotion, centrally located in the psychic structure of the person's life as to represent the person in a single event. Through this integration of both the single event and the summarized memory, the purpose and meaning of the person is fleshed out. They represent what Loevinger (1976) and McAdams (1993) noted as the highest stage of ego development. They are the most representational meaning in self-definition the person has about themselves. McAdams noted:

> In rare moments in our lives during a long intimate conversation with someone from whom we seek understanding or validation ... as part of a ... group or after an excruciating painful defeat or loss, we might step back and demand such narrative unity from our memory. What each of these moments has in common ... is a commitment to articulate one's knowledge of one's self, to ask and attempt to answer the question 'who am I'. (p. 160)

Later in the book we label the SDM as a positive core memory (PCM). We believe that it has considerable curative value.

Growth

Tedsechi and Park (1998) discussed PTG (post-traumatic growth). This is a process that represents a beneficial change in the cognitive and emotional life of a person who has had a trauma. In recent decades there was a plethora of writings in this area. This involved people who suffered from chronic illnesses, HIV infection, bereavement, heart attacks, health problems of children, among others (see Tedeschi, Park, & Calhoun, 1998). Personality or coping constructs that have addressed this issue include hardiness, sense of coherence, resilience, stress inoculation, and toughening, to name a few. In effect, there is a perception of self as a survivor, one who is self-reliant, and not vulnerable; an ability to be open to others; an appreciation of life; and a spiritual awakening that can even be "wise." The individual copes in a problem-focused way and has a change in their perspective in life. A dispositional optimism results.

Calhoun and Tedeschi (1998) posited a model of change that involves several features. The pretrauma factors that influence growth involve the way people process information. This involves hope and optimism, as well as an open and cognitively complex style. The person in a sense can indulge in chaotic cognition that allows uncertainty and chaos to unfold. The person is an ordered thinker who has been unhappy for life periods and now is influenced by the trauma. Rumination overcomes the person and is itself overcome by deliberation. Finally, the narrative becomes conscious. This may be the first conscious realization of the life story.

PTG is not an easy process. The process is slow and incremental. The initial response is adaptive, followed by low psychological growth. As part of this process, the survivor has a period of decrement. The variables that subserve the growth are many, often personality based. However personality is only the platform from which a newly constructed meaning is launched. Perhaps the proclivity to perceive growth from traumatic coping transactions bespeaks of a broader coping style. The tendency to find growth then may be a stable personality tendency.

The way the trauma was reacted to and handled will be used as a memory for growth. What is told about the trauma before and after the trauma is now salient. This was the moment. Perhaps wisdom results.

Just Aging (and Trauma)

Trauma and later life interact in many ways. In fact, the issues of age and trauma appear similar. Post-traumatic states and specific developmental problems belonging to aging interact and interfere with each other. Aarts and Op den Velde (1996) argued that aging is a risk factor for previously traumatized individuals and suggested that the developmental tasks on the one hand and post-traumatic sequelae on the other interact to cause problems. Survivors of trauma have to deal not only with the losses accompanying older age, but the losses and a changed self at the time of the traumatization.

Post-traumatic states and specific developmental problems belonging to aging do interfere with each other. Acceptance of one's past and present states is a necessary component for the adequate adaptation to aging and for trauma recovery. Establishment and maintenance of a sense of self-coherence and feeling of continuity is required. This of course is difficult in trauma survivors because of the rupture in the self-perceptions and the sense of self-continuity. In later life, health professionals, however, should not misconstrue post-traumatic symptoms as part and parcel of the degenerative process of aging.

Aarts and Velde (1995) outlined five factors in successful adaptation to aging as related to the trauma responses. Aging and trauma interact in some way, mostly for the better. First is the mourning for losses. The mourning for previous losses is rarely completed and new losses may trigger suppressed or postponed grief. In fact, anxiety arousing reminiscing of a traumatic past can be a serious hindrance in the mourning process. The second component is giving meaning to experiences and accepting the past and the present to facilitate ego integration. Again, it is important for individuals to be able to accept the course of their lives as inevitably their own. Giving a meaning, of course, involves cognitive events but also more. Equal in merit are emotional schema that are important. More than simply cognitive efforts are necessary.

Re-establishing self-coherence and self-continuity is the third feature. Both are essential to feeling that one is a whole person. *Self-coherence* refers to the integration of the here and now; *self-continuity* refers to the feelings of integrity in retrospect over the entire lifespan. Each loss can be a problem for both. Achieving ego integration is the fourth adaptive phase. It is no puzzle that trauma experts consider pathology of the self to be the main adverse phenomenon in trauma patients. Focus of treatment, therefore, is on the integration of the self and restoration of the sense of self-coherence. Fifth, culture and social support, generally not considered, are important. When the culture is not strong and when the identity is not placed on hard ground and relationships are lost, life becomes unpredictable. In some sense, trauma is viewed as the product of a combination of the severity of the stress and the support and capabilities of the environment.

Aging and trauma combine to produce something beyond each other. The course of one's development is really a series of transformations leading to a reordering of dimensions, an elaboration or simplification of the narrative. At various life stages or for various situational reasons, the person is disrupted and a transformation of the narrative is required. These are the "teachable moments" in a person's life. We do well in transitions to pay attention to what is strange, whatever breaks routine. Fresh energy ascends. We are moved along a dimension of time with change in a backdrop of constancy.

In sum, these five "models" seem to be naturally flowing processes for the older person. There are many similarities. They can be used to place memories in the context of the total "older" person. Often this is for pleasure, to experience and enhance self-image. It can also be for self-understanding. If older people are offered more opportunity to shape the content and process of their memories, at least some may choose very different events and activities from those available in a pre-packaged form. As a result of adopting a more reflexive and open approach to the selection of reminiscence content, it is possible that older people may come to radically different conclusions both about which past experiences they regard as important and also about the sense they now make both of their history and their present lives.

Skeptics

Not everyone benefits from the acquisition of core memories. For some, it seems pointless or depressing (Coleman, 1986): "Reminiscence can be a sign of successful aging and high morale, and so can the absence of reminiscence" (Coleman, 1994, p. 133). Garland (1994) also held that for some people there may be negative outcomes. Kastenbaum (1987), however, seemed to ask the best question: "Under what circumstances ... is life review a valuable form of prevention, and under what circumstances is it useless or potentially harmful?" (p. 325). Molinari and Reichlin's (1984–1985) issues about reminiscence are those requisite psychological questions that require ultimate answers:

> What is the optimal time, ideal frequency of sessions, type of content? What processes lead to what kind of positive (or negative) outcome? What older people can benefit? Does the nature of life-review vary according to age? How is life-review experienced from the client's perspective? How does life-review affect reactions to ongoing problems? Is reminiscence important in the process of aging?

Coleman (1986) studied older people and identified two verbal and two nonverbal groups. Of the two verbal groups, the first group enjoyed talking and were well-adjusted. For them creative reminiscence was easy. The second group were the compulsive reminiscers. This group talked a lot but often brooded and were very troubled. The task of their therapy was to see (in a cognitive behavioral way) how justified and rational the past was. In the two nonverbal groups, one of these saw no value in talking. They were simply too busy. It was viewed as best to leave this group alone because they are well-adjusted. The fourth group, on the other hand, did not want to reminisce because the past was so bad. These people were chronically depressed. Again, the use of grief therapy and perhaps cognitive behavioral therapy can be applied to these people. Many people in later life do not normally talk: A life-review is also hard work.

Although the autobiographical impulse may seem natural, life review itself is not natural nor universal. Some events cannot be repaired so easily, no matter how much life review. Here depression, guilt, anger, panic, and obsessional rumination may ensue. For some, the distance is too great. Looking back before the trauma, some older victims say "Was that even me?" Here management may be the goal. Additionally, in old age the keeper of the archives can suspend reality requirements just long enough to make it work. Reality can be bent because "who would know?"

If very old age is reached, truth is altered in even different ways. The old-old tend to give up the quest for a youthful self concept: They feel old, become less introspective, and focus on the practicalities of death. The old-old change the idea of being old to one of being a person, about which there are many things, including life's accomplishments. Across all this time, the state of self follows health status: All things being equal, if you are healthy and active, so are your memories.

☐ Internal Organization

The critical issues become: How did memories come together? Are they random or do they have some connection? and How is the complex self system of the person linked by affect, context, and goals? What is the glue that provides order here? We seek a friendly "conceptual base camp" (Mahoney, 1991) from which to observe the workings of memory. This is not a replacement for the understanding of the person described by McAdams in the previous chapter. Rather it addresses the workings of the memory.

Trauma memories organize themselves at many levels; perception, attention, memory, thought, and language. It is facilitated by complex organized internal modules or schemas that automatically act on and organize incoming information and outgoing responses. Human beings house this information automatically out of awareness and organize information into internal schemas. People possess different ways of knowing and have a capacity to be guided by feelings they know they cannot say. Automatic processing occurs all the time. Core schemas are "person" positions or cognitions that are most central to the person. In the words of cognitive behavioral therapists they are "compelling" to the person, even when latent.

In turn, schemas unfold, giving rise to personality styles or traits. Somewhere in the developmental sequence, "security operations" (Sullivan, 1953) are required for protection. Adler (1939) labeled these safeguards or "methods of operation." They are "me–you patterns" (Sullivan, 1953), experiential invariants (Stern, 1985), or structured schemas (Young, 1991) of the person. Millon (1984) described these structural attributes as "images and inclinations that provide a template of imprinted residues which guide and transform the nature of ongoing life events" (p. 460). The personality protects the cognitive and affective substrate that is quasi-permanent, containing the residues of the past in the form of memories, intrapsychic constructs, and self-images. The personality protects schemas. Schemas select and synthesize incoming data, direct actions, and organize patterns of the person. In our previous book (Hyer, 1994), we viewed this process this way.

Schemas→Personality→Memories

Emotions too play the key role in providing information about the readiness of our biological machinery to interact with specific events in the environment and in integrating abstract cortical functions with perceptual motor reflexes (Plutchik & Kellerman, 1990). This "person-part" allows people to act in an integrated fashion. Emotions recruit cognitions and organize information. Emotions then are intrinsically involved in memory; they help to code our experience of the world and to access certain episodic memories. Emotions are thus a form of meaning and have particular significance for the person as each experiences and expresses them differently. A central goal of affective-oriented therapy is evoking organized cognitive-affective associative structures to either motivate change or to restructure the affective schemas themselves. Therapists pay close attention to emotions, as these are the "white heat of relevance."

So we have schemas, personality, and symptoms. Where is the memory? The memory is everywhere. Adler (1927) held that individual memories are at the center of understanding the person. The person establishes core goals in life that are driven by memories. In turn, the person develops schemas as a filter and a personality for protective mechanisms. It all works.

For us, the autobiographical or core memories provide the meaning and content of this process. We are less concerned with how this happens, than the fact that it does. Tomkins (1987) believed that the links to these memories are in scripts, a psychological magnification of a connection of similar memories through a shared thematic content. A strong bonding material is effect. In time, memories stimulate other memories effect assists. The result is a template of memories, a life story that is measured by schema and personality.

☐ Conclusion

We discussed the autobiographical memory. This is the core of the person and the part that influences and is influenced by choices in life. In later life, it has some "decline" problems but seems robust and accurate. It has become part of the person. We have also discussed ways that this memory can be accessed. These are the memories that are often hidden, can be positive or negative, and can be curative.

The life review then is important for the person: it is central for the person in trauma. We discussed several methods or contexts of the excavation of memory. Remembering an autobiographical memory is really an active process characterized by shifting interpretations and new life situations attaching to an ongoing life narrative. In this way, the delayed recall of the trauma, common in many older victims, is understandable. People protect their selves well even with trauma. The likelihood is that an "awakening" unfolds over time rather than after a single event and that it ascends most commonly in the context of a life's crisis or a developmental milestone. Trauma reminders serve as triggers. Herman and Harvey (1997) showed that the events that most lead to psychotherapy are recent life crises/milestones, a change in a close relationship, intrusion of memories, idiosyncratic occurrences, and abstinence of drugs and alcohol.

Everyone experiences trauma. The most typical trauma response is one of reasonable coping, followed by shock, numbing, and persistent intrusions. This is normal. These last two components recycle over time, and may never be fully worked through but not lead to problems with trauma. When trauma is not handled, however, incoming stimuli are rudely treated and the normal learning processes of assimilation and accommodation cannot continue. Initially, the person attempts to assimilate new information into the existing schemas. Given severe trauma, attempted assimilation fails. Accommodation, the effort to rearrange existing schemas, then proceeds. With severe trauma, this too fails. Wachtel (1984) suggested that a neurotic stuckness occurs (because assimilation/accommodation does not occur). One might even say that at this point the stressor becomes a trauma. Symptoms evolve.

Over time and when age applies itself to an unresolved trauma(s), recurrent and intrusive recollections of the trauma age too and represent a low level of accessible repetitive dysfunction in the person. The poor performance of many treatment modalities may suggest that the initial conditioned fear responses become indelible and inaccessible to desensitization (Shalev et al., 1992); or the poor reaction may also be something else. In the chronic forms of the disorder, often the associated disability is more a response to the distress and disruption caused by the symptoms of the disorder than by the primary reactions to the experience of the traumatic event.

This is, of course, trauma of a more chronic nature. However even in acute trauma the person develops a working narrative and comprehends "facts" and stressors according to this story, with all those influences of the various life stages. This is done quickly. Therapy has its job cut out for it.

CHAPTER 5

Treatment: PTSD and Beyond

"Psychoanalysis does not set out to make pathological reactions impossible,
but to give patients ego freedom to decide one way or the other"
Sigmund Freud

Therapy is what we say it is (Watzlawick, 1990). Ways to describe psychotherapy and its proscriptions are plentiful. To say that a psychotherapy is successful with depressives and not with phobics belies the nature of the process. Isolating its processes is only a convenient fiction, though a necessary one for our understanding and monitoring requirements. Whatever one's stance is regarding psychotherapy, the goal is to optimize the status of the client as being accessible, expressive, compliant, and increasingly psychologically minded. Bugental (1987) advocated for the pursuit of the inner orientation as the compass course of care. This certainly seems to apply to PTSD victims.

We are awash in studies that show that this or that therapy works. However these are not done with typical clinical patients, much less older patients. To our knowledge, virtually all quantitative reviews of therapy outcome studies have concluded that study participants who receive therapy have equal or better outcomes on the average than those participants who do not receive therapy. If you are anxious or depressed or are having problems with people in your environment and you can talk to someone you trust, chances are that you will feel better (Strupp, 1996). The report of over 7,000 readers of *Consumer Reports* (1994) indicated that, of the readers who had psychotherapy, most were satisfied and improved the quality of their lives: Talk therapy worked and training made a difference.

In this chapter we look at PTSD. We address treatment in general. We then consider PTSD treatment and later draw conclusions on the best treatment components of care. Finally, we consider treatment for older people.

☐ Overall Treatment

The Mess

The attribution of change due to psychotherapy is a difficult one, because there are so many influences in real lives. There is no consensus regarding what outcome measures to administer, how samples should be chosen, and who would pay the cost of administering instruments and analyzing results. Variation among client samples must be addressed for profiling. Demographic characteristics, such as age, sex, and socio-economic status certainly affect outcomes. Even more important, clinical characteristics, including diagnosis, chronicity, severity of illness, and comorbidity, may lead to differential outcomes. With older people, external factors, such as level of family support, stability of housing, and stressful life events, may affect outcome. Failure to adjust for case mix and risk factors can lead to erroneous conclusions about treatment outcome (Iezzoni et al., 1992).

Also there are practical problems. Frances et al. (1984), for example, noted that research shows that patients are 10 times more likely to initiate "no-treatment" decisions than are clinicians who offer it. Psychotherapy research indicates that any specific form of psychotherapy helps only about two-thirds of the people to whom it is applied (Smith, Glass, & Miller, 1980), decreasing for continuance (6 months) and further for maintenance (Snyder, Wills, & Grady-Fletcher, 1991). As a rule, clients try to hide negative reactions from therapists.

Directly referencing PTSD, problems amplify. Elliott and Briere (1992) found that intrusive thoughts were the central impediment to therapy participants. As we have implied on several occasions treatment is more than the remission of symptoms. Beutler and Hill (1992) have stated that symptom characteristics are of little value in the planning of specific treatment plans that are effective. Some reviewers of the psychotherapy literature have concluded that change occurs in waves, with symptom relief preceding movement on more trait-like dimensions (Barber & Crits-Christoph, 1995; Steenbarger, 1992). If this is the process, then treatment needs to address both symptoms and traits.

The possible mapping between causes and effects in psychotherapy can be one-to-one (linear), many-to-one, one-to-many, and many-to-many. Any of these contingencies may lead recursively to changes in causal conditions themselves (negative feedback loops). There can be multiple levels of change and interdependencies between the levels. Hypothesis-testing is meant to test the validity of ideas generated in the practice environment. Although good designs at least have the virtue of direction and specificity, they contain one important failing—they lack ecological validity. Real therapy simply isn't like that. Therapy design implicitly assumes that the experimental and control groups are homogeneous with respect to their pathologies, that patients are therapeutically interchangeable. This is never true. The possibility that some combination of interventions might prove synergistic if tailored to the individual patient is neglected. Millon and Davis (1995) noted:

> In order for this kind of design to make a valuable contribution to psychotherapy research, the latent pathology or disease process "present" in each patient would need to so dominate, coerce, or canalize other variables into a characteristic expression during the development of the disease that its interaction with premorbid individual differences could be almost completely neglected. Only then could every client be treated in the same way."

In fact, two separate worlds coexist, often in cold war mentality: Academic scientists evaluate validity by the rigor of the methods used, the consistency of treatment applications across patients, and the replicability of the results, whereas practitioners tend to evaluate a treatment's value by the usefulness of the theory, the nature of the process, and the sensitivity of the treatment to individual patient differences. Practitioners produce ideas and advances in techniques and interventions at a rate much greater than researchers can investigate them (Stiles, 1994). Smyth (1995) noted that clinicians tend to operate from what might be termed an *implicit idiographic data analysis set* that results in them finding value in clinical strategies and techniques that may be highly valuable for a small subset of clients even though the technique may not be of much value for the average client. Clinical researchers, on the other hand, operate more from what might be termed an *implicit nomothetic data analysis set* established by the conventional research. These statistical procedures tend to lead clinical researchers to value only techniques that are of benefit to the average client. Scientific and empirical frameworks constitute only one way to approach human suffering.

Recently, there has been a switch from the pure science efficacy research (internal validity) to a more real world approach to theory and effectiveness (external validity). There is a clear lesson to be learned. Singly demonstrating efficacy under ideal conditions, or even effectiveness in a real world setting, is not sufficient for intervention to be successfully diffused within the existing system.

Most clinicians are aware of the gap between the global findings of research and the usual specific nature of clinical dilemmas: how to treat patients who suffer from more than one Axis I disorder (which is more typical in a case of chronic PTSD); why a treatment works, the mechanisms and processes other than those outlined by the specific brand name treatments; and how to treat underlying personality issues and other determinants or dynamics that may be directly related to symptoms. Goldfried and Wolfe (1996) noted that it is no longer tenable to hold positions that these issues do not exist. The treatment of PTSD is both sobering and empowering. We need to listen to its wisdom of our confusion.

Finally, we highlight the model proposed by McHugh and Stavney (1999). It speaks to the overall problem of the limitations of the major conceptual models in psychiatry. The clinician must simultaneously understand the patient's troubles in terms of life circumstances and human responses to adversity, basic principles of behavioral and learning theory, and biological processes operating outside of the patient's awareness that might not be altered by a therapeutic experience. Clinicians are forced to be renaissance thinkers and integrationists. This applies nowhere in a more apt way than PTSD.

This is, of course, just a way to say that psychotherapy is messy and its evaluation often too precise for realistic or practical answers. Generally, each form of psychotherapy is most effective when applied to its domain of expertise. Most psychotherapeutic errors involve the application outside of its domain of expertise. This means that even within their domains of expertise, specific approaches do not help a substantial number of patients.

Directions

There are perhaps two ways out of this mess. The first is through better research. Foa and Meadows (1997) have given us the gold standard of PTSD research. These authors have applied a series of seven standards for appropriate research on trauma. Maxfield and Hyer (in press) added three additional criteria. All are given in Table 5-1. These represent a consensus in psychotherapy research and can be used as such.

Few studies have met these criteria. In fact, Foa and Meadows (1997) have the scientific audacity to again remind us that it is "readily apparent that research on the efficacy of psychosocial treatments for PTSD has only recently begun to approach these standards" (p. 474). As the pursuit of the ideal is noble and would perhaps "prove" that one technique is better than others in defined conditions and with

---

TABLE 5-1. Gold Standard (GS) Scale (Adapted from Foa and Meadows, 1997)

GS #1 Clearly defined target symptoms.
    0: no clear diagnosis, symptoms not clearly defined
    .5: not all subjects with PTSD, clear defined symptoms
    1: all subjects with PTSD

GS #2 Reliable and valid measures.
    0: did not use reliable and valid measures
    .5: measures used inadequate to measure change
    1: reliable, valid, and adequate measures

GS #3 Use of blind independent assessor.
    0: assessor was therapist
    .5: assessor was not blind
    1: assessor was blind and independent

GS #4 Assessor reliability.
    0: no training in administration of instruments used in the study
    .5: training in administration of instruments used in the study
    1: training with performance supervision, or reliability checks

GS #5 Manualized, replicable, specific treatment.
    0: treatment was not replicable or specific
    1: treatment followed EMDR training manual, Shapiro 1995

GS #6 Unbiased assignment to treatment.
    0: assignment not randomized
    .5: only one therapist, OR other semi-randomized designs
    1: unbiased assignment to treatment

GS #7 Treatment adherence.
    0: treatment fidelity poor
    .5: treatment fidelity unknown, or variable
    1: treatment fidelity checked & adequate

Additional Items Added to GS Scale to Create Expanded GS Scale

---

GS #8 No confounded conditions.
    0: most subjects receiving concurrent psychotherapy
    .5: a few subjects receiving concurrent psychotherapy, or unspecified and
        no exclusion for concurrent treatment
    1: no subjects receiving concurrent psychotherapy

GS #9 Use of multi-modal measures:
    0: self-report measures only
    .5: self-report, plus interview or physiological or behavioral measures
    1: self-report plus two or more other types of measures

GS #10 Length of treatment for civilian participant studies
    0: 1–2 sessions
    .5: 3–4 sessions
    1: 5+ sessions

---

defined samples, it is quixotic at best to assume that this will be helpful in the short run for our client needs. It's a good thing that we are not held hostage to them.

Fortunately, a mass of less scientific studies, older and established methods in treatment (as case studies and multiple baselines), as well as newer methods, are slowly but determinedly parsing apart the influence of patient attributes and treatment characteristics to differentially predict the benefits of different interventions. These newer methods of psychotherapy research include aptitude × treatment, and event process, as well as newer hierarchical linear models. What therapists do to either facilitate or impede certain change processes in the patient, and the relationship between these change processes and ultimate therapeutic outcome, provides another important study question. How do clients change during the course of therapy? The identification of the change mechanisms associated with the various treatments, be they similar across orientations or unique to a specific approach, constitutes the target issue. To this end, psychotherapy process researchers use a research approach whereby they explore and attempt to specify the "essential mechanisms of client change" (Rice & Greenberg, 1984). This so-called second generation of researchers study clinical phenomenena, then, in context.

Extant studies of psychotherapy do tell us something (Box 5-1), however. Treatment is by and large efficacious. However we are not sure whether our data do much more than tell us this. It has not disaggragated the ingredients that result in change and for whom. It cannot tell us what to do clinically in most circumstances. Our psychotherapy technology lies somewhere between a "psychological placebo" and clear-cut evidence that is "incontrovertible" (Barlow, 1996). Goldfried and Wolfe (1996) noted: "In many respects, our dilemma may be thought of as reflecting a conflict between a wish and a fear. Our wish is that therapy interventions be based on psychotherapy research; our fear, however, is that they might" (p. 1007).

Second, we know that something like the diathesis stress model applies to PTSD: A pathophysiological diathesis must be triggered by some environmental or physical stressor. The person must act on the stimulus and in turn is acted upon by the stimulus. The efficacy of any therapy is mediated by variables, not just the obvious ones like age and sex. Whatever the efficacy of one intervention alone, once used, it is likely that highly significant psychological and psychosocial issues will be put in motion. At the least other acts/thoughts/feelings will be performed by the patient. Some may lead to change. Nowhere was this more evident than in the review by DeRublies and

---

Box 5-1
Overall Treatment Facts

Treatment is better than no treatment—at least in some areas.

You will probably like your treatment.

Early success is important in care.

Like any form of medical treatment, success is optimal if there is client involvement, a placebo effect, or strong alliance, and a limited measured technology.

No current data that effective treatment in one area of the trauma will have a positive effect on others. Does effective resolution of intrusions eliminate distractibility, for example?

Hollon (1995). They summarized several studies conducted in the Cognitive Behavioral Treatment Project. They were interested in attributional style (internal, stable, and global, suggesting intransigent styles), those who learn how to deflect problems as a result of better thinking. Clients who were trained in attributional style in the first 6 weeks of treatment got better, this group improved in attributional style directly as a result of cognitive therapy. Those who received medication got better but did not evidence changes in their attributions. Miller and Silberman (1996) too found that 42% of an older sample reported that to recover from their depressive episodes, they needed to resolve interpersonal conflict. Finally, Kopta et al. (1994) showed that, as a result of therapy, acute stress abated quickly, chronic stress remitted after about 11 sessions, and interpersonal problems did not lessen after 50 sessions. Different interventions were required for each change.

In each example, clients improved as a result of thinking changes or interpersonal improvements and (in one case) did so over time.

It is the clinician and client who work on issues. A careful case formulation, even a goal attainment formulation of care, is implied in all therapies. The therapist who targets thinking and interpersonal issues according to the person's profile achieves results. There is a person between the therapist and the outcome.

☐ PTSD Treatment

Theoretical models of PTSD vary considerably. As we noted in Chapter 2 these include behavioral, cognitive, information processing, psychodynamic, and psychosocial models. It has been argued also that such conceptual frameworks have been developed to the neglect of an organized treatment (Loo, 1993). In a review on the treatment of PTSD, Shalev, Galai, and Eth (1993) believed that an integrated model involves combining biological, psychological, and psychosocial treatment. This integrated care is perhaps the best form of treatment. This group also believed that rehabilitative goals should replace curative techniques in those patients with chronic PTSD. As if disgusted with traditional treatment, Johnson et al. (1994) also argued that treatment should focus on the cognitive, social, vocational, and academic deficits that have become functionally autonomous (of PTSD) over the course of time. Hobfoll et al. (1991) stated that "the best treatment of PTSD has not been established."

On the whole, the systematic integration of treatment models has assisted thinking about the sequencing and type of treatment of PTSD. These have involved a sequencing of symptoms so that the initial problem-based issues are addressed first, followed by dysfunctional beliefs and dysfunctional emotions, and leading to the trauma memory interventions. van der Kolk, McFarlane, and van der Hart (1996) divide the treatment of PTSD into five stages: (a) stabilization, overcoming the fear of trauma related emotions; (b) deconditioning of the traumatic memories, an attack on the trauma memories themselves often translated into narrative format; (c) reconstructing of the trauma-related cognitive schemes, overcoming the fear of life itself; (d) re-establishment of secure social connections and interpersonal efficacy, fostering emotional attachment; and (e) the accumulation of restituted emotional experiences must be addressed, experiencing mastery and pleasure. To be successful, use of such a model requires that the client's active contribution to the healing process not evaporate to be replaced by the therapists.

In an interesting model of stages of decompensation (for PTSD), Wang, Wilson, and Mason (1996) reminded us that PTSD is not one disorder, and the clinician must do different things at different stages. They highlighted the repeating cycle of stages indicating a wide range of functioning from adaptive to totally dysfunctional PTSD core symptoms, as well as several other dimensions of clinical functioning, such as affect regulation, defenses, ego states, interactions with the environment, capacity for self-destruction (suicide), and a capacity for attachment and insight. Stages include (a) adaptive functioning, (b) survival that includes moderate to severe symptoms, (c) decompensation where there is a severe disregulated discharge state with very poor functioning (sensation-seeking and avoidance subtypes), and (d) depression/hopelessness that is a disregulated affective state, clinically unstable, and poor functioning (re-grouping or giving-up subtypes). If there is any merit to this and similar models, older victims have had ample opportunity to cycle through several of these stages.

Boldly, Valent (1999) outlined a complete treatment package for trauma survivors. It is an anchoring framework. It is a dialectic of life and trauma, meaning and pain. Coordinated axes are provided that serve as a skeleton for care, a care model. Normal and moral people are abused by a trauma. They are disrupted. The trauma response is the best that the person can do. This cannot be captured in a medical model. Treatment starts with a recognition of the event and proceeds with a taxonomy of care, connecting symptoms with sources of awareness. This taxonomy includes three axes: (a) process axis, in which the biological, psychological, and social aspects of the stress are accounted for; (b) parameter axis, in which each disaster phase is addressed and planned for (beginning, middle, and end); and (c) depth axis, in which the meaning aspects of the person are considered (a readiness to respond to the injustice and person aspects of meaning making).

We are, of course, dealing with some complexity regarding the care of PTSD. Harvey (1996) noted that trauma victims come in several varieties: Those who have received clinical care and have psychologically recovered from their experience; victims who have received clinical care but have not benefited and have not recovered; survivors who have recovered without benefit of clinical intervention; and those who have not received clinical care and have not recovered. We know considerably less about the latter two groups. In addition, many people respond to trauma with subthreshold levels of PTSD. There is evidence that intrusive and avoidant phenomena are quite common in response to traumatic stress and they represent a normal response to the situation (Blank, 1994). Also, reactions to trauma alter over time, making it necessary that a simple inventory of symptoms give way to a model that can describe the processes involved. Treatment models of PTSD are just that, models. The psychosynergy (Millon, 2000) involved is an approximation.

Types of Treatment

In a much cited review paper on treatment studies of PTSD (in general), Solomon, Gerrity, and Muff (1992) identified only 11 outcome studies that used random assignment to treatment and control groups. None involved older people. Overall, the active therapeutic ingredients for the treatment of PTSD were striking. These included systematic desensitization and cognitive-behavioral therapy (Frank et al., 1988; Resick & Schnicke, 1992), exposure therapy (Boudewyns & Hyer, 1990; Cooper & Clum, 1989; Foa, Rothbaum, Riggs, & Murdock, 1991; Keane, Fairbank, Caddell, & Zimering, 1989; Kilpatrick & Veronen, 1983), and several general factors, including support and skills training (Resick, Jordan, Girelli, Hutter, & Marhoefer-Dvorak, 1988). The combination of anxiety management training (AMT) or stress inoculation training (SIT), along with prolonged exposure, seemed to constitute the treatments of choice for chronic PTSD (Foa et al., 1994; Resick & Schnicke, 1992).

Combat Veterans

Regarding inpatient programs of mostly combat victims, two treatment ideas evolved: treatment works for selective symptoms in the context of the milieu and they require methods other than exposure. Regarding PTSD combat milieu programs, there are many benefits but over time they dissipate (Rosenheck & Fontana, 1993). Patients tend to like the treatment program and exposure has advantages over non-exposure. Self-esteem, interpersonal relationships, numbing, and arousal decreased during the treatment. Often little change occurs in PTSD symptoms; anger may even increase. Rehospitalization rates and employment improves. Interpersonal actions and morale improve. There may also be a decrease in family problems and violence: at 1 year, only decrease in violence held. Regarding outpatient treatment, there appears to be a "movement" and "stabilization" phase in which different changes occur. Symptom improvement occurs during the movement phase, followed by recidivism. There is no change in symptoms over 3 years.

With this population, the PTSD focus is best directed to the management of the process of stages of decline; different interventions at different times. Intrusive memories may be the centerpiece of PTSD, but real-life changes percolate at the margins. Other features of care need be addressed. As noted above, rehabilitative goals replace trauma-specific techniques in those patients with chronic PTSD (Johnson et al., 1994). Often too more problems are caused by the symptoms of PTSD than the primary reactions to the stressor.

Prolonged Exposure (PE) and Stress Inoculation Therapy (SIT)

Applying most of the methods of Foa and Meadows (1997), the Foa group treated rape victims who were at least 3 months out of the trauma, using an independent assessor and a standard measure of PTSD, with carefully defined treatment. Treatment consisted of prolonged exposure (PE) and stress inoculation therapy (SIT). Exposure involved 9 weekly individual sessions including information gathering, treatment rationale, treatment planning, as well as reliving in imagery the traumatic experiences described as if it were happening now. Exposure continued for about 60 minutes and was tape-recorded so that the victims could practice imaginal exposure or homework by listening to a tape.

In this first study (Foa et al., 1991), PE was compared with SIT, supportive counseling, and a wait-list control. All treatments were delivered in the same biweekly individual format. Results showed that immediately after treatment victims who received PE improved on all three clusters of PTSD symptoms. Victims in the supportive counseling and wait-list conditions had evidence of improvement on arousal symptoms but not on avoidance or re-experiencing symptoms. Three and a half months following treatment, PE proved to be the superior treatment. However, the superiority of PE was evident only on a measure of PTSD symptoms and not on other measures of psychopathology. At follow-up, 50% of the clients who received SIT and 55% of those who received PE did not meet criteria for PTSD.

In a second study, PE, SIT, a combination of these two, and a wait-list control condition were compared (Foa et al., 1991). Again, PE was more effective than the wait-list control. At post-treatment, only 29% of the victims who received PE retained their PTSD symptoms versus 100% of the victims on the wait-list control; 68% of the victims on the PE also evidence at least 50% improvement of PTSD symptoms as compared with 7% of controls.

Similarly, SIT programs have been found to be effective. Again it was the Foa group conducting the studies (Foa et al., 1991; Foa et al., 1994). Coping skills included deep muscle relaxation and differential relaxation, thought stopping, cognitive reconstructing, preparing for a stressor, covert modeling, and role play. In one study SIT produced significantly more improvement of PTSD symptoms than did the wait-list control immediately following treatment.

The success of PE and SIT is noteworthy. There were many benefits to the use of PE, but patients did best with exposure and coping techniques. Of importance, clients who had PE did not drop out of treatment. Also rather important was the fact that clients who were reluctant to engage in the reliving of the trauma or had a problem with association were first applied doses of anxiety management training (AMT). In this respect, the treatment of a combination of PE and AMT seems to offer victims ways to manage the extreme stress and anxiety while learning to confront the feared memories and clues. Additionally, therapists who were convinced that short-term suffering would lead to long-term benefit tended to do better, also the therapist had to be willing to hear the traumatic stories (Rothbaum & Foa, 1996).

These findings appear to have merit for older trauma victims. Intensive exposure methods may not be productive. This serves to increase the level of autonomic arousal, with adverse effects on cognitive performance (McFarlane & Yehuda, 1996). AMT and SIT do not do this: The former seeks to manage the anxiety as it occurs, and SIT represents the giving of tools as well as the perception of control to tolerate trauma memories and the belief that one can cope. Gradual exposure is implied in both methods. AMT provides a user-friendly atmosphere, where the client feels in control. The trauma memory is approached gradually at first, becoming more aggressive at the direction of the client. The autonomic nervous system is activated at a moderate range and new and incongruent data are added. Just as exposure is provided in a dosed way, altered cognitions or behavior interventions are introduced when the naturalness of the intervention is less effective. The latter has been labeled *assimilation work* (Smyth, 1995). Anxiety then is managed within the treatment context of AMT (Box 5-2).

Integrations

Variously termed assimilative techniques, cognitive restructuring (Foy, 1992; Foa & Kosak, 1986), cognitive processing (Resick & Schnicke, 1992) or emotional processing (Foa, Hearst, et al., 1994), mix with exposure. It is instructive to look at three studies that apply these methods and then look again at the work of Foa. Resick and Schnicke (1992) used a 12-session treatment called CPT. It includes "everything." It has exposure (clients are asked to write and rewrite their account of the trauma), education (about PTSD), assimilative techniques (ABC cognitive challenges and schemas). (Chard et al., 1997, has applied this same method [CPT-SA] for sexual abuse cases.) Second, Falsetti (1997) also applied a loosely structured method in which they start with education, orienting the client to the diagnosis; then apply coping skills treatment, as in SIT; then exposure is given (if trauma-related fear is present); and finally, cognitive restructuring, addressing faulty beliefs especially guilt and shame. Third, Friedman and Schnurr (1995) assessed a technique labeled *trauma focus group therapy* (TFGT). This method consists of small groups of patients. The "focus" is the trauma memory that is exposed in front of the group. Group members validate and assist in the cognitive restructuring of the memory. Relapse prevention strategies are then developed. Interestingly, a developmental perspective is also used.

Box 5-2
Tenets of EMDR

Accessing associative networks is unique for each person, as EMDR is not a "cookie cutter."

Growth motives (of the client) ultimately control the process of EMDR.

The central goal of EMDR is movement (processing), connecting between nodes of information. In trauma these have been blocked, and EMDR is a natural method to process these. Problems (resistance) are immediately apparent from this perspective.

EMDR is nondirective in content.

EMDR uses the power of treatment expectations.

In the unearthing of trauma, EMDR uses clean language.

EMDR uses a mixture of both processing and meta-communication on the client-governed content, a chunking of data necessary for change.

Cognition is crucial to the therapeutic process. EMDR uses traditional cognitive techniques, especially the identification of positive and negative cognitions, challenging evidence, and the "downward arrow," to access information *and* crystallize change.

No change is possible without affect. EMDR optimizes the "now" experiencing of past targets, a "focusing" technique that increases processing capacity.

The role of the therapist in EMDR is to be an active "blank screen," simply being responsive to the client's inner life and the renarrative process (narrative attunement), but also at times facilitating the process (doing therapy).

It can be seen that exposure of the memory serves as the focal point for the other therapy components. The use of a multi-method approach in the care of severely abused patients is now the norm.

Eye Movement Desensitization and Reprocessing (EMDR)

One more treatment method is called for. EMDR (Shapiro, 1995) is a newer method of therapy that uses both exposure (i.e., "desensitization") and cognitive processing of the traumatic memories. Despite critical reviews (e.g., Acierno et al., 1994), EMDR is one other technique that shows promise (see Boudewyns & Hyer, 1997), especially for older victims (Hyer, 1995). This procedure too is a phenomenological method that provides a dosed exposure and targets state-specific information related to the problem. An unusual aspect of the technique is that it also involves having the patient engage in reciprocally inhibiting, therapist-directed, stocastic eye movements during the treatment procedure. Over time, the role of the eye movements has altered from one that was crucial (Shapiro, 1989b) to one where they serve as key "orienting or dual stimuli" for a fast paced task of memory change (Shapiro, 1995). Recent studies would appear to indicate that replacing eye movements with finger tapping (Pitman et al., 1993; Pitman et al., 1995) or eliminating them altogether (Boudewyns et al., 1994; Boudewyns et al., 1995) had little effect on outcome.

Maxfield and Hyer (in press) reviewed twelve controlled studies that investigated the efficacy of EMDR with PTSD subjects. They applied these studies to the first seven gold standards (Table 5-1). Nine studies met 5 or more of the 7 methodological gold standards and found EMDR effective. Three studies met only 4 or less of the gold standards, and found EMDR noneffective or minimally effective. In the more rigorous studies, the EMDR pre-post effect sizes ranged from 0.67 to 2.22, with an average effect size of 1.45. The treatment control conditions had an average pre-post effect size of 0.58. When EMDR was compared to other treatments, the average comparison effect size was 0.89, indicating that EMDR generally outperformed the other therapeufic interventions. When EMDR was compared to wait-list the average effect size was 1.86. In the three studies with less rigorous methodology, the EMDR pre-post effect sizes had an average effect size of 0.21. The treatment control conditions had an average pre-post effect size of 0.27. When EMDR was compared to other treatments, the average comparison effect size was 0.23. Only one study calculated the decrease in PTSD diagnosis in the EMDR groups; this was minimal, 18%. In sum, the discrepancy between the effect sizes of the studies becomes apparent when they are grouped according to methodological strength. The more rigorous methodological studies show larger effect sizes.

Interestingly too, recent results suggest that both patients and therapists prefer EMDR over exposure (Boudewyns et. al, 1994). As a treatment for anxiety disorders, a major advantage of EMDR may be that it does not seek to increase exposure beyond what the patient volunteers and therefore does not engender as high a level of initial anxiety during the treatment as do direct exposure methods (Lipke, 1995; Boudewyns et al., 1995). In this regard the eye movements may act as buffers or inhibiting stimuli that break up the exposure process into trials or "doses," making the exposure more tolerable to the patient (and perhaps to the therapist also).

Procedurally (in EMDR), the client is requested to just talk with self regarding the trauma, to "stay with that." The therapeutic emphasis is movement of information. When stuck, other modalities are used—emotions, sensations, cognitions, images, and contrived experiments—or other interventions (guided imagery). Unlike AMT though, EMDR guides the client when information is blocked but at the same time provides both exposure and assimilation components necessary for trauma repair. Hyer and Brandsma (1997) identified 10 reasons why EMDR has applicability in psychotherapy. At base is the idea that EMDR applies sound principles of treatment (Box 5-2).

Finally, we note that Taylor et al. (in press) performed a meta-analysis of PTSD studies (Table 5-2), CBT, and EMDR, as well as the SSRIs were compared. Placebo was also included. CBT and EMDR are in a dead heat. Medication lags behind. Placebo has a .51 effect size. The factors that suggest treatment completion are younger age, being in a relationship, higher income, lower initial severity of PTSD, lower initial anxiety, depression and guilt, less severe trauma, and working full time. Factors associated with a good outcome were perception of treatment as credible, high motivation, high attendance, regular attendance, and absence of ongoing stress.

In sum so far, exposure is the treatment of choice. The fear memory must be activated and processed with newer information. Overall, results show that a more gradual program that included confrontations with the feared stimuli in combination with SIT skills, would enhance treatment effects. The task is to activate the ANS at a moderate range with important and incongruent data being reprocessed in conscious awareness. EMDR seems to do these same tasks but more quickly and is more appreciated by the patient. See Box 5-3.

TABLE 5-2. Effect Size of EMDR, CBT, Medications, and Nonspecific Therapeutic Factors

Treatment	Effect size
Psychotherapy	
CBT (13 trials)	1.27
EMDR (11 trials)	1.24
Relaxation (1 trial)	.45
Hypnosis (1 trial)	.94
Dynamic psychotherapy (1 trial)	.90
Medication	
TCA	.54
Benzodiazepines	.49
MAOI	.61
SSRI	1.38
Pill placebo	.51
Supportive psychotherapy	.34
Controls	.43

Virtually no studies exist on patient characteristics that interact either positively or negatively with exposure treatment. In fact, the working parameters of exposure are also unknown. It has not been determined, for example, whether exposure is better than other treatments, such as relaxation training, stress inoculation, and pharmacological options. Comparisons have not been made (Frueh, Turner, & Beidel, 1995). Must exposure address each event for anxiety reduction or will it generalize with the use of core fears? What is the length of exposure necessary as well as other procedural parameters? How do compensation-seeking or symptom over-reporting affect treatment? Although it is commonly believed that characteristics—such as comorbid diagnoses, especially substance abuse, psychosis or cognitive deficits, Axis II pathology (particularly borderline or antisocial), history of treatment, noncompliance and inability to image and unresolved life crisis, as well as poor physical health—are negative characteristics of treatment (Litz, Blake, Gerardi, & Keane, 1990), these have not been carefully studied.

We emphasize: *There are no carefully controlled studies of trauma of older victims.*

☐ Information Processing

We have other data too. That the cognitive processing of memories is important in the treatment of PTSD is suggested by several studies. We are above all else thinkers. We consider the salient entrails of the trauma memory as an information system to contextualize the problems of therapy.

Secondary Process

Resnick and Schnicke (1992) treated sexual assault survivors who received cognitive processing therapy (CPT), over 12 weekly sessions in a group format. Exposure con-

---

Box 5-3
Components of Exposure and AMT/SIT/EMDR

Established ideas (form exposure):
  Processing of information
    Fear memory be activated
    New information added
    Repeated exposure resulting in habituation within and across sessions
    Change in threat appraisals
Key Ideas:
  Anxiety management training
    Variety of procedures, including biofeedback, relaxation, cognitive restruc-
      turing. Manage the anxiety as it occurs→not fear activation so much as
      the giving of tools to handle these. Use exposure for re-experiencing and
      structured cognitions or behavior interventions for avoidance
  Stress inoculation training
    More direct application on self schema than on story renarration
    Multiple coping techniques
    Perception of Control→tolerate the trauma memories longer
    Coping focus→reduces the negative valence by dosed exposure and assim-
      ilation work
        Challenge but not overwhelm
        Manage anxiety within the AMT, never escape or avoidance
        Practice
  EMDR
    Key treatment ideas and tenets of EMDR:
      Fast paced
      Equal to other treatments
      User friendly

---

sisted of writing a detailed account of the assault and reading it out loud to the treatment group. Cognitive restructuring was based on the model of the treatment for depression. It focused on areas of functioning thought to be disrupted by victimization according to McCann and Pearlman (1990). Cognitive processing clients improved significantly from pre- to post-treatment on PTSD and depression ratings and maintained their improvement throughout a 6-month follow-up period. These findings are significant despite problems with the study (not randomly assigned clients or therapists).

Tromp, Koss, Figueredo, and Tharan (1995) used a mailed survey of women employees of a medical center ($n = 1,037$) and a university ($n = 2,142$). Pleasant and unpleasant memories were differentiated by feelings, consequences, and level of unexpectedness. The most powerful discriminator of rape from other unpleasant memories was the degree to which they were less clear and vivid, contained a less meaningful order, were less well-remembered, and were less thought and talked about.

Memories of trauma adhere to the person in vague and integrated ways. Change involves an assimilative process that recognizes the patchwork quilt of the rogue memory system.

Attentional Bias

Considerable work has been done on depression that applies to PTSD. We can see how the processing of trauma causes problems for both conditions as well as their similarities. Some of the boundary and critical questions of this disorder follow:

1. Do depressed/PTSD clients think more negatively than nondepressed comparisons? Is negative thinking causative of depression/PTSD? Are dysfunctional cognitions state dependent?
2. When PTSD/depressive thinking is primed, do vulnerable individuals become PTSD/depressed? Are emotions and cognitions in bed with one another?
3. Are negative cognitions specific to PTSD/depression rather than other forms of pathology?
4. Does meaning affect PTSD/depression?

The answers to these questions are "yes."

For starters, several theories of depression advocate for a model in which depression occurs as a result of acute generalized stress and this condition fails to return to its normal state. Gold, Goodwin, and Chrousos (1988) speculated that the brain is sensitized as a result of early, acute exposure to stress. In adulthood, reactions are readily activated even by mild or symbolic representations of stress precipitants. Lockwood et al. (2000) went further and noted that after repeated episodes of depression the person has an altered brain at the cellular level and changes in the sensitivity to stress is evident.

What happens at the psychological level? Perhaps the most appealing model that reflects this thinking is learned helplessness (Seligman, 1975). This serves as a reflector of how memory works in the context of traumatic incidents. People subjected to uncontrollable, repeated trauma develop images of themselves as powerless and helpless. A deep sense of futility is internalized after numerous unsuccessful attempts to avoid the trauma. This reaction remains even after the threat has passed. With trauma survivors the world is assessed as a threatening and inhospitable place. Teasdale and colleagues (e.g., Teasdale & Barnard, 1993) have hypothesized that what gets activated in trauma or depression is an entire mental model of cognitions and affects, not a set of individual cognitions. This results in a global and negative view of self activated largely by moods. Popular stress-diathesis models extend this to include the interaction of attributions and stressors. Depression or PTSD or both result.

As we have noted, PTSD does not develop in the immediate aftermath of a traumatic event. It emerges out of a pattern of the acute distress triggered by the event. The unique feature of PTSD involves a memory that is stuck or undifferentiated or both. In several studies this is born out. The Foa group showed that the narrative changed over time as a result of processing (Brewin & Lennard, 1999; Foa, Molnar, & Cashman, 1995). Narrative length increased from pre- to post-treatment, percentage of actions and dialogue decreased as did the percentage of thoughts and feelings, particularly thoughts reflecting attempts to organize the trauma memory. An increase in organized thoughts was correlated negatively with depression.

This group showed also that PTSD has its own fear structure (as do the other anxiety disorders). This involves negative schemas or beliefs, such as the world is dangerous and the self cannot handle problems. The result is a disorganized narrative. Memory is activated by simple, every day events. New information cannot be meaningfully added, due to the negative schemas and repeated threat appraisals that become further consolidated. As a result, the processing of information or restructuring, rearranging, or reorganizing the past stuck memory does not occur. Additionally, those who have been exposed to potentially traumatizing events (e.g., a war zone), and who develop some degree of PTSD symptoms, are at risk for unwittingly having their attention drawn to personally salient, highly threatening stimuli in the environment.

Litz and colleagues (Litz et al., 1996) expanded on these ideas, especially as regards the generalization effects of the trauma memory. This group argued that (a) trauma-related experiences are stored in memory in a hierarchically organized network or schema; (b) they are easily triggered by trauma-related cues, resulting in greater accessibility of trauma memories and integrated programs of conditioned emotional responses (e.g., physiological reactivity); and (c) there exists a preferential allocation of attention to potentially threatening stimuli in the environment. In effect, the trauma-network is distinguished from other organized self-relevant knowledge by virtue of its hyperaccessibility (i.e., ease of activation) and the type of responses that are produced subsequent to activation (e.g., hypervigilance, conditioned emotional responses, etc.) There is a response bias toward trauma-related stimuli during memory retrieval.

Litz et al. (1996) assessed Vietnam veterans with current PTSD. A PTSD group, a group with other Axis I disorders, and with no Axis I disorders were studied. Participants were given tasks such as the modified Stroop procedure, the standard Stroop procedure, recognition memory tasks and a threat-rating task. Physiological responses are recorded, as well as other outcome measures. Results of the study supported several predictions derived from informational processing models of PTSD. PTSD participants exhibited greater modified Stroop procedure interference to high-threat words in both comparison groups and a liberal response bias toward recognizing military-related words. This was in contrast to Foa et al. (1991) who found only specific interference effects in rape victims with PTSD.

Whether the effect is generalized or specific, attentional bias for high-threat stimuli is the order of the day. Data support the view that the distinguishing feature of the trauma-related network in chronic PTSD is its interconnected and highly generalized character. Perhaps in chronic PTSD the trauma-network becomes more generalized over time, encompassing a variety of threat-related stimuli.

Memory Retrieval

Lurko, Macklin, & Pitman (1995) identified difficulties in retrieving specific autobiographic memories. He studied Vietnam veterans with PTSD and found problems with the retrieval of personal memories in response to positive and neutral cue words relative to healthy controls. This appears to be due to exposure to trauma memories. In other words the preoccupation with trauma memories makes it a problem to use memory in an adaptive fashion. Negative traits or attributes relative to positive ones dominate self schemas of PTSD victims. Positive autobiographoical memories are more difficult to retrieve. An "overgeneralized" memory may contribute to a failure to recover from depression and to poor problem solving: Emotional priming appears related to its specificity. One other feature may be that an inability to retrieve positive memories contributes to problems in the activation of positive affect.

Supporting this is a dual model of the traumatic experience provided by Brewin, Dalgleish, and Joseph (1997). Based on work by Epstein (1990, 1991), this group believed that people appear to respond in two different fundamental ways to trauma, one more intuitive (experiential) and the other more deliberate (rational). One involves verbally accessible memories and the other situational accessible memories. The verbally accessible memories contain information about the sensory features of the situation, emotional physiological reactions experienced, and a perceptual meaning of the event. They represent an accessible knowledge of the autobiographical memory that can be progressively edited. After trauma, these memories are likely to be dominated by detailed information concerning the conscious perception of sensory material and of bodily experiences. Some attempt also involves an effort to assign verbally accessible constructs and categories as early meaning to the trauma. Symptoms attributed to the verbally accessible memory are intrusive memories of the conscious experience, emotions related to the trauma and its consequences and selective recall.

In contrast, the situationally accessible memories include overall representation of the stimulus information automatically coded for its ability to discriminate the trauma from other previous non-trauma situations, the meaning information derived from prior associative learning and information about the person's state of consciousness. These appear automatically when the person perceives the physical features and meanings similar to those of the traumatic situation. This may be internal or external. Symptoms evolving from the situational accessible trauma memories include flashbacks, trauma-specific emotions, selective recall, physiological arousal, and motor output.

What is most important here is that the clinician should consider factors from both memory systems. The verbally accessible memories may be edited in various ways; not so the situationally accessible memories. These latter memories tend to be highly detailed, repetitive ones that are difficult to edit because they are accompanied by emotional or physiological changes experienced during the trauma. Processing is inhibited also as the verbally accessible memory remains protected because of constant reactivation by the situational accessible memory. Individuals develop a repressive coping style, show attentional avoidance and an overall impaired memory. Some may "foreclose" and be unduly optimistic.

Traumatic experiences, therefore, are not incorporated into the coherent narrative of one's life. The role of linguistic processing is critical here. Poor processing indicators include repression and dissociation (that is the quality of processing during and after the trauma), divided attention and differential processing (the nature of the problem and the immediate attention for its recovery), emotional features (excessive emotionality in the processing), memory storage and retrieval (intact, implicit, deficient explicit memory), symptom intensity and type (flashbacks), cognitive complexity of the organism (whether a child or an adult), and perhaps neurophysiological problems (conditioned fear that is not integrated into the cerebral cortex). As we noted above, Smyth (1995) added that the primary therapeutic task in PTSD treatment becomes the activation of the traumatic memories while keeping autonomic nervous system arousal in the moderate range so that the secondary process program can effectively rewrite the original codes created by the automatic thinking program to classify the traumatic memories and/or the secondary process program can be used to revise the meta-cognitions that the traumatic material contradict.

"Need" to Rewrite Memory

Whether traumatic memories were retrieved initially in the form of dissociated sensory and affective elements of the traumatic experience, or were simply not narrativized, over time participants reported the gradual emergence of a personal narrative that can be properly referred to as "explicit memory." The narrative is the most common way to transport the contents of the autobiographical memory and the explicit memory is not intact. PTSD then may be a deficit of explicit memory: The implicit memory is intact. The trauma victim cannot recall the specifics of the trauma event but can be primed by its cues. The explicit memory is not organized or free to be recorded, restored, and retrieved in altered ways.

In this and the previous chapter we have argued that memories of trauma are not in explicit memory, not narrativized or consolidated. There is some consensus that the more the trauma memory is simply disclosed (Pennebaker, 1989) and validated (Murray & Segal, 1994), the more improvement occurs. But also, the more organized (Foa, Molnar, & Cashman, 1995), narrativized and placed into explicit memory (van der Kolk & Fisler, 1995), elaborated (Harvey, Orbuch, Chivalisz, & Garwood, 1991; Sewell, 1996), and retrieved as less summary and more positive (McNally, Lasko, Macklin, & Pitman, 1995), the more improvement occurs.

van der Kolk (1996) used the Traumatic Memory Inventory, which is a structured way of recording whether memories of traumatic experiences are retrieved differently from memories of personally significant but nontraumatic events. This group noted many interesting findings. When asked about their memories, PTSD participants reported that they initially had no narrative memories of the events. They did not recall the story of what happened regardless of whether they knew the trauma had happened or whether they were retrieving the trauma from a later date. Participants (regardless of age at which the trauma occurred) remembered the trauma as a somatosensory flashback experience. These flashbacks occurred in a variety of ways (visual, auditory, olfactory, affective) providing little integration. The traumatic memory was apparently dissociated and stored initially as sensory fragments. These have no linguistic components. It was only later that participants developed a narrative. In fact, even after a personal narrative was developed for the trauma experience, most reported that sensory experiences or affective states returned. So, even with the "wording" of the trauma, the complete eradication of flashbacks is unlikely. The narrative experience assists in the integration of the experience and result in improvement.

Role of Emotion

Harvey, in the account making study noted above, found that the more engaged the person is emotionally, the more and deeper "parts" of the memory are accessed and treated. The status of a person's emotional state is very important. In a summary of trauma memories Koss, Tromp, Figueredo and Tharan (1995) reminded us that emotion appears to facilitate the accuracy of recall of central details. Across a range of studies the greater the emotionality of the experience, the greater the vividness of the memory. This relationship increases over time in longitudinal research (Landou & Litwin, 2000). High emotion appears to slow forgetting. Also the suggestibility of emotional memories has been overstated.

To a considerable degree, emotional arousal influences memory strength. It has been argued that emotional memories allow for better retention of memories because of the physiological arousal, the pre-attentive processing that necessarily involves these kinds of memory, and elaborative (cognitive) processing that increases for events that are personally important. Once formed, emotional memories appear to be very hard to eliminate (LeDoux, 1992).

Conclusion of PTSD Studies

With trauma, information processing is compromised, becoming "comfortable" with patterns that reinforce the status quo (Litz & Keane, 1989). Memories of the traumatic events do not meaningfully fit in prior schemas and are not narrativized. Triggers from the implicit memory continue unabated. These include perceptual stimuli, emotional states, interpersonal context, and language clues. Implicit retrieval produces a subjective internal experience of trauma-related emotions by sensations, images, and the like. Traumatic memories are not "moving" or not where they should be, and are often disorganized and fragmented because they are encoded under extreme anxiety. The therapeutic task, therefore, is to allow for the implicit memories to be processed in an explicit manner, where desensitization and narrativization would be essential. Assimilative processes are essential here: Language-based interpretations are important.

Box 5-4 presents a summary of the key clinical elements of care. First is exposure. Most effective treatments then are some variant of the exposure model, whether direct exposure, dosed exposure, or some form of stress inoculation training where an effort is made to attack the schemas in an exposure format. Imaginative and in vivo exposure procedures including confrontation (with mild to moderate high levels of anxiety) remain the staples for the treatment of PTSD.

The second component involves exposure too, the moderate activation of the trauma memory. This is best done in the context of AMT. Now, the memory can be processed and placed into a passive or long-term memory system. Earlier studies on the treat-

---

Box 5-4
Summary of Trauma Memory and Treatment Ideas

Key Treatment ideas
  Expose and decondition the anxiety.
  Use the context of AMT or EMDR.
  Secondary process where cognitive codes are challenged.
  Rewrite the trauma. Renarrate and reframe the horror. Integrate the trauma.
    Get the trauma memory organized.
  Keep emotion alive but in check. Moderate activation of the trauma memory.
Probable Action
  Memories of the trauma events are not placed into prior schemas. They assert
    a bias on incoming information.
  They are not in explicit memory.
  They are not narrativized and consolidated in the cortex.
  Implicit retrieval produces a subjective experience of the trauma, emotions,
    bodily sensations, and sensations that are not sensed as self in the past.
  Triggers are perceptual stimuli, emotional states, and language cues.

ment of PTSD noted that a necessary condition for change involved the fear memory being activated and new information being provided. Excessive arousal, of course, might make a PTSD patient worse by interfering with the acquisition of the new information. Trauma memories will not be corrected but rather they will be confirmed, thus preventing extinction and fostering habituation. Meaningful monitors to this include habituation within and across exposure sessions as well as changes in the threat appraisals. AMT and EMDR do this.

Third, a secondary process is required in the change of memories. New information must be provided so that the individual is able to alter existing memories. This involves the assimilative process where "positive or reframed" data can be provided. One new datum at least is the fact that the patient is able to confront the trauma memory in the presence of trusted therapist. The trusted therapist appears to be important. AMT and EMDR do this.

The use of AMT/EMDR along with traditional methods of CBT, as well as the methods applied to the narrative, are indicated then for trauma alteration of older victims. In a general way the techniques that appear to best accomplish the therapeutic task of PTSD symptom remission are the same techniques that have been found to be effective against generalized anxiety disorder, panic disorder, and phobias in general. These are exposure strategies coupled with CBT strategies that emphasize the importance of correcting "irrational" self-talk, such as SIT. After all, trauma healing is a continual retelling to self, shifting from previous negative narratives to more positive ones (van der Kolk & Fisler, 1995). With the combination, then, of assimilation (CBT and narrative work) and exposure work (AMT + exposure), trauma codes can become habituated (desensitized) *and* assimilated (corrective cognitive codes).

It is important to keep in mind that CBT strategies are effective because of their impact on cognitions, not because of their supposed impact on classically conditioned anxiety. It is also important to keep in mind too that once the codes have been corrected, recoded data must still be appropriately filed by conscious secondary process-dominated story telling. Also, it is likely that the particular technique used in helping patients confront their trauma memories is not the critical variable. Additionally, older people have the advantage that they can rework earlier stories "naturally," now older and as meta-historians.

It seems that the process for this is that the explicit memory is recast. Data stuck in the intermediate memory storage system (due to automatic thinking danger codes) can now be accessed into long-term memory via moderate levels of activation and "good" secondary process thinking. These codes are processed because they are habituated, and because of the impact of cognitions (corrective cognitive codes).

Fourth, we can rewrite trauma with the use of the therapies. People engage in account making when they are troubled and narrativize problems so that they can handle them. This can occur in many forms: helpful discussion with others, diary/journal recording, periods of private reflection about the event, as well as early and empathic response from a significant other.

For older people, interventions related to reminiscence (expose the story, unearth obvious distortions, and provide methods for alternative beliefs) and CBT (surface and core construals) actually emphasize this aspect of treatment. Reminiscence in this sense becomes not regressive but an adaptive way to rework problems (bad stories). As PTSD is a stuck story or an incoherent narrative, one that is ontologically locked and disorganized in fixed time and space, the therapeutic task is to repair the story and rewrite the biography of the person. At the least the task is to organize the story and provide a context for discovery and healing.

Fifth, the need to use emotion and to keep it in check are critical. The moderate level of activation is necessary for the person to process the trauma. The experience of emotion is necessary.

☐ Old Folks and Rx

"People do not just seek meaning in life: I think that what we're really seeking is an experience of being alive, so that our life experiences on the purely physical plane will have resonance within our innermost being and reality, so that we can actually feel the rapture of being alive."
Joseph Campbell

George Bernard Shaw once said something to the effect that Christianity has not failed, it has simply never been tried. While individual treatment of the elderly seems humane and potentially clinically appropriate, it ought not only to be tried, but also to be systematically studied. At age 37 Jung found his life disrupted by severe emotional turbulence—intense anxieties and depression—without knowing why. It is reported that he lacked a "myth," a framework of meaning, purpose, and direction in his life. He resigned his teaching position at a local university and undertook a 3-year series of experiential and meditative practices to "get to the bottom" of his loss of meaning in life. As he turned his attention to the symbolic life within his own psyche, and drew on and had dialogue with the images he experienced, he came to discover his own "myth," which he termed *individuation*, a transcendent function. The inner goal of his life, as he came to articulate it, was the conscious realization and expression of the "self." Life is a journey toward becoming a whole person, and shaping an outer life in harmony with one's true self. What do we know about the helping process in this journey?

It is hard to know where to begin when reviewing the efficacy of older people. In a recent conference on aging in Georgia, Michael Smyer (Hyer, 1998) noted that we may know that treatment works in a loose sense but we still don't have a good sense of the "particulars"—What are the most effective mental health treatments for older adults in a broad range of settings, as in long-term care? What do we know about depression/anxiety disorders in these places? What's the most effective and appropriate combination of pharmacological and psychotherapeutic intervention for older adults?

This statement does not come from a strange place. After Freud disavowed the treatment of the elderly as a group, Fenichel (1945) pointed out the value of neurosis to the chronically ill aged, and cautioned against tampering with the aged patient's defenses unless we are sure that we can provide adequate substitutes for them. Close on the heals of these offerings, Stieglitz (1952) used a teacher/student approach to patients, and Goldfarb (1955) encouraged the dependency of the aged as a therapeutic resource. In a further twist of this logic, Goldstein & Birnbom (1976) observed that the older patients tended to act passively ill in order to be taken care of, while staff tended to "push for" independence of functioning. The institutional version of this was a tacit agreement between staff and patients: As long as the patients were "good," the staff would not be "mean" and withhold basic social sustenance from them (Gatz, Siegler, & Dibner, 1979–1980). This has been called a "silent bargain" (see Gatz, Popkin, Pino, & van der Bor, 1985).

It was only somewhat later a spate of methodologically flawed studies showed that the elderly could be treated. Ingersoll and Silverman (1978), for example, compared the effects of a "there and then," reminiscence-oriented outpatient group to a "here and now," behaviorally oriented form of group intervention: "There and then" was better than "here and now." During the 1970s, several nonspecific factors were endorsed. Expectancy and efficacy have emerged as issues in virtually every type of intervention with older adults. Hope (Wolff, 1971), optimism (Verwoerdt, 1976), "symbolic giving," and bearing witness (Lewis & Butler, 1974), among others, are considered staples of good care with this population. Special psychologic needs of the elderly (Pfeiffer & Busse, 1973)—involving distinctive themes (e.g., loss, increased dependency, existential approach of death), age-specific reactions (e.g., survivor guilt at having outlasted others), and "aging" therapy needs (e.g., more limited goals, greater amount of positive benefit, as well as a slower pace and lack of determination), were proffered.

At about the same time several distinct therapies were practiced on older people, including remotivation, validation, reorientation, and the like. The notion of "excess disability" guided several attempts to show that older people can be treated. This represents the gap between existing and potential function in persons diagnosed as having organic brain dysfunction (Brody, Kleban, Lawton, & Silverman, 1971).

Cognitive Behavioral Therapy

"The aim of life is to be aware, joyously, drunkingly, serenely, divinely aware."
Henry Miller

Reviews

During the past 15 years, the use of the CBT model has proved effective with later life depression (Beutler et al., 1987; Gallagher & Thompson, 1981, 1982; Hyer et al., 1990; Hyer, Swanson, & Lefkowitz, 1990; McCarthy, Katz, & Foa, 1991; Thompson, Gallagher, & Breckenridge, 1987) and anxiety (Scogin, Rickard, Keith, Wilson, & McElreath, 1992), and has maintained treatment gains (Gallagher-Thompson, Hanley-Peterson, & Thompson, 1990). The same result applies to interpersonal psychotherapy (Hendrickson, 2000).

Early reviews by Garfield (1994) and Smith, Glass, and Miller (1980) show that at least some older adults can benefit from psychotherapy within the present system, certainly a short-term gain.

Recent reviews also indicate clearly and convincingly that psychotherapy with older people is effective (e.g., Gallagher-Thompson & Thompson, 1995; Gatz, 1994; Gatz, Popkin, Pino, & VandenBos, 1985; Knight, 1996; Schramke, 1997) on a wide variety of pathological areas (see Zeiss & Steffen, in press), even combined with medication (Thompson, Gallagher, Hansen, Gantz, & Steffen, 1991) or applied to more difficult problems (Hanley-Peterson et al., 1990; Thompson, Gallagher, & Czirr, 1988). Interestingly, these positive findings apply to older adults with cognitive decline (Snow et al., 1999).

Most reviews focus on depression. In their narrative review of six cognitive and behavioral therapies on depressed elderly, Morris and Morris (1991) indicated that older adults could benefit from these treatments. Robinson et al. (1990) in their review on the efficacy of psychotherapeutic treatment for depression found a high effect size ($d = .73$, $N = 37$). Scogin and McElreath (1994) conducted a meta-analysis of 17 studies on the efficacy of psychosocial treatments for geriatric depression. The overall effect size was positive ($d = .78$, $N = 23$). Finally, in one recent review

Engels and Vermey (1997) conducted a meta-analysis of 17 studies on the efficacy of nonmedical (psychological) treatments for depression in the elderly. Results revealed that treatment was more effective than placebo or no treatment. Effects were equal for mild and severe depression and proved to be maintained over time. The mean effect size ($d = .61$) was adequate. This result is in accordance with those of a number of other reviews (Engels et al., 1993; Prioleau et al., 1983; Robinson et al., 1990; Smith et al., 1980). (Effect sizes above about .6 indicate that the mean treated client was better off than 75% of the clients in control conditions.) Results apply less to group therapy (Robinson et al., 1990; Scogin et al., 1994; Smith et al., 1980). Although results have to be interpreted with caution (because of a conservative way of effect size estimation), Seogen and McElreath (1994) conclude:

> It can be concluded from this meta-analysis that nonpharmacological treatment for depressive complaints, including major depression, in elderly patients is possible and effective. Treatments seem to be equally effective for mild and severe depression. When assessed, benefits of psychological therapy were similar at posttreatment to those observed at later follow-up. Thus, pessimism with regard to psychological treatment of the elderly does not seem to be justified.

There is research also demonstrating the effectiveness of CBTs for other disorders; sexual dysfunction (e.g., Zeiss, Delmonico, Zeiss, & Dornbrand, 1991), sleep problems (e.g., Lichstein & Johnson, 1993), and tension (e.g., Scogin, Rickard, Keith, Wilson, & McElreath, 1992), both individually (Thompson, Gallagher, & Breckenridge, 1987) and with groups (Kemp et al., 1992), and in various venues (e.g., Carstensen, 1988). Positive results apply also to medical illness, with such factors as control/choice (Burish et al., 1984; Wallston et al., 1991), anxiety (Carey & Burish, 1988), relaxation training (Burish, Snyder, & Jenkins, 1991; Burish, Vasterline, Carey, Matt, & Krozely, 1988; Carey & Burish, 1987), conditioned responses (Burish & Carey, 1986; Burish, Carey, Krozely, & Greco, 1987), denial (Matt, Sementilli, & Burish, 1988), and different psychological effects associated with cancer chemotherapy (Arean, 2000; Carey & Burish, 1988; Nezu et al., 1998).

"Best" Studies

In perhaps the best conducted study on older folks, Gallagher and Thompson (Gallagher & Thompson, 1981, 1982; Thompson, Gallagher, & Breckenridge, 1987) followed more than 90 older adults diagnosed with a major depressive disorder. After receiving a course of cognitive, behavioral, or psychodynamic psychotherapy, 70% of the sample had improved considerably or were no longer clinically depressed. At a 1-year follow-up, no evidence of depression was found in 52% of the whole sample. Although no differences among the treatment groups were found at treatment time, the cognitive or behavioral group had less attrition and greater compliance (Thompson et al., 1986). A second study (Thompson et al., 1990) comparing the efficacy of cognitive, behavioral, and brief psychodynamic therapies revealed significant improvement for all three forms. One- and 2-year follow-ups showed a comparable extent of maintenance of treatment gains in all three groups (Gallagher-Thompson, Hanley-Peterson, & Thompson, 1990; Thompson, Gallagher, & Breckenridge, 1987).

These studies were important, because treatments were carefully noted, procedures manualized, patients randomized, measures specified, and patients followed for a year. A detailed summary of the efficacy of cognitive and behavioral therapies with clinically depressed elders (Teri, Curtis, Gallagher-Thompson, & Thompson, 1994) and a comprehensive review on the efficacy of psychotherapy with older adults (Gallagher-Thompson & Thompson, 1995) were now available.

The CBT elements that represent the core of the approach to therapy and are presumably some of the reasons for its demonstrated effectiveness are as follows: collaborative therapeutic relationship, a focus on a small number of clearly specified goals, emphasis on change, psychoeducational, length of therapy contracted and linked to goals, agenda set at each meeting, skill training (cognitive, behavioral, and interpersonal), and health status. Additionally, moderating conditions exist. Factors that may contribute negatively to treatment outcome include endogeneity, the presence of a personality disorder, severity of PTSD/depression at the onset of treatment, patient expectancies or commitment for change, and the patient's role in the development of the therapeutic alliance (Beckham, 1989; Gallagher & Thompson, 1983; Gaston, Marmar, Thompson, & Gallagher, 1988; Gaston, Marmar, Gallagher, & Thompson, 1989; Marmar et al., 1989).

Gallagher-Thompson and Thompson (1996) compared use of the tricyclic antidepressant drug desipramine alone with use of CBT alone, versus the two in combination, in a randomized design for a period of 16–20 sessions. Endpoint analysis (including dropouts) showed no difference in change in diagnoses of depression between CBT and the combined condition, but both of these showed significant improvement when compared with the desipramine-alone condition. As recent evidence suggests that antidepressant medications produce high levels of toxicity and are equal or less effective than CBT (Fisher & Greenbergen, 1989), this therapeutic approach becomes especially important.

There are virtually no studies on PTSD and aging. In one of the few studies that included stressor victims, Hyer et al. (1990) evaluated two groups of older clients, chronic PTSD or recent stress reactions due to loss, as well as a no-treatment control group. Two CBT components were identified and practiced—cognitive schemas/irrational beliefs and relaxation/anxiety management training (AMT). Each group received a 12-session CBT program and was evaluated on several psychological and behavioral outcome measures. Although objective repeated measures showed no differences among the groups (due to small numbers), subjective measures of outcome and individual change supported the treatment package. All participants believed they benefited from the cognitive therapy and the relaxation training along with the AMT. A subsequent study using anxiety and depression with older groups corroborated the importance of these two core factors with both objective and subjective measures (Hyer et al., 1990).

Above all, the CBT model allows for "narrative repair." The narrative memory subserves core schemas, forming a meaning system that is protected from influence. The person maintains identity by altering new information. Trauma does not allow this to be unperturbed. Narrative repair then involves an active approach and a reworking of adverse events. This entails a reinterpretation of the meaning of the event *and* behaving in ways that counteract unknown consequences. "Poor" cognitions consist largely of negative attributional styles and faulty interpretation (Mikulincer & Solomon, 1988), as well as negative world views ("assumptive worlds") (Epstein, 1991; Janoff-Bulman, 1989). Through an active therapeutic pursuit of the negative memory, then, the trauma is reprocessed and integrated.

Relaxation-based techniques are important. When used in combination (CBT and progressive muscle relaxation (PMR)), graded exposure in the form of systematic desensitization is likely to be helpful. As we noted earlier, with older trauma victims intensive exposure methods are countrproductive, tending to increase the level of autonomic arousal, with adverse effects on cognitive performance. The same applies to confrontational techniques (McCarthy, Katz, & Foa, 1991).

Finally, we highlight one other form of psychothrapy, interpersonal psychotherapy (IPT; Klerman, Weissman, Rounsaville, & Chevron, 1984). If you had to apply two forms of therapy for older people, you would want to use CBT or IPT. They have the most validation. The former addresses cognitions; the latter, the relationship. IPT has been used with older folks to good ends. This therapy focuses on here and now issues related to grief, interpersonal disputes, role transition, and role disputes. Hendrickson (2000) especially has built on the work of Frank and Spanier (1995) as well as Miller et al. (1998) and Reynolds (1997) for the application of this therapy to an older population. Results on older people show that the combination of IPT and medication is associated with the highest rate of treatment completion and efficacy for depression and bereavement in older people (Miller et al., 1997; Reynolds et al., 1999a; Reynolds et al., 1999b).

In sum, as always, even modest conclusions may be premature, because variations in such factors as systematic diagnosis, measurements, techniques used, and therapist's skill preclude comparison across studies. Also, no serious scientific studies on the effects of PTSD have been carried out on elders. Studies included the usual suspects: relaxation, cognitive therapy, psychodynamic therapy, biofeeedback, and life review. All seem to have some efficacy. Arguably it is reasonable to consider anxiety problems of older people as you would those of younger ones. The treatment of a panic attack, phobia, obsessive problem, general anxiety problems can be addressed with extant protocols used on patients of all ages (Schramke, 1997). At the risk of some scientific extension, relaxation—taught and practiced—has considerable merit (Linsansky & Cough, 1996).

For therapy to be successful it should provide a well-planned rationale, operationalized procedures, training in skills to conduct the interventions of therapy, reward the independent use of the skills by the patient outside therapy, and encourage the attribution of change to the patient. With older people, the therapist may wish to make some adjustments to traditional therapeutic techniques, such as being more active or task-focused with a few clearly outlined goals and using a psychoeducational label and collaborative approach (Zeiss & Steffen, in press). CBT and IPT do all this.

Medication

We briefly address one other form of treatment. We use medication frequently. It has many benefits. The SSRIs especially have positive effects on outcomes, are tolerated well, seem to result in a rather speedy response, and have a numerical advantage in improving depression and anxiety symptoms (American Psychiatry Alliance, 1997). But this has not been done with any regularity in PTSD and the above results are not without critics (Davidson, 1997).

Our concern is expectancy and psychological cost. Often the patient message is: "This is what I want/need, what I deserve/must have, and it is the only way for me." There is a pharmaceutical industry whose goal it is to convince people that this is the only way. They are like crash diets that "work," and then.... Many psychiatrists, after endless alterations of doses and types of medications, note that the only way for effective treatment is to be on meds forever. People go through life trying to outfox every unpleasant nuance. When that doesn't work, they are fast to note that it is not their fault—they have an affective disorder and the medication must be altered. This thinking "condemns" one to never finding a non-drug way of handling problems. The person is never taught to address their arousal threshold or stylistic pattern of activity. Worse, the patient identifies self as one who is mentally or emotionally ill.

Expectancy effects are critical to treatment outcomes. Kirsch and Saperstein (1999) reported the effect size for pre-treatment to post-treatment changes in depression in patients given antidepressant drugs is 1.55. This clearly suggests that these medications work. However the effect size for a response to placebo is 1.16. This indicates that 75% of the effect of antidepressant medication can be duplicated by administration of an inert placebo—but Kirsch and Saperstein go on. They have shown that the effect size for various medications is virtually the same. This included drugs that are not antidepressants. These data were replicated by Joffe, Sokolov, and Streiner (1996) and on chronic patients by Walach and Maidhof (1999). The reason that medication is so effective may be due to expectancy and not to the pharmacological properties of the drugs. Other data (Clay, 2000; Kahn, Warner, & Brown, 2000) also support this finding.

Unfortunately, perhaps due to a cohort effect, many older people prefer medication. We will consider this issue again. One thing, however, seems clear: Whatever the efficacy of medication alone, once used, it is likely that highly significant psychological and psychosocial issues will remain. Medication addresses symptoms. Both "reactive" and more character-based components are appropriately treated with psychotherapy or counseling (Beutler, 2000). Interestingly, there is limited evidence to suggest that combining CBT with antidepressant medication may be more effective than either CBT alone or medication alone (Barlow, 2000; Thompson, Gallagher, Hansen, Gantz, & Steffen, 1991). Decisions on what is the best combination of cognitive, behavioral, and pharmacotherapy elements are made on a case-by-case basis. Again, as long as age-related client characteristics are taken into consideration, psychotherapy for the aged is likely to be successful (Morris & Morris, 1991).

☐ Conclusion

Treatment of older adults is still relatively new, but optimism is the rule. The operative concern with the treatment of the elderly involves a melding of the differences that are specific to later life and those most relevant to issues of treatment in general. As noted above, when substantive compromises are required, change almost always involves alterations due to cognitive decline and personality. Otherwise, changes are situational and can be arrived at logically and adaptively. One particular strategy may fail in early applications and yet prove effective as it is modified and refined. Therapists need to be flexible.

In our review of mainstream literature on general therapeutic factors, we were impressed by the lack of attention to age or to developmental theory in writings. Few attempts have been made to use developmental theory to inform intervention. Baltes and Danish (1979) have defined life-span developmental theory in terms of the dynamic interplay between the individual and the environment and have drawn parallels between primary prevention and optimizing human development. Ultimately we argue that the identification of the curative properties of a treatment requires more careful specification of the theoretical model of the (older) person and of the problem from which the mechanisms must emerge. The exact extent to which these mechanisms of change also reflect processes of development is of course unknown.

Is there a model of change common to human growth and development and to psychological intervention? As the existential issues of trauma—loss, meaning-making, accepting reality, achieving ego integrity—are very close to those of aging, the treatment of trauma at later life seems to meld almost naturally with age. The wise clinician "treats" the person of the trauma victim at later life; ready to manage the victim or to facilitate a change of the trauma itself, or both. Again, any quick fix mentality of earlier ages may not be appropriate here. The trauma of an aging person is the story of a human being, who is a smorgasbord of resilience and vulnerability factors. The longitudinal course of PTSD is really a total person response.

Key Ingredients to Psychotherapy

Anxiety disorders can be viewed as representing different cognitive/affective structures filtered with both cognitions and affect. The presence of a relationship between certain situations and fear responses in simple phobics or obsessive compulsives indicates a disordered link among stimulus and response elements of their underlying fear structures. This difference in fear structure implies that for simple phobics the treatment focus is to promote activation and habituation of fear. For obsessive-compulsives, treatment encompasses variables that engage other mechanisms besides physiological activation and habituation, such as certain aspects of the meaning represented in that fear structure.

PTSD requires something else again. It requires a vision that a simple "main effects" model of care does not apply. One biomedical or psychological intervention is not likely to produce fruit. A diathesis stress model that can be triggered by internal and external stressors applies. This means that with trauma victims and with older folks therapists need to be aware of the probable active treatment ingredients, ones that we can be suspect about or use with some certainty. Whether we are seeking just a more comfortable narrative or major life changes, these treatment components are important.

There are conditions for change that are "more optimal" than others. In psychotherapy the task is to shift from the impulse to escape constraints (freedom from) to the positive desire to act. Mohr (1995) identified several interaction factors that bode well for outcome in psychotherapy. They include that the client have a (a) healthy anticipation of pain in the process, (b) non-suspicion of the therapist, (c) at least minimal interpersonal skills for psychotherapy, (d) a reasonable level of functioning (non-psychotic), (e) nondefensive attitude toward rating self as distressed, and (f) the ability to allow some control to pass to the therapist. There are others. What we focus on in this chapter are those that are most relevant for aging and PTSD.

Goldfried (2000) noted something rather important here: "I do not treat symptoms. I treat patients who have symptoms." This is always the case in psychotherapy whatever the problem. Good care of patients involves a procedural knowledge of therapy, the ability to do it with little effort. It also involves the ability of create certain relationship factors, a bond, a set of goals, and a plan for the intervention. Goldfried again noted that the patient must have the appropriate expectations, have an optimal alliance, be open to feedback, experience the corrective experience, and the ability to continue reality testing in an on-going way.

We focus on a set of curative factors or active ingredients, then, that drive the treatment of trauma-related memories. We treat curative factors as components of therapy that are both common (nonspecific) and unique (to a disorder). They involve the relationship as well as the down and dirty elements of the therapy for PTSD. We believe that they stand as important in their own right, reified components in the armamentarium of care. They provide a solid foundation in PTSD treatment. In a sense the previous chapters have led here. In our discussion also we note the extent to which each is supported by aging research and practice. Finally, we note that the reader can apply these to trauma (and other) patients as we apply the "how to" after each section. They stand on their own.

☐ Dosed Exposure

We begin with a heavyweight. For some time treatment outcome has been theorized to be a function of the amount of exposure the client's traumatic memories receive. Prolonged exposure (PE) techniques are thought to be more efficacious than other CBT techniques that emphasize briefer periods of exposure, e.g., SIT. In fact, PE interacting with a supportive and collaborative therapeutic relationship is believed to account for about 40% of the variance in treatment outcome (Horowitz, 1975). By exploring a particular situation as completely and fully as possible, people can access their fundamental, holistic models of the world, the models responsible for their experience of self. It is the full experience of a single instance of an experience that will bring forth the necessary elements of the actual experience from memory.

The amount and type of exposure have been a controversial issue for years. Exposure intensities vary from the very low intensity and graduated exposure of systematic desensitization to the very intense exposure of implosion and flooding procedures. The accumulated literature suggests that the exposure has to be at least intense enough to elicit the conditioned emotion. There is no need, however, for exposure to extreme situations. Instead, graduated exposure to increasingly emotion-arousing cues is easier on the patient and just as effective. Additionally, exposure should last long enough to elicit the aversive emotion at a relatively intense but still bearable level. Escaping or diverting attention before the emotion is elicited is unlikely to be beneficial. The patient should end the exposure voluntarily instead of allowing automatic processes (dissociating, depersonalizing, impulsively running away, attacking the therapist, etc.) to stop the process. When the emotion is fear (including fear of emotions), shame, or guilt, some reduction in the emotion should occur before exposure is ended. As PTSD patients often believe that emotions are uncontrollable and unending, the corrective use that this tactic provides is important (Linehan, 1993).

Hossack and Bentall (1996) have noted that few studies have investigated the impact of clinical strategies on intrusive images. We know that PE works. This comes from a long tradition and several cited studies we have covered. Case studies are always instructive. Schindler (1980) used a modified systematic desensitization procedure to successfully eliminate in six sessions intrusive nightmares following a trauma. Keane and Kaloupek (1982) reported the use of imaginal flooding to treat intrusive thoughts (nightmares and flashbacks) associated with a traumatic event, producing improvements in their patient which persisted at 12-month follow-up. Fairbank and Keane (1982) also used imaginal flooding to treat a Vietnam veteran's memory of a traumatic event; evidence of generalization of extinction to other trauma-related cues was reported. In the previous chapter we noted many controlled studies advocating for the efficacy of PE.

A spate of recent studies applied more novel dosed exposure techniques for trauma situations. The application of trauma resolution has been applied from a safe vantage point (e.g., thought field therapy [TFT]; Calahan & Calahan, 1992) and visual kinesthetic dissociation (VKD; Koziey & McCloud, 1987). Ochberg (1996) used a counting method for ameliorating traumatic memories. The memory is contained within an interval of 100 counts—less than 2 minutes. This constitutes a relatively brief dose of traumatic recollection, as well as control over the recollection process: The therapist counts and the client recounts. Ford (1995) too applied a guided trauma disclosure (GTD), which involves repeated oral reading of and brief imaginal exposure to a personalized trauma script in a group. The focus in GTD is a mastery of nonavoidant and nondissoicative coping by rehearsal and elaboration of a coherent affectively varied narrative trauma memory. Through the use of repeated brief (not prolonged) exposure episodes done once daily over several weeks, GTD does not directly target fear extinction but instead uses a differential reinforcement of another (DRO) response model. GTD interrupts the predominant inhibition pattern ("frozen hypervigilance") characterizing avoidance/numbing in chronic PTSD and shapes conscious constructive coping.

What to Do

There is every reason to believe that these studies apply to older victims. It especially makes sense that the older individual perceives trauma from a safer vantage point. It also makes sense that the older person is active, empowered, and feels safe.

Box 6-1
Therapeutic Exposure-Based Tasks

Orientation to exposure-based procedures and commitment to collaborate.

Client understands principles of exposure-based procedure.

New information about fear and anxiety-eliciting situations is received and processed.

For guilt and shame, use exposure-based procedures only when guilt and shame are unsupported by the situation.

Ensure that exposure actually takes place, by being alert for diversion tactics, keeping imagery skills in place, and by describing scenes in detail and in present tense.

Graduate exposure intensity.

Exposure lasts long enough for emotions to be elicited and for some reduction to occur, but not so long that the patient loses control.

Assess need for other change strategies (such as skills training and fading of supportive activities).

Block tendency to escape/avoid, hide, self-punish.

Escape from situations occurs voluntarily.

On the basis of studies from the previous chapter, we use PE in the form of AMT and EMDR. Evidence indicates that the combination of PE and AMT may constitute the treatment of choice for chronic PTSD. AMT again involves a variety of procedures, which attempt to manage the anxiety as it occurs. It de-emphasizes fear activation and provides tools to handle these. To recapitulate, the key treatment idea is to activate the ANS at a moderate level with important and incongruent data being reprocessed in conscious awareness, to use dosed exposure and assimilation work. This is best done by challenging but not overwhelming, managing anxiety within the AMT (never escape or avoidance), and practice.

With the guide that heavy exposure is not suitable for all trauma victims and that in some cases the technique needs to be amended (Foa & Meadows, 1997), and knowing that self capacities are enhanced as a client learns concrete coping skills (including SIT and assertiveness training) and that transforming events can occur with the massaging of positive memories (Horowitz, 1986; McCann & Pearlman, 1993a), the "dosing" of one's exposure to emotional discomfort or stressful events can proceed. Several tasks that foster therapeutic efficacy are given in Box 6-1.

☐ Goals

Goals are the (often) undisclosed underbelly of treatment. They are behind and influence everything in therapy but are given short shrift. Older folks often come with poor goals, social goals, or undoable goals. Clients often desire to have past life issues altered or an external situation changed. Bereaved elders hold that they will always be this way. Chronic health problems are also externalized.

Below the details of the surface narrative, below the niceties of communication and the social desirability, lies "the want." The phenomenology and epistemology of the want can be critical elements of treatment. In some ways they are the treatment. People in general, but certainly people in trauma, are disorderly in the translation of their trauma into coherence and workability. The task, then, of having the client struggle with the goal, the ambiguities, confusion, or assumed certainties, is a worthwhile search in and of itself. From the initial therapist inquiry "What do you want that might happen here," the real desire of the patient unfolds and approaches understanding and later care. In a very personal and existential sense, this placement of the problem in a conceptual container that is real is the therapy. The client is now in the moment, not in the memory.

Adler noted that everything is related to one's goal, the teleology of the person. This is the therapy. According to Adler, the goal of the person may be to connect, to be alone, to win, to lose, to foster some self ideal. For Adler this is always prepotent. Any deviation from this results in some form of resistance.

In therapy this can be critical. One way to expose this is to know the goal as never before. The therapist can be like the TV detective Colombo—slow, asking that extra question, keeping the inner ambivalence alive as it approaches understandablity. This inquiry alters the inner environment. It mutates problems to an epiphany. Eventually, the mirrored room of the therapy brings on a confession of the chaos. Now at least, the client possesses the problem as never before. The client senses the integrity of the want. They can also give it up. The client comes to know these inner concerns as "known." Probably for the first time, the client knows what is important and its demands on choice. At this point the client can reformulate the choice.

Clients come to psychotherapy to find solutions to their problems, *maybe*. Whereas therapists are purveyors of insight, many clients are supplicants of magic. They often describe presenting problems in vague, global, metaphoric terms. Walter and Peller (1992) held that the clinician should assume a constructivist rule of thumb when clients present problems: Never believe them! The problem is that this is simply how clients have experienced their issues. It is only their view, but there are other truths. In the throes of change there is a yin and a yang and a synthesis.

What to Do

The methods of CBT and solution-focused therapy assist in the formulation of treatment. CBT is logic bound and provides structure for subsequent activities in treatment; solution-focused therapy is technique-driven and becomes the therapy itself. In CBT, goals are established slowly and carefully (Box 6-2). A central feature of CBT has always been to help clients reconceptualize their predicament in problem-oriented terms that will lend themselves to solutions, to reshape vague negative accounts into specific problem-oriented statements, and to break up problems into smaller, discrete units that are more amenable to solutions. The CBT therapist is insistent on operationalizing goals and checking these out with clients.

Burns (1999) held that agenda (goal) setting is critical to treatment. Free choice and accountability are the staples for patient care: "I agree to do this and this is my responsibility." This is a matter-of-fact transaction, where there is no persuasion or cheerleading, only choice and follow-up. For Burns, there are no plans then for a "PTSD patient." Rather the plan of care is established by an individual agenda: specificity (person, place, and time), motivation (what are you willing to do?), conceptualization (individual mood, interpersonal, or habit problems), and methods (various techniques for care). Importantly, the value of specificity is so central that any discussion of a problem without the particulars of the person is impossible. From this position comes an eclectic barrage of techniques where the clinician can apply what works after several failures.

With older clients, at least one goal is set in the first four sessions. Often clients have multiple goals and the task is to prioritize these. Not infrequently with older trauma victims therapy goals become stalled. A renegotiating is then appropriate. It is necessary to identify and modify core beliefs. Gallagher-Thompson and Thompson (1975) believe that, if the client brings in other matters in response to these kinds of questions, it is generally good to pick up on the new topics until a specific problem is defined. However once a goal(s) is established, it is pursued with reasonable focus. Goals that keep changing are usually reflective of firmly entrenched personality issues. Problems often occur with dependent or avoidant personality features. For them, schema therapy would be the next step (Gallagher-Thompson & Thompson, 1995). For us, Stage 4 of the Model is applied (Chapter 8).

In therapy, goals can also shift to prepare the client to continue to use the skills learned. Gallagher and Thompson (1994) again used a written document (maintenance guide) that summarizes what has been learned in treatment and anticipates how it could be used to reduce negative reactions to future events. A working guide or flip chart can also be used in each session. This is a living document, one that "works" as an ongoing autobiography and summary of the client. It changes in each session. The progress of all therapy can be assessed after 10 sessions.

We recommend solution-oriented questions. This is performed in a purposeful manner by carefully assessing the client's cooperative response patterns and matching their questions with those patterns (Lipchik, 1988; Lipchik & de Shazer, 1986; O'Hanlon & Weiner-Davis, 1989; de Shazer, 1988, 1991). These are guiding questions that reframe problems (Figure 6-1). The "outcome question," for example, is often

Box 6-2
Key Questions

CBT

Before we begin, what would be realistic change for you? How would you do this?

What do we need to do first to alter the situation?

What minimal changes do you see happening as a result of coming here?

In what way is that a problem?

What will be the smallest sign that this is happening? What will be the first sign that this is happening?

I am sorry about ... , but in what way can you and I alter things in your life now (with you and me today)?

Under what circumstances are you unhappy? Is there anything going well?

How likely is it that four months from now we will have this change?

What sort of progress would satisfy you?

SFT

What is your goal in coming here? (goal frame)

Let me write this out and see if it fits.

What can I say positively about the client that can promote a positive atmosphere?

What things is the client doing that are already working, positive, or exceptional that I can highlight and encourage?

Is there anything about the context that I might want to normalize?

How can I give credit to the client for changing?

So this is a practical area to change that relates to the bigger goal that we identified.

This sounds like a very serious problem. How have you managed to cope? What have you been doing to fight off the urge to (let yourself be depressed, feel worse, commit suicide, etc.)?

How is it happening now? or When doesn't the problem happen? (exceptions frame)

How will you be doing your goal in the future?

I have a good picture of what happens when there are problems (mention the specific symptoms here). Now, in order to get a more complete picture of your situation, I need to know about when the (specific symptom) does not happen?

Suppose you go home tonight and while you are asleep, a miracle happens and your problem is solved, how will you be able to tell a miracle must have happened the next morning? (miracle question)

If you were on track to solving the problem, what would you be doing differently? (hypothetical solution frame)

Between now and the next time we meet, I would like you to observe, so that you can describe to me the next time, what happens that you want (or not want) to continue (stop from) happening.

DO

Observe what you do when you want to keep something.

Observe what you do when you resist the problem behavior.

Do something different.

Background

Presentation: _____

_____

Treatment

Hx: _____

_____

Goal Formulation:

1.

2.

3.

4.

Prognostic Indicators

1. Tx Expectation:

1	2	3	4	5	6	7	8	9	10

REALISTIC   UNREALISTIC

2. Tx Willingness:

1	2	3	4	5	6	7	8	9	10

Precontemplation   Contemplation   Decision   Action   Maintenance

3. Tx Capability:

1	2	3	4	5	6	7	8	9	10

Psychol-minded   Skill deficit   Resistant   Sabotage

FIGURE 6-1. Treatment Profile

4. Impediments:

Psychological problems _____

Social supports _____ _____

Medical _____ _____

Current stressors _____

Cognitive ability _____

Practical problems _____

5. Axis II

    1.

    2.

    3.

    Axis I

    1.

    2.

    3.

6. Problem List

    1.

    2.

    3.

    4.

    5.

    6.

    7.

FIGURE 6-1. (*Continued*)

7. Hypotheses

_____

_____

_____

8. Treatment Plan

_____

_____

_____

9. Obstacles to Treatment

_____

_____

_____

FIGURE 6-1. (_Continued_)

asked. Clients are asked to describe what will be different when the problem(s) has been successfully treated (Berg, 1990). Another question is the miracle question. Exception questions too inquire about times when the problem is either absent, less intense, or dealt with in a manner that was acceptable to the client. Calling attention to such exceptions reframes indirectly the meaning of problem-saturated stories. Clients almost always have assumed that a negative or stressful event is pervasive rather than proximal. Coping or externalization questions elicit discussion about how the client manages to cope with and endure their problem(s) on a day-to-day basis. In the process of answering such questions, the problem becomes a separate and distinct entity external to the client (White, 1986, 1988; White & Epston, 1990). This, in turn, serves to reframe the meaning frame of a trauma context.

Finally, it may also be helpful for the therapist to engage clients in a detailed review of all the potential pros and cons in changing a behavior prior to attempting to change (Burns, 1999). Therapeutic collaboration is facilitated when therapists show that they are willing to look at the pros and cons of change (Grilo, 1993). Tasking may also be advocated, if necessary; the client actually plays out the tape of the negative event in detail. The client, for example, may be asked to actually play out loud a potential suicide, all the details and ramifications.

☐ Relationship

Tang and DeRublies (1999) evaluated an interseting area of therapy: They looked at the phenomenon of sudden gains in CBT therapy. They were interested in those patients who improved after any session. In their study they identified patients who showed an average of 11 point gains on the Beck Depression Inventory between two sessions. This accounted for over 50% of the change of patients' total improvement. This gain was maintained over a long period of time. Interestingly, patients who showed these gains had previous sessions where there were substantial cognitive changes and improved therapeutic alliances. This suggested that the combination of cognitive techniques and a solid working relationship translates into therapy gains.

How people see their therapist is critical. The importance of the relationship is one of the stages of our model. In the two forms of therapy that most apply to older folks, CBT and IPT, the relationship is pivital. In CBT, it is labeled socialization; in IPT, it is the therapy, where nondirective exploration, affect, teaching, insight, and role-playing are applied.

Cognitive Behavioral Therapy (CBT) has been a (our) staple of the psychotherapies for older peole, especially for depression and anxiety. But there are limits. Recent data from younger therapy samples especially have indicated that the key components of CBT (e.g., importance of cognition) may be lessened with older groups. Additionally, the importance of the alliance has resurfaced in these samples. That is, the importance of the collaborative relationship has been restated.

CBT is also wanting in other ways. Goldfried noted seven ways.

1. CBT provides a fine-grained analysis of reactions to specific situations. They prevent a look at the big picture.
2. CBT is dedicated to the development and study of effective interventions. Manuals are too inflexible.
3. CBT is based on skills training orientation. This raises the question of manuals versus healing process. The therapist is more than a didactic teacher.
4. CBT focuses on the client's current situation. Therapies that address only the "now" are wanting.
5. CBT has emphasized the importance of psychotherapy outcomes. CBT does not look a process.
6. CBT has provided interventions for reducing symptoms. A view of self is lacking.
7. Role of emotion is downplayed. The first line of intervention is assimilative.

If we were to parse apart the salient components of the alliance, we would see that a connection early in treatment is most important (Loborsky, 1975). We would know also that a direct confrontation of the alliance and cognitive elements of therapy would often favor the alliance (Floyd & Scogin, 1998). In a CBT program of a head-to-head challenge between components of CBT and the alliance with older people with depression, Hyer, Sohnle, and Nielsen (2000) showed that the alliance components were rated most favorable. Barkham, Stiles, and Shapiro (1993) showed that among the components of the alliance, strength of association of change was related to different elements (of the alliance) as measured by the Working Alliance Inventory at different times. The elements of bond, partnership, confidence, openness, and client initiative were all important.

In the PTSD research, this component of the care equation has been universally endorsed. Chemtob, Hamada, Roitblat, and Muraoka (1994) even believed that the key to PTSD treatment is the relationship and the therapist's role as guardian of it. What this implies is that the alliance is the gorilla in the therapy room always: without it, there is no therapy.

What to Do

The second stage of the model addresses the "how to" of the relationship. Suffice it to say here that the therapist is in such a unique position that he/she must do three relationship tasks: (a) be liked/respected; (b) be believable (with a plan); (c) initiate some success. Without these, there is "no salvation." Again, we address these more in Stage 2 of the model.

☐ Relaxation

"I have learned that my total organismic sensing of a situation is more trustworthy than my intellect"
Carl Rogers

As a whole, few studies have addressed anxiety or the use of relaxation in the elderly. When done, relaxation training has been effective with the elderly (Bortz & O'Brien, 1997). In one study on anxiety, Scogin et al. (1992) reported on the effectiveness of progressive muscle relaxation training and imagery for elders with anxiety problems. They used a group of community-dwelling older adults. Progressive muscle relaxation and imagining muscle relaxation appear to be equally effective; results were maintained at a 1-year follow-up. Teri and colleagues (Teri & Uomota, 1991) even adapted traditional therapies for the treatment of anxiety and agitation for a demented population based on learning theory.

With older patients relaxation seems to help as with younger groups. The specific technique used for relaxation is less important than its constant practice. Typically the goal of relaxation training is to teach the individual to recognize signs of tension, to reverse them, and to achieve a state of deep relaxation at will. What is also important is that the technique is believed and is relatively easy for the client to learn and use. Progressive relaxation, autogenic training, biofeedback, and hypnotic induction are all useful in assisting older clients to learn to relax (Goldfried & Davison, 1976; Pelletier, 1977; Rimm & Masters, 1974).

In vivo relaxation seems to work with the elderly (Arean, 2000). As we know, the relaxation response is an integrated hypothalamic response that results in decreased sympathetic and probably increased parasympathetic activity (Benson, 1975). It is the opposite of a stress response. With the elderly, anxiety is often in the picture, at least as a predisposing factor in illness. These states, as well as insomnia, exhaustion, and worrying, exacerbate both acute and chronic illness. Older people may take longer to learn to relax (5–10 sessions) than younger adults (Cautela & Mansfield, 1977) or younger PTSD victims (Hyer et al., 1994). A standard progressive muscle relaxation (PMR) procedure is ideal, but most any are appropriate.

Once this skill is learned, briefer methods can be applied to various situations, like trauma. To date, only AMT (Hyer et al., 1990) and standard relaxation of CBT (Gallagher & Thompson, 1981) have been used with trauma victims. In AMT, for example, Suinn (1990) proffered that behavioral change must involve an active coping component, such as relaxation. He recommended that this active coping component be introduced at the very beginning of therapy, so that the client learns that it is possible to control the anxiety associated with the traumatic event. This component, then, forms the foundation for the other components. At least it allows other components to proceed.

What to Do

Relaxation is part of virtually every study on the use of exposure. This skill is one of the necessary coping strategies of care. Like any learned skill, it must be practiced and, even then, the person will sometimes be "on" and other times "off." It should also be fun. The relaxation response should be practiced a minimum of once daily, twice daily at first. Intrusive thoughts are to be expected. Bothersome, distracting thoughts are best handled by allowing them to pass in and then pass out of mind. With practice, intrusive thoughts are less likely to occur. Finally, clients should be instructed not to expect perfection. It is best to develop a wait-and-see attitude, allowing for error. As noted, older people may take longer for this element of care to take hold. If one is naturally anxious (high anxiety scale scores), the integration of the relaxation response into daily life is critical. With this patient, it is also problematic because anxiety has become a trait.

Some form of relaxation is required too in the overall attack on the trauma memory. As noted, in EMDR and AMT relaxation is initially learned so that the client can control the anxiety associated with the traumatic event. An audiotape can be used and the person is instructed to practice at least once daily (Hyer et al., 1994; Suinn, 1990).

We use a variety of approaches and try to "tailor" the approach to the client as much as possible. We allow the person to sample several techniques including simple diaphragmatic breathing, breathing to a count (e.g., in for 4 seconds, out for 5, pause for 1), or while reciting a self-chosen mantra. We also instruct in autogenic training and do imagery exercises.

Jonathan Smith (1999) provided an excellent approach for surveying several techniques quickly through a "Grand Tour" of relaxation. It cannot be overemphasized that the relaxation method that works wonders for one patient may be of little use— may even cause anxiety—for another patient. Personality even plays a role in how an individual relaxes (Sohnle, in press). Patients are often exposed to at least three or four methods to find the one that most effectively allows them a higher degree of control over their arousal. Smith (1999) gave an informative description of the varied relaxation states (R-States) as well.

Once the "best" technique is discovered, the patient must, as noted earlier, make regular practice a part of her/his life. One of the best ways to encourage compliance is with a personalized tape. Generic tapes are sometimes helpful, but a personalized tape helps the patient to internalize the process as "theirs" more quickly. We provide a 12-8-4-4-0 muscle relaxation exercise in Appendix D.

A Simple Model of Relaxation Training

1. Identify anxiety, physical manifestations (awareness).
2. Educate about the role and usefulness of relaxation methods.
3. Demonstrate (not just explanation) of a *variety* of methods.
4. Self-rate relaxation experience and response reported to treating professional *as or shortly after it occurs.*
5. Identify the technique that is most useful for the individual.
6. Make a tape of a relaxation session and encourage daily use.

☐ Assimilation

"The greatest weapon against stress is our ability to choose one thought over another."
William James

It is estimated that we have 60,000 thoughts/day. It has also been suggested further that these are the same 60,000 every day. Reality does not cause PTSD: negative thinking does. Foa (Rothbaum & Foa, 1996) said that cognitive restructuring is *the* promising candidate for enhancing the efficacy of prolonged exposure.

There appears to be almost universal acceptance that cognitions lie behind psychopathological disorders, especially depression, anxiety, and PTSD. The current issues involve what model to use (as in hopelessness, Abramson, Metalsky, & Alloy, 1989, or negative attributions, Beck & Freeman, 1990), how to measure cognitions, and assorted other interactive influences, like the impact of avoidance (Livingston & Hill, 1993) and the importance of interpersonal conflicts (Miller & Silberman, 1996). Even in standard psychotherapy the proper application of assimilation strategies has something in common with interpretation, a new partialized idea of what is happening. This is what most therapists do.

There is some evidence to suggest that thinking errors may not be the "cause" of PTSD or depression problems. Although it appears that depression or PTSD is replete with negative thinking, when levels of depression or PTSD are controlled, negative thinking was not predictive of the disorder. This appears to have more to do with the mediational effect of cognitions as measured by traditional cognitive scales (e.g., DAS). This is weaker for older adults (Floyd & Scogin, 1998). Perhaps too the assimilative process is only curative when common psychotherapy factors (relationship) are in evidence. When confronted with the importance of thinking issues and the relationship, the therapist may be on guard as to whether to listen or confront. Tarrier et al. (1999), for example, found no differences between the two. They showed that either relationship or assimilative processes reduced PTSD symptoms. Again, this only shows the importance of both of these therapy constructs.

We believe that exposure to the trauma is effective because of its impact on appraisals or codes created by the automatic thinking program. Treatment outcome then would depend to a large extent on the client's ability to apply assimilative coping techniques to modulate the affective arousal provoked by exposure to their traumatic memories. Suppression of (negative) cognitive processes and "rational" appraisals of the client's distress are the two emotion-focused coping techniques thought to be more useful in this regard (Smyth, 1995). Clinicians, then, should have the ability to assist clients in the assimilation of information embedded in their traumatic memories that are discordant with prevailing beliefs they hold about themselves or the world. This requires the ability on the part of the clinician to recognize what aspects of the trauma the client is having trouble assimilating.

When meaning making occurs, several information segments are activated. For a good percentage of time, this is a process of differentiation of feelings and thoughts. This act leads to the emergence of new experience. One of the principles of cognitive or affective processing is that "one thing leads to another" (Greenberg & Safran, 1987; Polster & Polster, 1973). Processing affective/cognitive information by attending to it, symbolizing new features, and differentiating and integrating these new symbols leads to the creation of new meaning and to the emerging of new experience. Thus, the experience "I am angry" may evolve into "I feel some fear and annoyance" when new features of the experience are attended to. Meaning will metamorphize again (and again).

Most assimilation techniques are discrete forms of story repair. Here the client develops a theory of self, the tool for establishing a consistency to his/her own confirmatory bias. In effect, the client selectively tells self and others "stories" to fit his or her own theories. In this theory, cognitions are the information in this confirmatory bias process; emotions are the supports. If a victim sees self as a victim or a perpetrator, for example, the content of the narrative alters for the worse. If the victim blames self or assumes responsibility in the content of the story, the constructivist narrative so orders that felt experience.

Meichenbaum and Fitzpatrick (1991) have identified several cognitive processes of activation. These include both positive and negative features of the narrative's expressions of coping, appraisal, and attributional processes. Positive biases, positive illusions, the search for meaning, and a striving for coherence are more salutary components: Unfavorable comparisons, seeing self as victim, blaming others, incessant and compulsive meaning searches, a focusing on negative implications, and feeling vulnerable are examples of negative ones (Meichenbaum & Fitzpatrick, 1991). Those who construct positive narratives will, as a result of this, cope well with distress and vice versa. This is the victim's own "healing theory." Thinking makes it so.

CBT is, of course, quintessentially cognitive. Queries that are offered in the form of questions and metaphors delivered in a straight-forward didactic method or in a Socratic method are beneficial for older people. At some point the new thinking seems appealing. A rationale sets the table to educate the "irrational" automatic thinking portion by repetition. Addressing memories of older adults who were depressed, Fry (1983) applied reminiscence therapy to unhappy memories. These depressed adults were taught to identify depression memories and taught to cope with intrusions. They were taught to think differently. Compared with a group that did not have this training, the coping group showed greater reductions in self-reported depression and an increase in feelings of self confidence. In fact, just an attack on stable and global attributions on specific behaviors in depressive older caregivers produces positive results (Cook, Ahrens, & Pearson, 1995).

In sum, the healing of trauma memories occurs when the thinking is less dangerous and negative. Memories also become organized. The use of better thinking allows for the formation of new explicit memories. As we noted, data stuck in the intermediate memory storage system (implicit memory), due to automatic thinking danger codes, can be woven into long-term memory via moderate levels of activation and secondary process thinking. These codes are processed because they are habituated and because of the impact of cognitions (corrective cognitive codes).

What to Do

Any of the standard methods used by Beck (1995) are appropriate. The attack on the trauma can be cognitive and the management of life around the trauma can be cognitive. The component "thinking" must be viewed as important, a status equal to that of other treatments, as medication.

There are several ways to communicate the "attack" on the trauma. All involve education. Borkovec, for example, noted that anxiety comes in two forms: cognitive and somatic. The feeling of anxiety lasts much longer than the catecholamine surge with generalized adrenal and cortical stimulation. The important point is that the cognitive component is operating and must be activated to challenge the worrisome thoughts. As with depression, the act of negative or worry thinking prevents other (positive) thoughts. Consciously or not, the patient allows this or it would not work.

Another method (to discuss the importance of thinking) is also from a biochemical purview. Every thought sends out electrical signals in the brain. Thoughts have actual physical properties. They have a significant influence on every cell in the body. When the person is burdened with negative thinking, this affects the limbic system especially. Daniel Amen (1998) stated:

> You can train your thoughts to be positive and hopeful, or you can allow them to be negative and upset you. Once you learn about your thoughts, you can choose to think good thoughts and feel better, or you can choose to keep thoughts and feel lousy. That's right, it's up to you. You can learn how to change your thoughts, you can learn to change the way you feel. (p. 59)

This applies to memory. Whenever one thinks of an event, the brain releases chemicals exact to those that were around when the event first occurred. Consequently memory brings back a similar mood and feelings, so to change a memory takes time and effort. However the pursuit is worthwhile. After, it is a "real" change, at least for the person.

In a more straight-line cognitive intervention during trauma work, typical cognitions can be isolated. They include (a) habituation anxiety—"anxiety will not stay forever"; (b) discrimination between remembering and re-encountering; (c) differentiation of trauma from similar but safe events ("All the world is not dangerous"); (d) mastery experience ("I am competent"); and (e) organization of trauma narratives. The client is taught that the core beliefs are not true and can be challenged.

There are many ways for the client to manage life. The client can also develop a perspective on problems. At the least the therapist can have the client just watch for external and internal triggers. The client can commit with a coping contract: "I will pause when I notice my signals ..."; "I will tune into my signals and monitor these self statements"; "I will not say these negative self-statements"; "I will relax myself by ..."; "I will reward myself by ...".

Finally, everyone has an "inner voice" that can be "for the better or worse." This voice can be represented by the polarities in Box 6-3. In any situation the person can use the "good critic" and remind the self that they are bigger than the trauma and

---

Box 6-3
Stress Manager

"Good Critic"	"Bad Critic"
Fearful	Anxious/avoidant
Irritated	Excessively angry
Self-critical	Ashamed/self-defeat
Pessimistic	Depressed
Supportive	Avoid/dependent

can think about the situation appropriately. Being fearful, having irritations, and even resentments, being self-critical, pessimistic, and supportive in various situations are natural and healthy.

We do not want to oversimplify here. But we do seek simplicity: The patient can always carry out cognitive tasks. And, they are effective.

☐ Emotion: Keeping in the Zone

"All man's miseries derive from not being able to sit in a room alone."
Pascal

Daniel Goleman (1995), in his popular book *Emotional Intelligence*, stated that we have two minds—one thinks and one feels. In general, it is the emotional brain (emotional mind) that makes a difference in life; the complimentarity of the limbic system and neocortex that allows for an emotional intelligence.

With PTSD, first we have feelings, then thoughts. In the typical PTSD reaction, the situation is first experienced by means of the immediacy of emotional thinking. There is apparent chaos. The emotional mind is, to a large extent, state-specific determined by the dictates of the moment. Feeling is often the first reaction. But how a person feels later is determined by the thoughts, reactions, and even memories. In time, each emotion comes to possess its own repertoire of sensations, thoughts, feelings, and behaviors. In this way the memory serves as a organizer, a selective representation of affective/cognitive complex. Memories that ascend are ones that are most relevant to the situation as the person sees it. They are suffused with the particulars of the person. The task of therapy is to integrate memories, desensitize the "emotional" memories, or reshuffle memories so others compete favorably. All can work. Goleman (1995) wrote:

> The working of the emotional mind is to a large degree state-specific, dictated by the specific feeling ascendant at a given moment. How we think and act when we are feeling romantic is entirely different from how we behave when enraged or dejected; in the mechanisms of emotion each feeling has its own distinct repertoire of thoughts, reactions, even memories. These state-specific repertoires become most predominant in moments of intense emotion. (p. 296)

Individuals organize information then into units that guide processing. Once activated, schemes are seen as automatically directing attention, providing a framework to preserve information, combining generic and specific information with the other concrete events, and active in retrieving and editing material from memory. Within this frame, consciousness can be viewed as a higher level organizer that monitors and regulates the operation of lower level modular processes. That is why knowledge of emotions is critical. Brewin and Lennard (1999) indicated that the emotional processing stands behind this organization, either incomplete or poorly processed. At the extreme, this is a "phobia of memory."

We report the results of one important study (Ansorge, Litz, & Bergman, 1996). Evaluating trauma victims, these authors found that the "best position" about trauma work involves two factors: (a) a meta-experience of emotion (positive attitude to process), including acceptance (feelings are permissible), maintenance (sustain emotional effort), and repair (reconstruct emotional states); and (b) positive cognitive processes, including openness (available to moment-by-moment processing) and the ability to manage fleeting thoughts. The person must have some skills to deal with this.

In a sense, the task of therapy is to facilitate experiential processing (rather than conceptual processing). Therapy needs then to open people to more internal and external information and to stimulate and evoke the emotion schemes that generate the person's fundamental experience and that serve as the basis of emotional meaning. By exploring a particular situation as completely and fully as possible, people can access their fundamental models of the world, the models responsible for their experience of self. In fact, it is probably the full experience of a single instance of an experience that will bring forth all the elements of the actual experience from memory. Greenberg and Safran (1987) showed that it is the combination of relief after the expression of affect with the subsequent cognitive reorganization that leads to change. This arousal of affect and cognitive reorganization is a core of a set of interventions. In restructuring events, affectively charged emotional schemas are aroused to make them amenable to change.

To play off another metaphor, emotions are like a value-added tax: They are always influencing the actions of the participant, sometimes at multiple levels and depths. As a simple definition, they are action tendencies based on appraisals in relation to needs. They are whole person responses. They involve cognition and many other person features. Westen (1998) noted that affects recruit cognitions in the service of one's attributions toward oneself, and emotions tend to be the most honest and reflective of the ongoing processes. They are truly hot spots.

Where PTSD is concerned, this is important information. Many trauma victims come with too few (numbing) or too many emotions. These need to be addressed. Kennedy-Moore, Watson, and Safran (1999) in their book on emotions also provide a primer on the importance of the emotion, especially the interaction between them and thoughts. These authors hold that expressing emotions is only beneficial if it leads to the re-appraisal of the maladaptive cognitions. In fact, expressing unpleasant feelings might lead to adaptive cognitions. These authors argue further that the "best" process is to experience emotions at moderate levels while in control. So, the idea is to express emotions at moderate levels (not catharsis), to "think" about the meaning of the emotions, whether suppressed or not.

Where older folks are concerned, we are less firm. On the one hand, there is scant data on the application of emotion-focused therapies and the aged. On the other, we know little about emotional changes across the decades. Are there age-related changes in the structure, experience, and expression of emotion? We do not know. We do know from clinical lore and common sense that older people mellow. Lawton, Kleban, Rajagopal, and Dean (1992) compared younger and older adults of 11 dimensions of emotional self-monitoring. Older adults appear to become moderate and self-regulated in their emotional experiences. In a follow-up study on another scale, this group (Lawton, Keblan, & Dean, 1993) identified six factors common to all age groups. Again older people showed less emotional arousal than younger groups. Levenson, Carstensen, Friesen, and Elkman (1991) corroborated this with physiological data. Interestingly, positive emotions did not alter across time but negative ones did—older people had fewer.

It can be argued that PTSD is a thought disorder. Victims distort reality and are preoccupied with their distortions. PTSD clients may have less cognitive strength or ability to modulate affect when their traumatic memories are activated. Many victims also report frequent panic attacks, recent histories of impulsive violence, and report a loss of secondary process thinking at low levels of distress. In some ways too victims are obsessed; thoughts increase anxiety. They seek refuge in the environment or in the body. The latter is where emotions range and feel some degree of comfort. It is familiar. When a PTSD victim attempts suicide, he or she does so to "get out of their head." They are trying to escape the pain of emotions.

In sum, we know that cognition is not inherently rational, nor emotions inherently irrational. These processes are intertwined in complex ways. Emotions involve rapid processing; cognition slower processing. Consciously experienced feelings are complex syntheses of a variety of types and sources of information. They are physiologically based, somatically based, and verbally based conceptual systems. Emotions influence cognition in many different ways: They also influence by cognition. They are a unit.

What to Do

Change in psychotherapy is heightened when this is accompanied by emotional arousal and expression. A crucial task of therapy, then, is to facilitate experiential processing rather than just conceptual processing, to enable the person to process holistic, emotionally toned experience in more effective ways. As implied, clients change in therapy as a result of the exploration and articulation of their inner subjective sense of being, emotional schemes related to the person's fundamental experience. This more than anything serves as the basis of meaning, emotional meaning.

The tasks of emotion involve emotional self-awareness (recognize and name) and mood regulation, including managing emotions (better frustration tolerance, express emotions), harnessing emotional productivity (less impulsive), empathy (take another's perspective), and handling relationships (resolve conflicts). Of course people, people in trouble especially, are not able to parse apart their emotion, put a label on them, and act with temperance. Many do not have good mood awareness. But the good news is that mood awareness is stable and is teachable. The task with older folks often involves mood awareness. Once mood awareness is available, mood regulation is possible. What follows entails emotional awareness (largely) and experiencing, as well as the transition to regulation.

The patient can be aware of the somatic stimuli to assist in the processing of data, in the formation of less conscious feelings. Or, they can be engulfed by emotions, emotional illiterates if you will. The goal is emotional literacy. In this way, emotions are markers, like family rituals. They become rather disorganized and noisy when problems are present. But if the therapist listens, the logic of the heart can be persuasive at these times, with each emotion having its own biological signature. The task is to attune to emotions and become aware of the hallmarks of the emotional mind.

Specifically, where there is avoidance, let there be approach. Affect is an indication of accessing deeper parts of the person, an emotional schema. The therapist should seek genuine contact, a real contact with the person for internally exploring. This involves noticing, tracking, and nurturing the affect. The therapist slows down, validates the experience, and allows long pauses. The therapist focuses on the body, provides language stems ("and," "because," "but") so that the emotion is coaxed out and exposed.

The therapeutic use of emotional care is important. Therapists are wont to soothe patients, to arrest the emotions when they start. Therapists seek cognitive solutions: This is the way, now follow it. They ignore bodily expressions and give advice. They present theory and solve problems. They do not nurture the emotion: They do not nurture the now. They nurture the person: "Do not get upset." There is a balance.

The therapist also should affectively attune to the client; they support the primacy of the affect and allow it to build and confess its power and direction. The therapist prevents the choking off of the emotion, the talking about the emotion, and avoidance. The therapist asks the client to contract to "stay with that." The therapist keeps the ball rolling when the emotion is building (support the emotion). When the peak is reached, the therapist provides summary statements, cognitions, and interpretations. The therapist, in effect, follows the energy: Energy→action→meaning.

Box 6-4 provides treatment ideas. The key is to respect and nurture emotion. Thus learning to identify an emotional response is aided enormously if one can observe and describe: (a) the event prompting the emotion; (b) the interpretations of the event that prompt the emotion; (c) the phenomenological experience, including physical sensation, of the emotion; (d) the expressive behaviors associated with the emotion; and (e) the aftereffects of the emotion on one's own functioning. Linehan (1993) sought to develop the emotion and the mind as the way to modulate turmoil and find direction. Linehan identified several sound emotion-based techniques that use the emotion in a therapeutic way and cultivate safety procedures. These include (a) modulation and decreasing emotional reactivity; (b) increasing self-validation and reducing self-invalidation; (c) increasing realistic decision making and judgment, and reducing crisis-generating behaviors; (d) increasing emotional experiencing and decreasing inhibited grieving; (e) increasing active problem solving and a decreasing active-passivity behaviors; and (f) increasing accurate expression of emotions and competencies and decreasing mood dependency of behavior.

The therapist may apply a scale for emotion marking. Several scales exist that reflect the level of experiencing of older patients (e.g., EAS; Daldrup, Beutler, Engle,

---

Box 6-4
Facilitating Affect

I. Support emotion build-up: Respect and make contact—slow down and validate the experience. Focus on the body, provide connectors (*and, because, but*).
   1. Identify and label affect.
   2. Identify obstacles to changing emotions. Emotional behavior is functional to the individual.
   3. Provide language stems (*and*).
II. Prevent choking off the emotion, talking about the emotion, and avoidance.
   1. Facilitate patience: "Stay with that."
   2. Reinforce "emotion mind." People are more susceptible to emotional reactivity when they are under physical or environmental stress or if they are fearful of their efforts.
III. After peak is reached, provide summary statements and tentative meaning statements.
   1. Increase positive emotional events.
   2. Increase mindfulness to current emotion.
   3. Apply distress tolerance techniques.
   4. Take opposite action.

& Greenberg, 1988). One scale that is especially relevant is the Experiencing Scale (EXP; Figure 6-2; Hyer et al., 1994). This scale was used by Sherman (1991) to indicate a "working level of processing" for older persons struggling with issues of meaning. This is a 7-point rating device that is sensitive to a client's involvement in therapy within a single session. The levels of the scale are characterized on a continuum, from impersonal or superficial references, limited or externalized self references, to inwardly elaborate descriptions of feelings. The highest level of experiencing clients are involved in the exploration and new awareness leading to problem solving and greater self-understanding. Clients who are at Level 4 or greater have a sufficiently inward focus to address self issues in a change-based way. At this level they can tolerate ambiguity and deal with issues without ready-made answers.

And we note one more thing here. A perspective that we are wedded to, personality (Chap. 8), addresses this. Clients are addicted to a setpoint of affect. When the person is deprived of familiar affective experiences, he/she is motivated to seek them out. People are brought back to their personological affects, now operative within the parameters of the personality rules. This is a self-regulating process in which the person's emotional state is sought after within a range of familiarity. Individuals are so good at this that they pull for these affects in others (Messer, 2000). Dependent people seek to avoid the fear of being abandoned, avoidants seek to avoid negative evaluation, and narcissists to avoid criticism. The therapeutic response is to know this and not to trust this. This is emotional self-care. People are not their emotions; they are bigger than these and they can read and master these.

Shame may be a critical emotion because it becomes the final common pathway for perturbation problems. That is, shame attenuates fear without resolving it and in so doing results in a defensive posture like dissociation. In effect, any information processing is stopped. How this works is important. The person is motivated for an action. The interest builds and then at some point shame occurs ("I should not be doing this"). Usually this is normal as the person simply puts the brakes on activity. Shame is nature's way of saying "It is time to stop." It is a central inhibition and

EXP Stage	Content	Treatment
1	External events; refusal to participate	Impersonal, detached
2	External events; behavioral or intellectual self-description	Interest, personal, self-participation
3	Personal reactions to external events; limited self-descriptions; behavioral descriptions of feelings	Reactive, emotionally involved
4	Descriptions of feelings and personal experiences	Self-descriptive, associative
5	Problems or propositions about feelings and personal experiences	Exploratory; elaborative, hypothetical
6	Synthesis of readily accessible feelings and experiences to resolve personally significant issues	Feelings vividly expressed, integrative, conclusive, or affirmative
7	Full, easy presentation of experiencing; all elements confidently integrated	Expansive, illuminating, confident, buoyant

FIGURE 6-2. The Experiencing Scale

down-regulates the arousal system; however in more toxic shame something else happens. The shame intrudes and stops a fear reaction without any solution. In other words, the person does not feel fulfilled and the slights of life, through trauma or the vagaries of a poor environment or stress, accumulate causing a cascade of negative emotions.

So much about therapy is about education, as well as acceptance and reassurance. The therapist might do well to inform the patient that this is nature and it requires respect. "This is your nature," is a phrase that seldom crosses a *psycho*therapist's lips. This is not a terminal sentence. Quite the contrary, it is a statement of fact and hope. The person is told that, if they can accept and understand their emotional dispositions, then these can be managed and used for empowerment of actions. The person can organize, modulate, and balance their life. Temperament needs no cure.

☐ Presentness Power

"Awareness in itself is healing."
Fritz Perls

Following emotional sensitivity comes a respect for mindfulness, an awareness of the moment. Borysenko (1988) believed that events like trauma result in a "wound of unworthiness." For this to be understood and handled, the person must be engaged in the now: Epiphanies occur in dis-ease comfort of the now. Viscott (1996) notes that the ability to express yourself in the present is the single most important element in an emotional pain-free life. The build up of any emotional debt is prevented. Good therapy is not pleasure; it is work in the now.

Another way to view this is that we go back and forth between reality and the self-created version of reality. We "create our own moments." We carry around a load of this superimposed reality and we drop it onto every moment and interaction. In a strange way life keeps trying to show us the real reality and we keep trying to push it away. We feel safe in our imaginary reality. Our defenses work. We are only half-alive. Awareness of the moment allows relaxation.

In the treatment of PTSD, two aspects of client engagement—re-experiencing the narrative past and experiencing the present moment—are important ingredients for engaging clients to reorganize a new experience and construct a new meaning (Safran & Greenberg, 1991). Re-experiencing the past involves promoting the client's reconstruction and experiencing again the "past events in the present." In effect, when clients are talking about an important incident from the recent or more distant past, the therapist attempts to evoke the past feeling in the present. Or better, the therapist directs the client's attention to the current experience of what's occurring in the session without reference to reliving the past. Gendlin (1981) also noted that in the processing of the past it is not enough just to re-experience it as it was: A new present experiencing is needed. He said:

> The past is not a single set of formed or fixed happening. Every present does indeed include past experiences but the present is not simply a rearrangement of past experiences. The present is a new whole, a new event it gives the past a new function, a new role to play. In its new role the past is "sliced" differently. Not only is it interpreted differently, rather, it functions differently in the new present, even if the individual is unaware that there is a change. . . . Present experience changes the past. It discovers a new way in which it can be a past for the present. (p. 14–15)

In fact, Gendlin (1996) identified a complete method of the processing of confused information. He noted that the creation of meaning may be an intense emotional experience but is one that is an experientially based symbolization process. He starts from the position that the bodily or felt sense (tacit knowing) knows a great deal. How is it possible, Gendlin asked, for the body to have all this information? Focusing on a bodily felt sense can bring creative steps of new development and resolution. This is a way of describing a complex whole that is not yet known. In therapy a new deeply felt meaning emerges from the felt sense. There is no split between cognition and affect in this process of creating meaning. He emphasized the act of symbolizing the felt sense, the creation of a unified cognitive-affective structure, a new complex meaning, which in turn is part of a process of creating new feelings and thoughts. The key is in the symbolic label that is attached to the processing: the interplay between the felt bodily sense and the label produces knowledge.

PTSD sufferers do not stay in their mind. The PTSD victim has learned to cope with certain painful experiences by developing intricate psychological strategies to avoid the pain. However, in therapy people learn that fear is not weak, that pain will not kill, and that anger is not necessarily bad. PTSD clients inhibit emotion because it is experienced as too dangerous to express in a specific relationship. Old stuff hangs on, such as resentments, frustrations, hurts, guilt, and grief. These are all markers of the need to complete unfinished business. Whether an unfinished situation arrives from the distant past or is contemporary, it will clamor for attention until the expression is completed, the experience reprocessed, and the closure attained. Closure is brought about by reorganizing perceptions so that one no longer perceives the situation as thwarting one's attempts to achieve satisfaction. A re-enactment is often called for (Perls et al., 1947). This is done in the now, and emotions facilitate problem resolution.

What to Do

Respect presentness. "You are the music while the music lasts" (T.S. Elliot). Practice mindfulness as much as possible. The ideal therapeutic session is one that proceeds in small steps, escalating the degree of difficulty at a rate that taxes the patient's emotions but that never provokes him or her to abandon the task. Given minimal distress, tolerance, emotional regulation, interpersonal effectiveness, and self-management therapy communicates to the client that intuition and "now" knowledge can be as valid as empirically verifiable knowledge. This involves a sense of self-trust. This involves a sense of being in the here and now in a spontaneous and connected way. The therapist does well to foster this.

Jon Kabat Zin described mindfulness with seven attitudinal foundations; nonjudging, patience, a beginner's mind, trust, nonstriving, acceptance, and letting go. It is the ability to live in the moment. For an older person this means giving up old resentments, reducing stress, and enhancing relationships. It also means slowing down and reflecting, tasks honed at later life. It requests of the person that he/she identify with the distress and not try to escape. It attempts to quiet the mind by perspective and presentness. What a wonderful and simple human task, especially for trauma victims.

Focusing, the Gendlin technique, is listening to the body with compassion. There is a slowed down quality. It is a process that asks the body: "What wants my awareness now?" It is saying "Hello" to emotions. It is the trust in the self and the realization that feelings that are read are ones that can be changed. It is staying in the present. It is the wisdom of knowing and of not knowing. It is the closest way of knowing what is there now. It is really looking for an aha! experience that represents a "felt shift," a new understanding of the phenomenon. It takes the inner critic and gently requests what is the matter, where is the fear. The person can be requested to say:

"I am sensing into my body."
"What wants my awareness now?"
"I am checking back with my body."
"I am sitting with it, with interested curiosity."
"I am asking what it needs."
"I am sensing how it feels from its point of view."
"I am asking the body to show me that it is OK."
"I am thanking my body."
"I am asking if it is OK to stop."
"What is the edge of the experience?"
"Just sit with it."

☐ The Marker/Reflexiveness

Affect, presentness, and this section are related. Consciousness is a great unsolved problem. It is an internal narrative whose processes supply comment on thoughts. In consciousness, the here and now are flanked by the past that illuminates them and by the anticipated future. The drama of life comes from consciousness and that makes life, life. It is reflection. Primary reflection is a way to solve problems in the now: secondary reflection allows for a discovery of the abstract connections, unity, wholeness of meaning. It honors meaning by noticing. Rennie (1994) highlights reflexivity, defined as self-awareness and agency within self-awareness: both are linked to change.

In CBT there are three levels of cognition: the automatic level (fleeting but accessible to intervention), the conscious level ("That is what I mean"), and the metacognitive level (realistic or adaptive reflections). The metacognitive level selects, evaluates, and monitors further development of schemas for particular situations, tasks, or problems. The metacognitive level allows the person to monitor problems of content and processing errors (arbitrary inference, mind reading, etc.).

Let us take a step back and set the scene here as well as to operationalize this aspect of care around the client's puzzlement of self. If you ask the client what he/she was just doing, each will tell you what he/she was saying as well as what was not said. It is the understanding of this reflexive component that is most human and curative in treatment.

Something interesting occurs in this process: The client is aware of his/her own reaction. Clients benefit in therapy in part because they not only had thoughts and feelings, they also had thoughts about their thoughts, feelings about their feelings, desires about their desires, and various combinations of these modes. Reflexivity is something that clients work within and something that they have (Rorty, 1976b). The objectification within self-awareness of the activity of telling a story, we believe, is best represented in the client's reaction to self. It is the reaction to one's processing that occurs frequently in trauma recall. In our view, a majority of therapy categories constituting the taxonomy of the client's experience of the therapy hour are expressions of their reflexivity. Accordingly, we have conceptualized the client's reflexivity as the core (i.e., most central, unifying) category in the trauma analysis.

We believe that change occurs not so much because the repressed memory of the early experiences (leading to unconscious motivation or defensive mechanisms) is activated, but because present functioning is distorted as a result of rigid schemes being maintained. Relevant new experiences are repeatedly processed through these dysfunctional tacit schemes that are automatically applied to the situation. New experiences are distorted and assimilated into the old structure, and change does not take place. Tacit schemes then fall apart: They guide perceptions and generate external and internal reactions in inappropriate ways.

This reflective process is "natural" for older people. At the risk of being ageist, it is what comes naturally. In some sense it is the core of what reminiscence is about. It is also the core of meaning making.

What to Do

The overall process is simple. The therapist queries reflexively ("What does that say about you as a person?") and nonreflexively ("Stay with that"). Although represented in the past, the memory enhancement process is created in a present context. With this balance the victim can identify agency/communication elements that foster change. This is distinctly therapeutic. The emphasis is on "now" experiencing and the process of meaning changing. In effect, the trauma victim is "compelled" to apperceive the past to conform to the ongoing identity and "compelled" to conform the present to the ongoing past. Past indeed is prologue, but so is present. To paraphrase Henry Miller's dictum: "Everybody becomes a healer the moment he attends to himself."

The rest of this section involves a combination of the corrective emotional experience and experiential processing. When there is a recognition or re-experiencing of any puzzling reaction between scheme and current event, the therapist has something of value. This reaction, a puzzling client marker, can lead to accessing, re-examining, and ultimately to reorganization of the relevant tacit schemes, and thus to basic changes in one's conscious experience of self. This has been treated by any of the case formulation methods, as systematic evocative unfolding of problematic reaction (Weiss, 1971) or as a patient marker (Greenberg, Rice, & Elliot, 1993). It is also a most important element of therapy for trauma victims.

Good therapy means that clients become aware of the ways in which they interrupt their emerging experience. At some point in therapy the client becomes aware of feelings and needs that are not "just right." Even with little awareness or expression of these orgasmic feelings and needs, there is usually some small sign of an interruptive process. When the victim becomes aware of the fact that she/he is interrupting him/herself and how they idiosyncratically interrupt themselves, a significant moment in therapy has occurred. What is being interrupted slowly becomes more available to awareness.

Greenberg, Rice, and Elliot (1993) have noted that problematic reactions may involve either an external, behavioral reaction or an internal response such as a strong emotion. The marker that signifies client's readiness for engaging in the experiential search required in the unfolding of the problematic reaction should contain two elements: First, the client recounts an instance of a reaction in a situation; and, second, the reaction that is felt as problematic is the client's own, not that of someone else.

Some aspect of the person's current attentional allocation and processing capacities remain involved in either the reliving of the experience, in misperceiving, or overreacting to current situations in terms of the unfinished business. The art is encouraging the person sufficiently until the feeling flows spontaneously and then facilitating this authentic expression. The therapist needs to shift between directing the client to ac-

---

Box 6-5
The Marker

Event: The client is experiencing a negative self-related feeling and is puzzled by it. The feeling deepens in response to empathic affirmation from therapist. Empathic affirmation is followed by some reduction in anxiety. Puzzlement continues.

Interventions

I. Identify relevant marker
   Verify problematic aspect
   Heighten idiosyncratic meanings
II. Ground client in experience
   Maintain client's focus on sensations/emotions/reactions to stimulus
III. Provide client with reasons for this behavior—"You learned this"; "We can see how this applies to you, given what you have been through."
IV. Facilitate broader self-exploration: Point out generalizability
   "Would you like to see if we can change this typical reaction?"
   Acknowledge and focus on client's spontaneous recognition of meaning
   Acknowledge the pain involved and the desire to change
   Facilitate client's re-examination of self-schemes
   Acknowledge and focus on client's new understanding of own scheme-guided dysfunctional styles and the new implications for self-change

---

tively express and helping the person try to attend to the experience. The oscillation between expressing and attending helps to bring the emotional experience alive.

The goal here is to reach a spontaneous recognition that this way of functioning is really an instance of a more pervasive mode, one that now feels inconsistent with their own self-expectations, satisfactions, and goals (Box 6-5). This self-recognition usually provides the stimulus for a self-guided search process that is much more than an intellectual analysis. Resolution is reached when clients achieve a new awareness of their own mode of functioning in a way that restructures the issue. The client has a sense of what they want to change and a sense that they have already begun to change. This resolution point is usually accompanied by an upward mood shift.

The therapist needs to be responsive, not only to the initial marker but also to the nature of the client's responses to the therapist's empathic reflections. If there is a sense of the client's retreating and clamping down on the feelings, then the therapist may want to back off. At this point the genuine empathic affirmation by the therapist should continue but without emotional arousal. When the client begins to feel more integrated and a sense of agency or energy emerges, the therapist recognizes this and follows with a growth-oriented reflection picking up the new sense of possibility.

☐ Integration

There are three aspects here. The first involves PTSD and the direction treatment, especially inpatient, has taken. Therapy programs of PTSD are effective when used as an integrative program. Newer programs addressing PTSD have advocated for a more holistic and integrated approach. In recent separate clinical trials, Falestti (1997) and Ford et al. (1995) have adapted structured therapy programs for trauma care, applying many forms of care. The tasks involve a client-centered beginning, an education session(s), followed by trauma narration, cognitive restructuring, and some form of coping or problem solving. Falsetti, for example, adapted a complete treatment program; cognitive processing therapy (CPT; Resick & Schnicke, 1992), stress inoculation therapy (SIT; Kilatrick & Veronen, 1983), and the anxiety-based treatments of Barlow (Barlow & Craske, 1988).

This treatment addresses the total PTSD problem in a concerted way. Exposure to traumatic memories is conducted through writing assignments of the trauma events. Writing provides more detail than verbal reports (Resick & Schnicke, 1992). Exposure is also addressed through the behavioral channel by in vivo exposure to conditioned cues of the trauma. Also, challenges are conducted to beliefs and errors in thinking, catastrophizing, overgeneralizing, emotional thinking, and the like. Additionally, this aspect of care involves education and coping. This is a total treatment approach.

Second, good therapy itself is integrative. Psychotherapy of any form requires an order, more so with PTSD as there is such variance. Janet, an early PTSD theoritician, noted that trauma must be accessed and then mourning occurs. It is in the venues of the interactive/intrapsychic/biosocial/cognitive/affective patterns directed by the person that a holistic sense evolves. It is best done with a vision of the person and goals that are serving this end. This is possible because the person is a covariance structure of domains that are integrated: If A is present, then B follows, etc. For some, just some movement is necessary. An intervention at any point in the system is all that is required to start the ball rolling. Movement in the most salient areas (related to the personological integrity of the person) is best. Haste is made slowly. This is a most important strategy also, because most therapies do not hold in the long run: Important change requires planning.

To expand, in developing an integrative focus, the therapist is not just allowed but required to consider both a symptomatic and a personal perspective. As a mutually supportive relationship between the two goals is established, the integrative focus converts the symptoms into a logic that dictates the course of care. Each goal implies the other, symptomatic work becoming charged with personal overtones, and personal work with symptomatic ones. The integrative focus thus offers a grasp on both the personal and the symptomatic motivational handles, leading to a therapy with higher levels of commitment.

Therapy will always depend on choices by the therapist, the integration of care principles that are far from simple but far from unknown. There are not extensive studies assessing this aspect of care. Sadavoy (1994) emphasized the "therapeutic necessity of using treatment strategies with older adults that are both interactive and integrative." His model (Figure 6-3) starts with assessment of the psychodynamic, interpersonal, and cognitive behavioral issues. The key element is the process of joining and the building of a therapeutic alliance. Diagnoses are then formed on the basis of the DSM and also cognitive distortions, roles, relations, and developmental defenses. Next come triage factors. Treatment is based on accessibility (determined by mental frailty and the ability to overcome attitudinal and environmental treatment barriers), need (determined by the immediacy of the intervention), and availability (determined by the treatments at hand). Treatment then is integrative, the careful and studied application of care principles to complexity—but one that is based on extant data and core psychotherapy tenets.

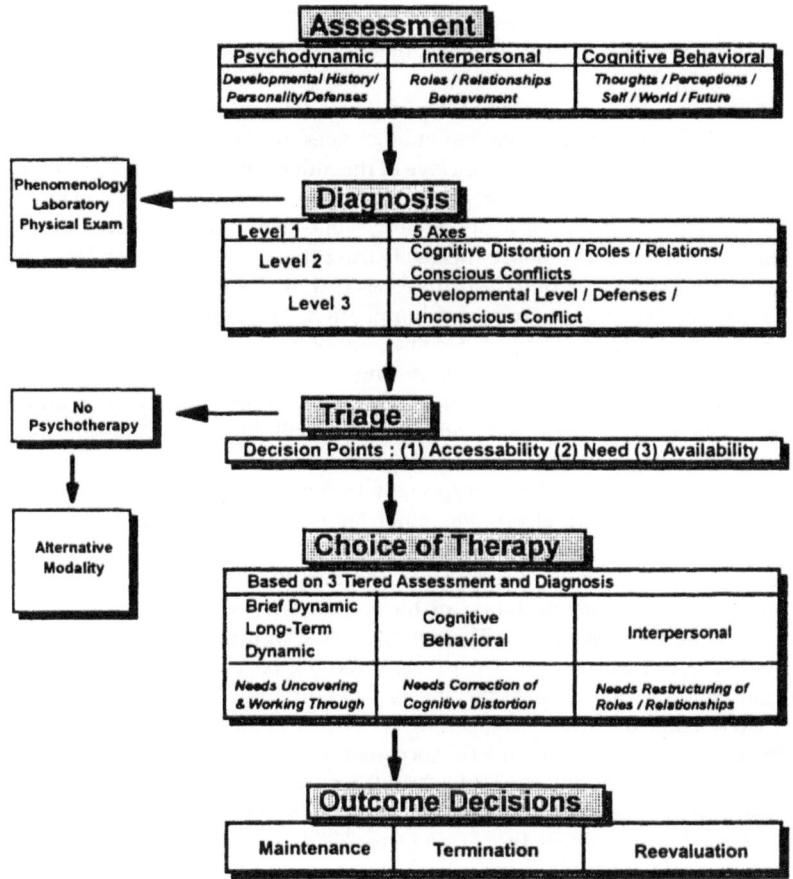

FIGURE 6-3. Sadavoy's psychotherapy decision pathway.

There are "tensions" that pervade the formulation of any psychotherapy plan. This is the case formulation. It requires a balance between the now and the complete, the simple and the complex, among others (Eells, 1998). There are several essential tensions of case formulation (Immediacy vs. Comprehensiveness, Complexity vs. Simplicity, Clinician Bias vs. Objectivity, Observer vs. Inference, and Individual vs. General Formulation). These are the grist for the ultimate formulation of the case, the case formulation.

This is the single most important element of care with the elderly. Case formulation is a deliberative and conjoint effort of identifying the etiological, precipitant, and maintaining problems of the person. It represents the formulation of theory into practice. It is integrative and dynamic. It looks for the whole picture. Symptoms are placed in the context of cyclic patterns, both internally and externally driven. The patient becomes a participant observer, becomes informed about the therapy, and generally assists in the care process. It is in this process that the whole of treatment is informed and decided. It is here that we can tell if "treatment receipt" (is the client getting what is called for?) and "treatment enactment" (is the patient doing what is requested?) are set down. And, it is equally important that the patient be totally informed about therapy. In effect, they become participant observers and active collaborators in their care.

Third, we must know the overall picture of PTSD for older patients. Overall, recovery at later life is much like that at other ages: the process of recovery generally occurs within 1 year. One way to conceive of the influence of trauma is in terms of time (early, middle, and late). In the early stages the issue is safety and meeting basic needs. Usually the pattern is one of acute anxiety, some depression, perhaps dissociation, and many emergent and practical needs. During this time too, "secondary" stressors can be incurred. Other secondary features ascend, including safety, control, possible reoccurrence of the trauma, trust, and humiliation. The telling of the story can seem cruel and often is. Social support becomes important. Just allowing people to have symptoms can be therapeutic. This is during the first month when the acute stress disorder (ASD) applies: If one has an ASD, then later problems can be anticipated. Most often, however, the influence of the trauma will dissipate.

As a loose strategy during this early stage, we want to stress that the biology of the disorder takes precedence. This is especially true with older people who are victims. This includes depression, sleep, and other "noise" in the system: Can the person negotiate the day-to-day happenings of life?

In the middle stage (next 3–6 months), the therapist can follow PTSD prognostic indicators. Here, the manifestation of the intrusion-avoidance dynamic is evident. Usual exposure therapies apply. There may be special problems with sleep, phobias, and grief. These must be attended to. Here too the psychological issues of care are important. Initially this involves the effects of conditioning, most notable by problems of intrusion. Later this involves meaning (Why me? Who am I?).

In the last phase, the reality of PTSD becomes apparent, as well as depression. Probably comorbidity is modal: probably Axis II problems exist. Here the psychological issues of care are prepotent. The treatment concern here is management and social clarity—"Am I a part of society?" "Can I trust?" "Am I a spiritual person?" The issue of social clarity is honorable survival.

What to Do

The basic structure of case formulation includes those features outlined by Persons and Thompkins (1997). They include (a) identifying information, (b) problem list, (c) personality (core beliefs), (d) current precipitants, (e) etiology, (f) hypotheses, (g) treatment plan, and (h) obstacles to treatment. In the next chapter we provide our version of this formulation. We follow a model of care, but it is based on the case formulation approach. In effect this guides the treatment.

In addition to the issues raised here we are interested in the "usual suspects": treatment history, presentation (precipitating, predisposing, and perpetuating factors), and so on. We use the form given below (Sperry, 1995). It includes all the moderating variables noted in Chapter 1 as well as the relevant issues discussed here. Queries are directed to treatment expectations from very unrealistic to very realistic (older people do better if they have appropriate expectations); willingness for treatment (Prochaska & DiClemente, 1986)—older people do better if they are or have done something in the treatment plan; treatment capability based on psychological mindedness—older people do better with a greater amount of openness and ego strength; impediments, including psychological impairment (degree of PTSD problems and comorbidity, especially depression), social support (degree of support), medical status (psychological debility), medical status (physical debility), current problem stressors (current irritants), cognitive ability, and practical problems. The all important problem list follows, along with hypotheses, treatment plan, and obstacles to care.

Finally, we note the obvious: PTSD is a problem of anxiety (mostly). The patient often rebuffs interventions, making a planned program essential. But, even here, the issue is slippery, as the patient provides the therapist with many other fronts that surround the core problem. Patients sometime present with one problem but mean something else. It is often helpful to "interpret it," in the way that self-theory would dictate, but the therapist with a vision or focus can address many issues of care and always return to the focus of care, the case formulation.

☐ Little and Big Stuff

"Go ahead and throw some seeds of your own. In the end there is one dance you'll do alone."
Jackson Browne

Little in life is linear except aging. With age comes stuff. With some patients the status quo is all there is and all there will be. That is fine. With many patients, however, there is an awareness of the problems of living that may give way to the problems of being. For them, there is always the danger that "reality" may break through and the person regress as this world-view is too honest and is beyond the level of acceptance. This lietmotif of the person is most vulnerable at older ages. Over time also, many may develop a "deconstructed awareness," manifest by a sense of meaninglessness or a practical focus, concrete thinking, and a distorted sense of time (Baumeister, 1990). This is avoidance and it works for many. But for the troubled, this does not work. Fortunately, the therapeutic frame can endure this where the person may not be able to.

Aging then encompasses the best of times or the worst of times. For the latter group the issues of life for the therapist can be big or little. It may be a strange twist of fate that the gods have ordained: When one gets older, the small issues of living *and* the big issues of living (being) become very important.

We do not address the little stuff here. This comes out in the first three stages of the model. We note, however, that the little tasks of life are often the only ones for many older people. Joan Erikson, Erik's daughter, maintained that the last stage of living is more a problem than he had intended earlier. In effect, she revisits the work of her father and concludes that older people are at risk of an onslaught of life, societal and biological. Turner (1995) noted that the aging process is a contradictory relationship between the subjective sense of inner youthfulness and the outer realities of biological aging. The aging person must feel shaky and protect the self against uncertainty. Because the older person is at the mercy of society and an aging body, the only solutions rest in the skills that are different at later life, a selected maturity of the aging process itself. At times the only reality of care involves the application of "little stuff."

Now for the big stuff. We have a bias in this book, noted in other chapters: Older people have creative things to say/do/seek that are part of growing older. It is independent of psychopathology but influences it. Those at later life can march to a different drummer; gerotranscendence, postformal operations, interiority, an autobiographical impulse, integrity-seeking (loss of egocentrism), and wisdom. Teachable moments are real for this group. It has been suggested that meaning is discovered by doing the deed, by experiencing a value, and by suffering. The first is achievement-based; the second involves an awareness of the suffering of another human being; and the third entails an attitude that holds that suffering in life is meaning making. This last issue involves what is important in life for the individual (Kalish, 1985). It is also this last task that most applies to older folks who have been victims of trauma.

"Good aging" represents a shift away from the external world and toward inner life, disengagement of everyday life, commitment to virtuous behavior, increase to a higher transpersonal level of awareness, and a desire to give back to the world. Moody and Carroll (1997) reminded us that this is a process that includes a search—a quest for guidance, the "correct" compelling path, a struggle—the actual passage and its cosmic/human trials, and a breakthrough—making the leap a logical and spiritual one, an inner awakening that illuminates the way, as well as a return—a translation of the new way with the ordinariness of life and the silent language of reality. When people commit from the depth of these issues, or even if they just toy with them, they transform other life issues. After all, a stress response is just the body and mind's coping response to an abnormal situation. This "bigger" pursuit engineers a psychologically minded person who has the ability to struggle nondefensively. They can place symptoms in perspective, can establish boundaries between self and others, and are not beset with the daily taunts of PTSD—avoidance, anxiety/pain, and non-commitment to the care of others. They are bigger than the problem. They are oriented to hope.

In later life if one does not seek to safeguard the necessities of coping, the person starts to "shrink." Like arteries that have been abused, one's comfort zone shrinks. People do "use it or lose it." They must choose. Milan Kundera, in *The Unbearable Lightness of Being* (1984), stated:

> The heavier the burden, the closer our lives to the earth, the more real and truthful they become. Conversely, the absolute absence of a burden causes man to be lighter than air, to soar into the heights, take leave of the earth and his earthly being, and become only half real, his movements free as they are insignificant. What then shall we choose? Weight or lightness? (p. 5)

People can make the reality of heaviness in the only life lived a "lightness of being."

Lest we think that psychopathology is our enemy, Havens (1999) reminds us: "pathology is inevitable in life. No one can truly understand themselves. What we do is discover felicity, what Joseph Conrad called the "jewel set in the iron of failures and shorcomings." (p. 28)

What to Do

Just a word about the day-to-day activities. Data exist arguing that the older one is, and the more severe the mental problem, the more the person has trouble with activities of daily living, especially functional ones. Although this screeches in the chronically mentally ill, it also has some applicability for the run-of-the-mill trauma victim who is older. The mental health provider should attend to the "vagaries of the normalcy trance" with older trauma victims by simple questioning or the application of an activity of daily living scale. This includes functional tasks, such as check writing and problem solving living tasks. At times this can be most revealing. Again, we address this in the first three parts of the model.

Box 6-6
Tasks of Living

Task	Question
Waking up	What wake up calls does your body/mind give you?
	What death events/births are present for you?
Embracing sorrow	What is the deepest loss in your life?
	Are you denying loss/grief?
Savoring blessedness	What are your best memories?
	When did you know you were sacred?
Re-imaging work	Where do you get your rewards now?
	What soul work do you need to do?
Nurturing intimacy	What intimacy memories do you treasure?
	What risks will you take now for intimacy?
Seeking forgiveness	Whom do you need to ask forgiveness?
	Whom are you willing to forgive?
Taking on the mystery	Where does you soul sing?
	What stories need to be told yet?

Although there may be no protection here, especially if very frail or poor, an endpoint of the vexatious requirements of living can be stabilized by an attitudinal set that allows for comfort and peace. Raines (1997) outlined this for older folks. He asked the question: Is it possible to have an older hero? Might there be a sunrise in the context of a sunset? Raines, along with many others, answered with a resounding "yes." He raised seven tasks in living at later life (Box 6-6). They are as good as any at later life.

These tasks echo a "time to live," a balance between healing and defining, between integrating and ripening, between getting there and being there, between a commitment to others and a responsibility to self, and between forevermore and now. These issues are understood in a paradigm of living a life that is partner to authentic being. Fear at the edges is faced and a covenant of self is made. When the older victim can trust self, each can know how to live.

☐ Conclusion

"My own youth is locked somewhere in this stiller body"
Roger Rosenblatt (1999, p. 22)

We have presented a disparate mix of important treatment components. They may seem unconnected. If anything this flies against the tide as integration is the byword. Williams and Sommer (1994), for example, advocate for a four part model of treatment: (a) safe environment and good relationship, education, as well as control over the environment; (b) working with the trauma memories; (c) working with maladaptive beliefs and social skills/emotional intimacy; and (d) finding spiritual and intellectual meaning in the trauma and initiating social responses, as well as termination. Of course this is where we are going, but all integrative formulations have a building blocks.

Burns (1999) held that it takes, on average, 15 treatment strategies to initiate change (i.e., there are 14 failures for every hit). So, in the mix of contact with the patient, the therapist applies both joining issues (empathy) and working issues (change strategies). This is a highly individual process. Often patients "feel better" but do not "get better." The corrective therapeutic experience, however, is one that allows for both. If this is to occur, the "correct" profile of key ingredients must be applied.

If these components are at all responsible for change, the victim must shift the discourse and move a stuck narrative that can entertain healthy mental components (e.g., insight, mindfulness, modesty, discretion, confidence, composure, nonattachment, adaptability, or proficiency; see Goldstein, 1994). In fact, it is this shift in discourse that is common to all therapies. It is the development, depending on the therapy, of an observing ego, a cognitive reframing or restructuring, or a second-order shift. It is also often a move from an either/or position to a both/and or neither/nor position. The individual who moves to a healthy view makes a shift, either by changing to a new narrative or by examining the former one from a distance. That is, the individual takes a reflexive stance to an earlier discourse.

We have provided, then, overlapping ingredients in the care of patients with PTSD. In a sense this is an optimistic view because so much works. The elements themselves include those that engage the person, activate the autonomic nervous system, and foster a friendly presentness of affect and now experiencing, and allow for the correct context to ascend for a better translation of living. This provides for the person to alter the narrative, the one truth that (in PTSD) is most noxious. The person takes command and thinks differently. Now we become specific and discuss changing the memories themselves.

7

CHAPTER

Treatment Model: Early Stages

"All models are wrong; some are useful."
John Tukey

In structuralism, the principles by which the entire phenomenon is organized are first viewed and then an interpretation of the elements of the structure is made according to the relationships to the whole. Often the organism seeks an equilibrium and operates around a set pattern of safety. What is important is not whether an answer is right or wrong, but how the structure of the organism is set so as to solve the issue at hand. Best results occur with integration. Our model is about integration, what to do when. Importantly, the trauma memory is only a last consideration.

With PTSD and older people, this is an appealing model. It applies most to more chronic PTSD, but also to acute PTSD. We know that the existence of PTSD is less a continuation of an acute stress response and more a distinct state that developed from a host of factors in addition to trauma severity. In "normal" PTSD it is probable that the constellation of symptoms changes over the course of a lifetime. Older victims may even recapitulate their trauma at all life cycle points. In more insidious forms of PTSD the experience is worse. In fact, the course of chronic PTSD is one that gravitates to rigidity—not a worsening of symptoms. Jonathan Shay (1994) stated that there is a process of change (in PTSD): It begins with a betrayal of what's right and this encourages a survival mode of a narrower focus on what is important. What develops is an "undoing of character."

With this idea we seek to understand PTSD by providing structure for its care. In our model we provide structure with flexibility: first, care directed at perturbation, then coping/social supports, and then issues specific to trauma. In trauma therapy, always a balance is necessary between self-capacity and exposure to the traumatic memory so as not exceed the therapeutic window (Briere, 1992). Like any other map, it is a modest mediator between the known and the unknown, a nondogmatic vision open to interpretation, a touchstone around which flexibility can fluorish. Recall too that vast majority of psychotherapy gains in older people come from common sense input with cognitive and behavioral alterations or monitoring. We seek this balance.

Realizing then that the map is not the territory, we present a model for therapy for older trauma victims. We lament at the outset that we may understand much about PTSD and not a thing about any one trauma victim. This is what models do. Our treatment model has six parts (Box 7-1). In this and the next three chapters we present this model. Here we address the model itself as well as the first three components.

First, the task is to stabilize symptoms, including the treatment of comorbid disorders and current stressors (including health). This is an important component in the treatment of older people (Gatz, 1994) and for trauma, in particular (McFarlane & Yehuda, 1996). Symptoms must be treated initially, both because they are important by themselves and because only by a reduction of symptoms can later components of care be provided (Cummings & Sayama, 1995). This may especially apply for depression, which may require a focused dose of CBT or medication or both (Hyer & Stanger, 1997; see Gallagher-Thompson & Thompson, 1995). Clinical depression reduces the ability to access memories in a therapeutic way (Shapiro, 1995); and first impressions matter.

Second is the relationship itself. This is really an extension of the first model feature. No other component of therapy is more accepted than this second treatment factor, the glue of therapeutic attachment that unfolds in a working alliance between client and therapist (Kahn, 1991). Can the therapist let the client know that he/she is doing the best to understand the way the situation looks to the client (empathy; Yehuda et al., 1995)? In Judith Herman's ground breaking work the elements of change consist of attaining a sense of safety, remembering the details of the trauma, and nourishing a normal life. All gains come from safety. Traumas can reoccur even in therapy and with trauma victims.

In a larger sense, the relationship extends itself and involves the whole orchestration of care, the ability to balance therapy needs requiring stroking and therapy needs requiring the work of therapy. The therapist joins and works in therapy. On the one side, Howard (1991) noted therapy is only done by the therapist who can enter/join the core issues of client's stories and provide the appropriate word repair. Brandsma

---

Box 7-1
Treatment Model

1. Stabilize symptoms → Treat co-morbid disorders or stressors (including health).
2. Relationship building → Build trust, the ability to confront trauma with a trusted therapist. Respect the narcissistic alliance (what he/she needs to have stroked).
3. Attend to necessary developmental and treatment and education (normalization) factors → Assure social supports, daily coping, and social skills and treatment compliance.
4. If avoidance/other symptoms persists: Use tactics of personality style.
5. Build on positive core memories → Foster a renarration of self with core memories that can generalize to current life situations. The self-defining memory is a core life story, an identity that can assist in the balance of life.
6. If intrusions: Decondition trauma memories → Apply AMT or EMDR.

(1998) saw this as a covenant, a contract beyond the medical/legal commitment of mutual care. On the other side, patient and therapist conjoin in problem solving, focus on work, and bond for change.

The third task of trauma therapy is to attend to necessary developmental and treatment factors. The major issues are to assure social supports, daily coping, and social skills and treatment compliance on a bed of treatment expectation and acceptance. If trauma is intense and if social support and coping mechanisms are inadequate following the trauma, the "total" resources of victims (social roles, possessions, self- and world views, and energy) become depleted (Freedy, Shaw, Jarrell, & Masters, 1992).

This is a special problem for older folks. With them, this is often the most salient model stage. This requires an active stance by the therapist that shapes the direction of a life. This stance is as much a significant intervention as any in therapy. This is perhaps the one major difference between younger and older victims. Much of this involves everyday problems, both structural tasks and individual empowerment for action. Therapeutically, the older person must come to know what to do and have sufficient internal (coping and social skills, as well as treatment compliance) and external (social supports) skills to appreciate the therapy. A significant portion of change is attainable by social skills training, social supports, coping, and skill building.

The fourth task is easy to explain but difficult to apply: If resistance or avoidance symptoms predominate, the therapist can use tactics of personality style. The idea here is that an analysis of personality is the best vehicle available to improve the outcomes of psychotherapy, to understand entrenched patterns of coping (Ruegg & Frances, 1995). Evidence exists that among patients with PTSD ingrained patterns of personality are more resistant to change (Fontana & Rosenheck, 1994; Frueh, Turner, Beidel, Mirabella, & Jones, 1996), and that a knowledge of these assists in treatment (Reugg & Francis, 1995). PTSD in many victims is chronic and relapsing. A comprehensive awareness, then, of the structural integrity of personality (behaviors, thoughts, emotions, interpersonal and biological patterns) serves the clinician well. Clinicians have the most to gain in this understanding as an integrative therapy is opened.

The last two components of the model are about memories. Both apply *after* other issues are considered and both can occur at the same time. Component 5 represents the positive side of the treatment process. These are the stories of victim's that are self-representational. One label that has been applied is *self-defining memories* (SDMs; Singer & Salovey, 1993). We use the term *positive core memories* (PCMs). They are a blended summary/single event memory of something important to the self. Each person has such a collection of autobiographical memories, a core set of slides in the person's carousel. They are episodes in the person's life repeatedly considered and if strung together can form a script or personality. In therapy, they can assist in the balance of life and can generalize to current life situations. In therapy (or life) too, these memories can be used to understand personal meaning and assist in present demands.

The last (and complement of the fifth) component involves the trauma memory. We have discussed the trauma memory. It represents rogue events that do not fit into prior schemas and are not narrativized (McFarlane & van der Kolk, 1996). The therapeutic task is to bring this implicit memory (easily triggered by emotional states, interpersonal contexts, external stimuli, and language cues) to be experienced as self-as-past, that is, into language in the form of a narrative. In our model, trauma memories are reconditioned by the application of anxiety management or EMDR techniques. These are efficient methods that allow for the care of the trauma memory. We can effectively target the target memory, its intensity, negative and positive cognitions, emotions, and salient sensations.

☐ Integration

It was Adolf Meyer, the psychiatrist at Johns Hopkins, who held that the diagnostic checklists of the DSM-III and beyond would obscure what was meaningful to patients. He believed that clinicians should work at case formulations and not diagnoses. This may especially apply to older people as there are few therapy virgins (Friedman, 1999). With older people, management is most critical at the beginning of therapy. *With older people who have trauma, acute or chronic, the need to plan care is critical: what do we do first, second, third.*

Therapists think about the therapy, the case. Again, the clinician is asked to plan, to decide if the trauma memory is relevant to the care of this older person, and to manage care. Overall, preliminary ideas that are important are the following:

1. What does the patient need? Does this person require psychotherapy? If so, what form? Can this person be helped in other ways? Does this require management only? What modules need to be implemented first? What keeps a person doing what they are doing?
2. Can the need be met? What do I need to do here?
3. What is the outcome? What are the workable goals (vague goals, vague outcomes)?

An outline of a case formulation follows (Box 7-2). It was developed from the work of Persons (Persons & Tompkins, 1997). It posits that the formulation of care depends on this thinking, all the time. Any choice of intervention requires a response to the formulation. The treatment plan is seen as a working understanding of the person addressing problems tempered by core beliefs.

The therapist's role is as a "therapy manager," initially and foremost with annoying symptoms and then with the scaffold features of personality and negative beliefs. The integrated therapist influences healing, behavior change, and skill enhancement. Often operative tasks are basic: keeping the trauma victim in treatment, being supportive during difficult periods, maintaining appropriate arousal levels, and, in general, assuring commitment to the goals of therapy. The more pathological the victim is, the more influenced by trauma symptoms, the more the therapeutic tasks relate to the beginning parts of the model. The therapist needs to obtain some stability. The less the victim is impacted by the trauma, the more the therapist can address the latter parts of the model for more lasting change.

We know that success in therapy depends on a considered working knowledge of the patient. Directive treatments (cognitive therapy), for example, are more effective among patients who have low resistance traits, whereas nondirective treatments (supportive/self directed) are superior for those who are highly resistant. Similarly, symptom-focused interventions (cognitive therapy) are often more effective among patients who are impulsive and extroverted, whereas insight-oriented interventions (supportive) exert stronger effects among those who are introspective and introverted. However, we must know the patient first. This occurs early in therapy. To the extent that use of services reflects the course of the disorder, results of studies suggest that remissions are usually followed by relapse: The absence of symptoms does not mean that the disorder has run its course (Ronis et al., 1996). There is substantial idiographic

---

Box 7-2
Case Components and Model Stages for Interventions

1. Identifying Information—Age, race, education, previous psych hx, lifestyle problems (smoking, alcohol, etc.).
2. Problem List—5–10 short descriptions of problem. Probe all domains (interpersonal, biologic, intrapsyschic, and behavioral.
3. Current Precipitants—Both practically in the day-to-day activity and dynamically (core issues). Can you think of recent situations that apply here? What were you thinking/feeling when this happened?
4. Etiology—Salient learnings. Do a developmental history. Get time line information complete with memories and incidents.
5. Personality (Core Beliefs)—Core beliefs and salient personality patterns. What does this say about you? Has does this apply to you?
6. Obstacles to treatment—Personality patterns and practical problems that impede change. Therapy interfering behaviors?
7. Hypotheses—A story of the whole pattern. What is your best guess? What are the mechanisms at play?
8. Reformulate Plan

(individual-level) stability of patterns of use, suggesting both a recurrence and a high persistence of use over the years.

Ultimately we seek to deconstruct the trauma experience. However we attempt to finesse the ongoing conscious construction of meaning by being theoretical and formulative, as well as practical and preventative—forcing a dialectical change (Components 1,2,3,4) and psychotherapeutic change—activating emotional schemes (Components 5 and 6).

In our model that follows, treatment should be front-end loaded. Outcome especially will determine the course of treatment—long-term, short-term, symptom remission, life change. What is most important will dictate the care. If the short-term symptom reduction is all, then medication and management is applied: If longer term quality is at issue, then the application of several of the model components (including 4, 5, and 6) apply.

We believe that the choice to manage care only occurs in 50% of victims. That is, the first four elements of the model apply. This entails a plan of management, knowledge of cyclic maladaptive patterns, a focus on the externals of adaptation, and a simple coping strategy for intrusions. The application of the positive core memory (Stage 5) also is in order. The choice to treat the memory (Stage 6) occurs in the other 50%. Here all stages are considered, but Stage 6 is applied in some form. Again, the case formulation will dictate the organization of care.

Finally, we note that psychological reductionism is a problem in therapy. Reductionism often follows an ease of formulation, as models provide. It raises red flags about everything not anchored to absolutes. Treatment of traumatized individuals needs to be paced and to be directed by a clinician, requiring a skilled reading of the individual's capacities and the work that needs consideration. In this model clinicians are requested to be both passive and active, to listen and to be in a position to explore and to address the effects of trauma on perceptions and decision-making processes. Therapeutic activism alone involves the danger of accepting the clients' helplessness as inevitable, and of taking over control where clients need to learn to establish control themselves (van der Kolk, McFarlane, & Weisaeth, 1996). Always there is a needed balance.

☐ Stage 1: Stabilize the Client

"We must cultivate our garden."
Voltaire

We have to know what to do and what we cannot do. How do we treat this person in front of us? It starts with a loving clinical ear that has to communicate the message that enduring the unendurable is a task for understanding and working with. *It can be made better.* The selling of this belief is critical. Older people especially must see that the therapy will make a difference. This is performed with an understanding of the person's needs in the context of the trauma experience.

This process is initially addressed through the stabilization of symptoms. Often the focus on the somatic symptoms is helpful (e.g., sleep). van der Kolk, McFarlane, and van der Hart (1996) noted that the treatment must first control and master physiological and biological stress reactions. This includes the treatment of comorbid disorders and current stressors (including health). This is a central component in the treatment of older people (Gatz, 1994) and for trauma particularly (McFarlane & Yehuda, 1996). Symptoms must be treated because only by a reduction of symptoms can later components of care be provided (Cummings & Sayama, 1995). Early stabilization is necessary as a patient is likely to leave therapy if not attended to, and impairment with many symptoms interferes with attempts to adjust at other levels. Clients in turmoil leave therapy if they have not connected and made some change by the third session.

Often the moment of commitment for an older victim involves a paradigm shift and one that older people make slowly. Older people maintain a cautious attitude regarding use of services for mental health. In fact, the likelihood of walking into a mental health clinic after an acute response is small, unless symptoms are high. They are likely to see a primary care physician. With younger trauma victims, use of mental health services is higher but is usually episodic. In general, older people come to therapy because many of the normal events associated with aging are stressful (Gallagher-Thompson, 1994). Four common presenting problems of older adults seeking psychotherapy (life-style changes, bereavement, relationship problems, and health-related difficulties, especially) have been noted (Schramke, 1997), and the "correlates of aging" (lifestyle changes; Schnurr, Aldwin, Spiro, Stukel, & Keane, 1997) interact with aging itself to create conflicts. Retirement and a chronic illness are modal examples. Blazer (1998) addressed this issue around the DSM disorders, the traditional ones of memory loss, depression, and anxiety, plus suspiciousness, agitation, and hypochondriasis.

Whatever the issue that brings the older client to care, as a general rule the therapist must use clinical judgment and redirect the patient's focus to "here and now" problems, ones that brought him or her into therapy. The point is that older adults seeking psychotherapy arrive due to lifestyle changes resulting from these events. Trauma makes this measurably worse.

Several issues deserve consideration. None of these require an exhaustive evaluation, but not to consider them is ripe for problems.

Health Beliefs

The issue of the older person's model of health is apt. From a society perspective a tension exists between the psychosocial identity and the aging body. The technological advances are recoding the body and thus solving the contradictions of a world of older people. In this way the person is body-centered. The mind has yet to catch up, and there is a pull by "typical" aging features, physical frailty, low income, stigma, lack of education, and cohort features, independence emphasis, not psychological mindedness, to resist psychological care.

Box 7-3 identifies four areas related to health beliefs. The first addresses research considerations. Among the elderly, predisposing and enabling factors are stronger predictors of service use than need (George, 1981). In practical ways older people cannot or will not come to therapy. As an alternative in-home psychotherapy, telephone services, psycho-educational modules, optimizing social contact or religious coping, as well as the judicious use of a case manager, have been advocated. The creative alteration of the typical therapy session with other labels, alternative settings, and the extra pursuit of the client are most often suggested (Zarit & Knight, 1996). Older people also do not possess the flexibility, openness, range, and attitude to avail themselves of psychological care (Box 7-3 research dimensions).

Older people then do not have the "correct" cohort attitudes or beliefs of pscho-therapy. Evidence exists (Gurin, Veroff, & Feld, 1960) that older people go through a three-stage process before a decision: Is the problem a psychological or physical one? Do I seek help? Do I decide to seek professional psychological help? Older people tend to have problems with the first of these. Often it is not seen as a psychological one. Having decided to seek help, however, many will go to a physician or a self-help group rather than see a psychotherapist. This applies to physical disorders also where psychological problems complicate treatment (Gallagher-Thompson & Thompson, 1996). As a rule, then, older people are less likely than younger adults to label problems as psychological. Many do not classify the problem at all but simply try not to think about it. As implied, beliefs at each stage are important in any decision for care.

Convincing a person that he/she should make changes in the presence of a psychiatric disorder is a challenge. Leventhal (1999) has several suggestions. The clinician must get into the frame of the person, how he/she perceives health threats. At its simplest, this requires mild arousal (a perceived threat) and a plan ("This is what you do"): The person is motivated and has a method of action. As people are active problem solvers and common sense biologists/physicians, the plan must be relevant to the situation. The patient then must have a clear image of care, be motivated, and have a plan: "This sleep problem is caused by PTSD, a treatable disorder, that we can change with your help, largely beliefs and behavior." Viney (1987) noted examples of negative thinking: "I am a burden," or "The future is bleak and I will fail alone." Positive beliefs about therapy may have to be fostered (Box 7-1).

One other perspective is provided by Spiegle and Classen (1999). He used knowledge of the person's model of care to good advantage regarding cancer. To have a psychologically minded person (personal/psychological beliefs) is the ideal. Whatever the variant, however, the therapy must be adjusted for care. A knowledgeable read of this state provides an important entry into care. The dimension that seems

Box 7-3
Conditions to be Considered for Psychological Care

1. Research Conditions
    Predisposing (e.g., demographic, social, beliefs)
    Enabling (e.g., health insurance, accessibility)
    Illness, level of need factors (e.g., perceived symptoms)
   Research Dimensions
    Breadth—flexibility of belief in mental illness
    Openness—seek help for a variety of issues
    Range—inclusive estimate of the scope of problems that can be treated
    Bias—more positive attitudes toward care
2. Overall Questions
    Is the problem a psychological or physical one?
    Do I seek help?
    Do I seek professional psychological help?
3. Health Beliefs*
    Fatalistic—"This has beaten me." Often older people are prisoners of their
     own positive thinking. They are upbeat but fatalistic. They will not commit
     or act on their own behalf.
    Religious thinking—"Prayer is the only answer". Most older people are reli-
     gious and prayer is a helpful coping method. However many will simply
     allow nature to take its course ("PTSD will never change and I must suf-
     fer").
    Medical thinking—"Give me medication." Here too there are problems, as
     the personal acts or mastery are not present. There is no internal locus of
     control.
    Personal/psychological beliefs—"I can make a difference." This attitude
     should be fostered.
4. Helpful Beliefs
    Belief that the patient can improve PTSD/quality of life.
    Belief that problems are common and treatable.
    Belief that the person can accurately identify problems.
    Belief that patient can make a difference.
    Belief that working on tasks can lead to empowerment.
    Belief that medication helps but is part of only effective treatment com-
     ponent.
    Belief that people with a positive orientation can make a difference on the
     course of treatment.
    Belief that the journey from victim to survivor is a journey and made easier
     with tools of therapy.
    Belief that the person can always "stop and think" or rate problem state and
     then make choices in life.
5. Two Key Health Belief Questions
    What is your theory of your problem?
    What is your theory of how you can be helped?

*Extrapolated from Spiegle.

helpful with older people with PTSD is locus of control: Can I make a difference or do others determine my change capacity? With the more internally controlled, the clinician can take liberties and make suggestions; with the externally controlled, less so.

But there may be good news. Where the younger population might ignore or delay seeking care for symptoms of illness, the older group (70 plus) seeks care to define and treat health threats, apparently as a mechanism to reduce emotional distress. Increasingly, older folks are motivated to reduce the emotional distress that is caused by threats to their health. Fortunately for physical health, older people have self-regulation strategies that are more risk-averse and involve conservation. Unfortunately, the vehicle of mental problems is through the body. For elders who have minor problems it may be that depression and like problems are discovered through body problems. Unresolved mental health problems lead to further health problems. However as stress reduction interventions are increasingly making a difference in therapy and newer cohorts are more open to these interventions, the increased use of mental health services may be forthcoming (Leventhal, Leventhal, & Schaefer, 1992).

The patient is told then that PTSD has been diagnosed, as well as any comorbid problems. The person is told that the symptoms are the result of PTSD; that the lack of sleep, intrusions, and avoidance, and so on, are a direct result of this disorder. Other symptoms are heaped on: "This is all part of the clinical picture of PTSD"; "You may even feel hopeless"; and "all the relationship problems, that we discussed are also a part of this disorder." In addition, it may be said that PTSD is common, that it affects about 15–20% of people depending on the trauma, and that it is not "your fault." This disorder also responds to treatment and chances of recovery are good. The disorder is made the villian. Comorbid diagnoses are also discussed in this way. The patient is told further that changes in symptoms can be expected within a short time. So, we give the patient the "sick role," and we create the expectation of change.

Medication

In *Of Two Minds*, Luhrmann (2000) highlights that a gap exists between psychotherapy and pharmacotherapy. Clients are viewed as "fixable forms." This needs to be overcome. Most chronic victims of PTSD have been on several medications. This is certainly the case if they have seen a psychiatrist. With PTSD, medication trials to date have shown moderate results, with a significant proportion of patients rated as improved but not recovered (Box 7-4). A subgroup of PTSD patients will develop chronic refractory illness that requires long-term treatment. Avoidance symptoms and consequent numbing, which can be quite disabling in PTSD, respond more readily to psychotherapy, or to the combination of psychotherapy with medication, than to pharmacotherapy alone. For this group a careful medication strategy is called for. Blazer (1998) noted that this is best done with a firm attitude that "other factors" (psychological) must be in the brew. This applies especially with older patients where neuroticism, the personality trait, is present.

Davidson and van der Kolk (1996) noted that the purposes of the medications for PTSD are numerous: (a) reduction of the frequency and severity of intrusive symptoms, (b) reduction in the tendency to interpret incoming stimuli as recurrences of the trauma, (c) reduction in conditioned hyperarousal to stimuli reminiscence of the trauma, (d) reduction of avoidance behavior, (e) improvement in depression and numbing, (f) reduction in psychotic and dissociated symptoms, and (g) reduction of impulsive aggression against self and others. Unfortunately there exists little hard evidence for these in the context of the older (or younger for that matter) trauma victim. There is evidence for a positive effect on using both pharmacological and

---

Box 7-4
Pharmocotherapy Principles for PTSD

1. Only a few drugs have been effective
2. Symptom or comorbidity focus
3. Acute trauma effects—decrease autonomic arousal and prevent kindling
4. Often leads to polypharmacy or high doses
5. Dependency leads to chronic treatment
6. Goals of use: Target symptoms that are dysfunctional; avoid short- and long-term side effects; improve functioning; and use as an adjunct in psychotherapy

---

psychotherapeutic interventions on patients (see Engels & Vermey, 1997). Davidson and van der Kolk again believe that trauma needs to be treated differently at different phases of people's lives following the trauma. Drugs that decrease autonomic arousal will decrease nightmares and flashbacks, will promote sleep, and may prevent the limbic kindling that is thought to underlie the long-term establishment of PTSD symptomatology.

However, given PTSD and the passage of time, medications have at best a palliative function. The questions arise somewhere in treatment: "What are we treating?" and "What is the role of medication really in the treatment of this disorder?" Many older people see the mental health provider as a physician extender. They need education about the role of therapy.

Although there are few absolutes here or anywhere, the clinician may well choose to apply medication but this works best only for a period and only with the expectation that treatment requires personal work (Gallagher-Thompson & Thompson, 1998). Under the worst of circumstances, medications are a seductive form of care for many older victims, which can lead to a biological reductionism with less focus on the "work" of psychotherapy. They are "dumb chemicals" and will not work for any long-term change for PTSD symptoms without other interventions. On the other hand, PTSD interventions may be anemic without medication, at least for a period.

The patient is then evaluated for medication. If the patient has sleep problems, severe intrusions, and of course depression or another anxiety disorder, he/she is told that medication will be used and that its use will assist in the important work of psychotherapy. We are not averse to medications, but we recommend that the interaction of these two forms of treatment be made clear to patient and consultant. Otherwise the psychosocial treatment will likely fail (Gitlin, 1996). They will be focused on short-term change and will use avoidance as a care strategy. They will also be rather passive in the care process. If not, the patient will monitor change by severity of symptoms only. For therapy to proceed in the model, the relationship between clinician and psychiatrist—consultative, collaborative, supervisory—must, then, be decided.

Physical Health

Knowing the older adult client's physical health status and medication regimen is a necessity for psychotherapy. It affects everything. Anxiety and health status are inversely related, and anxiety does not dissipate over time. It stays. The clinician should obtain a medical history and confer with the patient's primary physician about current health status and medications (Myers, 1991).

We have addressed this issue elsewhere. It is our belief that the somatic arena is often the battleground for problems of living in older people. It is the message center for emotional problems. Regardless, it is also one area of life that, if compromised, will alter all psychological interventions.

Nezu and colleagues (1998) addressed this issue with cancer patients. They advocated for a problem-solving procedure for somatic issues as these relate to cancer. The patient with (real) cancer is taught a problem-solving method of coping. What is of interest is that the cancer is considered a major life stressor, that a careful rationale is provided for the need of problem-solving coping, and behavioral methods are applied for treatment. The patient is told that the problem-solving method has been shown to be effective, that the added stress of an emotional problem causes emotional problem-solving and not rational problem-solving, that added stress causes the "first" problem of the disease to become worse (lower immune system, etc.), and that the disease impacts the whole person. As in other forms of psychosomatic treatment, careful goals are formulated, the patient's beliefs are addressed, moods are monitored, and outcomes are assessed.

Health problems are the gorilla in the room. Often an activity of daily living index done informally can be helpful as health frailty will confess its presence in many ways. If the patient remains fixed on a somatic focus, the treatment is slowed down and a reconceptualization is in order. That is, the "place" of the physical problem must be understood to be a result of the disorder. PTSD must be addressed for this to be addressed.

Symptom Reduction

Just under 50% of patients dropout of therapy for one reason or other. The most sighted reasons include poor alliance, low SES, poor expectations, reduced satisfaction, client likability, and client preparation. The important point here is that the sense of well-being and a positive attitude toward self and therapy is initiated. Symptom reduction will follow. Howard, Kopta, Krause, and Orlinsky (1986) found that just the changed subjective well-being of the patient in the first few sessions was enough to assure compliance.

Our clinical experience and that of others (Smyth, 1995) suggests that a reduction of symptoms of at least 50% is a good target. This information is received from the patient. The use of the SUDS (Subjective Units of Distress Scale) scale, the Beck Depression Inventory (BDI), or a PTSD/anxiety scale can be used. We routinely use the BDI. It monitors success in older depressives (Gallagher-Thompson & Thompson, 1995) and, we think, PTSD. Once the patient believes that they can make a difference, that mastery is possible, *along with* medication, the task of care becomes easier.

As noted, the patient is given the expectation that symptoms will remit in a short time, given compliance and commitment to treatment.

Special Symptoms and Comorbidity

Some symptoms are more equal than others. They must be attacked or massaged. As noted elsewhere, the therapist is wise to address sleep problems, panic anxiety, depression, substance abuse, and psychotic symptoms, especially. With the possible exception of sleep, these symptoms may become functionally autonomous. We have learned that around 80% of PTSD patients (of a chronic nature) receive an additional diagnosis (McFarlane, 1992). PTSD also involves abnormalities in a number of domains within the individual, such as memory, mood, bodily experience, interpersonal relatedness, emotion, and behavior. Those that result in perturbation are of most interest initially.

According to Smyth (1995), the chief complications (for the treatment of PTSD) include (a) the presence of resistance to treatment; (b) the presence of an active substance abuse disorder; (c) the presence of a personality disorder; (d) the presence of additional anxiety disorders and mood disorders to include phobia, panic disorder, generalized anxiety disorder, dysthymia, and major depressive disorder; and (f) the presence of psychosocial stressors in the form of legal, financial, marital/family, health, or employment problems. Traditional internal barriers to treatment of PTSD include avoidance, especially issues of shame (where special problems regarding the acquisition of trauma memories are involved), alienation, personal constructions, and even the significant connotations about the relationship between the traumatized individual and professional and cultural factors (Turner, McFarlane, & van der Kolk, 1996).

Although much of this applies to older people, we believe that it is best to treat other comorbid anxiety disorders that are functionally related to the PTSD simultaneously with the PTSD (especially social phobia and panic disorder), as these are kindred brothers and the common territory can be addressed. Substance abuse, severe depression, psychotic states, and severe problems of sleep should be attended to prior to PTSD. They are comorbid disorders that are functionally autonomous from the PTSD and are best treated separately as they inhibit the care of PTSD.

We are especially concerned about depression. Depression should be treated early as this state functions as an opaque filter preventing light in the needed illumination of care. Depression may require a focused dose of CBT or medication, or both (Hyer & Stanger, 1997; see Gallagher-Thompson & Thompson, 1995). Clinical depression reduces the ability to access memories in a therapeutic way (Shapiro, 1995). The clinical task is to get depression down to a subthreshold level before (or during) the treatment of PTSD.

One clinical rule of thumb is that when depression is but part of PTSD (subthreshold), then treat the PTSD: If a distinct syndrome, then treat the depression. If the person meets criteria for clinical depression (major depressive disorder or dysthymia), then treat this with CBT or medication or both. Depression is that important. Here it is especially important to use the BDI (as a depression measure).

Finally, the clinician needs to attack sleep problems. A brief history and understanding of the effects of sleep problems are in order. Sleep interventions occur in six areas: sleep hygiene (habits around sleep), stimulus control (discriminative stimuli of the bed and bed room), sleep restriction (limiting time in bed to slightly more than the actual amount of time the person is able to sleep), relaxation, cognitive therapy (re-examine validity of worry), and multicomponent interventions (Morin, 1993; Pallesen, Nordhus, & Kvale, 1998). The application of standard sleep hygiene is especially helpful, along with the application of sleep efficiency model (Morgan & Clark, 1997; Morin, Culbert, & Schwartz, 1994). The patient is trained to sleep in the bed at 85% efficiency by the simple methods of getting up at the same time, varying time for sleep onset, getting up at night if not sleeping (and returning when tired), as well as the better habits of sleep hygiene. An important point here is what to do with intrusive thoughts, the cognitive element of sleep problems. Intrusive thoughts require focused attention by the use of sensations produced by relaxation. A shift of attention away from worry thoughts works (Goleman, 1995).

As noted above, the presence of any of these problems leads to other problems—PTSD is then not treatable. As noted above also, the task of the therapist is to assess these and to outline these for the patient, just as done for PTSD. Once again, the patient is given the "sick role."

Cognitive Decline

This issue raises its ugly head at later life, especially when there is comorbid anxiety or depression. Older people experience cognitive decline that influences the processing of information. Often a pre-existing PTSD is exacerbated by the onset of a neurological condition. This is a special problem. Exacerbation may result from the added effects of neurological conditions to the existing trauma symptoms, direct triggering of trauma content, or indirectly as a threat to health that having a disease implies. Also, such a disease process may diminish the patient's capabilities for suppressing negatively balanced memories and affect.

It is helpful to evaluate cognitive functioning. This information is crucial to designing an appropriate treatment plan because both the in-session work and homework rely heavily on the person's ability to comprehend, remember, and produce material in oral and written formats. Many treatment modifications can be made (Snow, 1999). Some clinicians (Gallagher-Thompson & Thompson, 1995) routinely administer the Mini-Mental State Examination (MMSE; Folstein, Folstein, & Mc Hugh, 1975), which has been shown to be a valid and reliable screening measure to detect cognitive impairment in the elderly. In this way, clients can be referred for further neuropsychological testing if needed, and treatment planning can be done with knowledge at least regarding certain aspects of the older person's cognitive capabilities.

Factors related to cerebral functioning, therefore, might be a cause of other PTSD-related problems and co-produce mood and panic problems as well as other symptoms. Knight (1997) concluded that obtaining a good neuropsychological history "cannot be stressed enough" (p. 467). Box 7-5 provides necessary neuropsychological questions in the context of PTSD. Like depression, this area of human functioning at later life should always be addressed. Cognitive changes may be similar in people with a specific disorder (e.g., Alzheimer's disease), but each person loses abilities differently and each responds differently to interventions (Siegler, 1994).

Belief/Expectancy Formulation

While this issue was considered in the more general area of health beliefs we also consider it here. It is that important. Patients must believe in the therapy. If they do not, the therapy will not move. This means that they must be convinced that what is here works (can work), and that they can make a difference. Patients need to see that the situation is challenging, have to exert a moderate degree of effort, the client sees that he/she is making an improvement, that the client feels control over the situation, and that success is attributable to the client.

Patients need a sense that they will not make things worse and that they can do minimal things. For most, these involve the following:

1. Not making a problem with the problem.
2. Appropriate attitude on justice: What is fairness in life?
3. Perspective on preferences and wishes versus demands.

Box 7-5
Distinguishing PTSD from Neuropsychological Problems

Consideration of the following questions can be of help in differentiating PTSD from other neuropsychological involvement:

1. Do neuropsychological deficits exist?
2. What deficits are present and what are patterns—localized, lateralized, or diffused; qualitative performance of the features?
3. Is the pattern of deficits similar to other disorders (e.g., dementia) or is this pattern typical of PTSD populations?
4. Is the clinical testing process free of the effects of unintended affective priming when the individual who has PTSD becomes emotional due to the problem?
5. Do cognitive problems at the time of the testing represent an exacerbation of existing symptoms typical of the phasic variation of PTSD or do they represent a stable level of symptoms for the PTSD patient?
6. Do "special" neuropsychological signs of aging exist? (Examples include rapid forgetting: episodic memory deficit, intrusion errors, retrograde amnesia, and semantic memory deficits.)

---

4. Willing to take minimal risks—are they willing to . . .
5. No or little self pity—everybody has it.
6. Tolerance for discomfort anxiety—tolerate ambiguity.
7. Exposition of the "fear": success, consequences, conflict, disapproval.
8. Compassion not competition.
9. Ability to enjoy self—some observing ego.
10. Minimal skills for problem solving and living.

Often just an educative and normalizing of these issues are sufficient for change. A "psychological" understanding that change is possible and that the person can make a difference are then requisite. The therapist too needs to have an attitude to begin at the beginning, to assume little, and to assist in the management of a life, an older life. This is the integrative therapy offered here. The older person is besieged with the character traits of life and the vagaries of age. The request is for information of the stressor experience. The clinician gets a sense of the whole life of the person and what are the presenting issues. This is the time to be the thorough clinician.

Goal Setting

Initially therapists listen to the patient. They are seeking goals. They observe the background of the patient, listening to the symptoms, and making a list of complaints and problems. Therapists are most behavioral in the pursuit of care. Only problems that exist can be solved, and all problems are specific. Burns (1999) says that depressed patients try to convince you that there is no hope: Anxiety patients that there is no solution. PTSD patients do both. Therapists need goals to have a direction.

Box 7-6
Goal Formulation and Working Clinical Issues

Process
1. Elicit target complaints.
   What is the complaint?
   When does it occur?
   What does the patient see as the cause?
   What are strengths?
   Rate severity.
2. Translate complaints into goals.
   These must be important, time-limited, specific, realistic, positive, and measurable.
   Solution-focused queries apply.
3. Elicit cooperation and commitment.
4. Teach the model of care to patient.
   What is patient/therapist role?

Key Questions
   Was this your idea to come for treatment?
   How serious is the problem for you?
   What do you know about PTSD?
   Are you willing to alter aspects of your life to reduce problems of PTSD?
   How much do you believe that what we do will make a difference?
   How much do you trust us?
   What have you been successful with to date?
   What are the barriers that prevent you from making changes?

We apply many of the ideas presented in the previous chapter on goals (Box 7-6).

We offer one technique that assists in this query. In the previous book (Hyer et al., 1994) we advocated a timeline. We have not been able to improve on this method of unearthing events/meanings/life experiences across the life-span, but we do add that the timeline that identifies periods across life does one thing especially. We are attempting to identify evidence that supports the way the person is/was. In this way we maximize empathy as we can say to the patient "Now we can both see why it is that you are that way." Although time consuming, it can be worth the commitment.

Strengths: Do Not Forget Seligman

A learned optimism is a desired goal. Seligman (1998) believes that this belief is a special trait toward optimal health. The person says: "I can do this." In the development of this, the therapist should not forget the assets of the person. The best predictors of well-being are the person's meaningful outlook and goals. In addition to the suggestions of Seligman and others on the importance of self-efficacy, patients can be given the Pleasant Events Schedule or activity schedule (see below) as well as a careful inquiry into the day-to-day events of the person. This solution-focused thinking can be the target of much discussion.

Conclusion

The ball must be put in motion carefully. Some success or optimism must be experienced early. Always this means an aggressive management of the early symptoms. Perturbation, therefore, must be addressed early. For older people the issue is "Can I be helped?" and the focus is selling possibility and titrating person-based concerns with the needs of therapy. The therapist must be especially sensitive to themes of a somatic focus, losing control, as well as those of loss, meaning, and death (Blazer, 1997). The therapist must "hear" and validate these.

In effect, the therapist needs to "socialize" the client into treatment. They must fight against the tendency to blunt or underrepresent their condition. Many are practiced at avoidance and do not want to be informed. Many will not return (Gallagher-Thompson & Thompson, 1996). Such responses are directly related to the person's perceptions of the meaning of therapy in the context of these major life events. Poor thinking patterns feed off the these triggers. In turn, they cause poor behavior and feelings. We will address socialization again under Stage 2 as there should be a seamless connection between the two stages.

☐ Stage 2: Relationship

"The notes I handle no better than any pianist. But the pauses between the notes—ah, that is where the art resides!"
Arthur Schnabel

If Stage 1 is about management, Stage 2 is about understanding. In 1912 Freud suggested that patients and therapists band together in a therapeutic pact. Now we know that this is more than anyone imagined. No therapy is done without the feel of *empathy*. So, none of the stages are pursued if this aspect of therapy is awry. In fact, we return to it regularly when the patient becomes annoyed/angry with the therapy.

Symptoms may have brought the client to treatment, but the reduction of turmoil is ultimately not the goal. The work of therapy involves the person of the victim, the problem-based infrastructure that subserves the symptoms. This is approached best by the necessary meandering of something messy in psychotherapy, the relationship. This is best measured by the therapeutic alliance, which clients rate consistently as the best reflection of clinical outcome. The therapeutic relationship is a fuzzy set of connectors that really connect. We believe that the best treatment for the older trauma victim may well be the preparation for the treatment. This is the true "good enough mother" and holding environment for the patient.

As previously suggested, a review of the outcome research suggests that 30% of outcome variance is accounted for by the common factors (variables found in a variety of therapies regardless of the therapist's theoretical orientation). It has been estimated that techniques (factors unique to specific therapies) only account for about 15% of the variance of treatment efficacy. There is now a considerable amount of evidence demonstrating the quality of a therapeutic alliance as one of the better predictors of outcome regardless of the particular type of therapy (Cartonguay, 2000). Models of the patterns of patient and therapist transactional sequences associated with improvement or not in the therapeutic alliance have also been developed (Safrin & Muran, 1996). In PTSD, work, this translates into safety (Rappoport, 1997).

Interestingly, through the years the essential features of Rogers and Perls have been that there is a discovery-oriented methodology that considers clients as experts in their own experience. Clients are viewed as having a privileged access to their own unique experience. There is a belief further in the fundamental motivation toward growth and development. Borden (1966), an early writer on therapy's touchstones, advocated a "universal change processes" that are common across theoretical models of psychotherapy. They involve five areas: therapeutic contract, therapeutic operations, therapeutic bond, therapeutic openness-involvement, and therapeutic realization (see Orlinsky et al., 1994). The therapeutic bond was especially relevant as it addressed questions of clients:

> Were you able to focus on what was a real concern for you?
> Was your therapist attentive to what you were trying to get across?
> How well did your therapist seem to understand what you were feeling and thinking?
> Was your therapist friendly and warm toward you?

More recently Linehan (1993) created a context of validating rather than blaming the patient. She did this with perhaps the most exasperating kind of patient, the borderline. Linehan even has a cute term for the therapeutic process of validation of the patient, *radical genuineness*. Additionally, she also holds that irreverence becomes part of this relationship process as the therapist now has the liberty to handle noncompliance. This is radical genuineness. Interestingly, a popular form of therapy for older people, validation therapy, was also founded on these ideas: explore individual's subjective reality (the who, what, when, and how of emotional focus) and respect the individual's sense of reality.

When you are in sync with clients, associations are on target, the situation is truly "in the zone." Here neural networks seem to make contact: Thoughts produce molecules (Amen, 1998; Brigham, 1994). As the clinician applies the biopsychosocial model, the mix of understanding and technique play out in sessions.

In the writings of PTSD, the the relationship is the most practiced element of therapy but the one that has received least attention. The careful therapist need only watch out for the "tyranny of the technique" (Mahoney, 1991). About possible problems with this on the part of the therapist, Egendorf (1995) stated:

> Whatever else we can say about it hearing people through their pain is most of all privilege. On the way we may fall into self inflation ("Look at what I can do")! or skirt the challenge out of fear ("I can't bear this!"), callousness ("Better him than me!"), counterprobia ("What a wonderful challenge!"), guilt ("How awful of me to get off on someone else suffering!"), and the various ways of erring by blurring or emerging ("He is me!"), rescuing ("She needs me!"), and romantic or pseudospiritual fusion ("We are one and our love is all"). But what path to this sublime is not paved with pitfalls. (p. 25)

"Damage" Listening and Safety

The recognition that the trauma event was beyond the control of the person and that actions that occurred were normal are perhaps the most curative elements of PTSD treatment. Many events are terrorizing, situations disgusting, and enemies loathful.

A recognition of these *by the therapist* is needed for client participation. Additionally, the client needs to have natural narcissism restored, that felt-entitled-feeling of just being human. The victim needs to be made to feel as an un-victim.

Although the primary damage is to the workings of the person in life, damage really occurs in the person's relation to internal objects, a pervasive loss of trust and, for many, a fear that aggressiveness will spill out of them. Victims become defensive quickly. They may resort to denial and un-attend to obvious distress; they may become enraged at the injustice of being a victim, thereby splitting and projecting impulses will-nilly; they may be chronically angry, in efforts to regain control; they may become guilty as a defense against helplessness; or they may dissociate as a way to foster distance from the trauma. How things go early in the therapy make a difference.

The essence of trauma is that the person loses faith that there is order and continuity in life. Eventually there is no safety except in the extreme caverns of life. Eventually learned helplessness evolves: You have no say in your life. Empathy seems and is a natural remedy for this disorder. Brandt (1981) distinguished between "technical" and "hermeneutic" psychologies. The former attempts to change others by interfering with observable behaviors; the latter seeks new meanings involving different perspectives and different reference systems. "Whereas technical psychology aims at power through controlling others, hermeneutic psychology aims at power through questioning the taken-for-granted" (p. 64). The key difference between the technical and hermeneutic approaches is in the implicit equivalence of psychologist and client. Better trauma repair involves a hermeneutic stance.

Reflection and unconditional positive regard are only rarely overused in an environment of dosed exposure. Again, this starts with safety. Referencing trauma, Weiss (1971) early identified three processes of psychotherapy that influence this variable: external circumstances, degree of control over defenses, and the therapeutic relationship. The relationship is, of course, integral to all three. The therapeutic relationship is the "that's me" personal communication that is both clear to all and impossible to define.

Turner, McFarlane, and van der Kolk (1996) noted that, if this stage is not reached, a serious dysychrony exists where the therapist becomes a potential enemy and is watched like a hawk. As PTSD patients seek security (Turner et al., 1996), they must do so without typical defenses that automatically arise in the session, as well as between sessions. A constant focus of the therapist and patient for an understanding of how the natural vulnerability of trauma distorts the curative actions of the therapy. Turner et al. (1996) noted:

> Much of the treatment of victims of trauma is intuitive. It depends on both a sensitive understanding of the unique issues that make every individual different from all others, and clinical knowledge about the accurate timing of appropriate interventions. What occurs between a patient and a therapist is a function not only of the particular diagnosis of the patient, but also of the unique and personal relationship between patient and therapist. Despite the fact that the nature of the therapeutic relationship and the appropriate timing of interventions form the backbone of all treatment, these factors can not easily be quantified, and probably can never be satisfactorily studied with acceptable scientific methodology. (p. 539)

Work of Therapy

There is a delicate balance here. At some point treatment must reach the place where it provides more than validation by the therapist and comes to include tolerance of conflicts and ambivalence that safety brings. The therapist helps. Gendlin (1991) stated:

> Whatever is really going to help must be the person's own. What then is the role of the helper? The helper must somehow point out what might help, and yet without taking over and directing the whole thing. Some activity of the helper is involved and yet the main process of the helping is the person's own process which must arise and continue.

However the therapist cannot be too active. As part of this problem (especially for older victims), Turner et al. (1996) stated:

> The less therapists are in a position to address and explore the effects of trauma on perception and decision-making processes, the more they may be tempted to do something to take over control or to pass control onto outside parties. Therapeutic activism involves the danger of accepting the patients' helplessness as inevitable, and of taking over control where patients need to learn to establish control themselves. When this tack fails, as it usually does, the price for trying to run the patients' lives is abandonment. (p. 555)

For many, education of the manifestations of PTSD actually encourages a positive revisionist thinking. At the least, this provides a more friendly superego in a more open client. Often this is sufficient for change. As humans we have only a few necessary existential illusions; world as benign, self as immortal, and others as safe. The saliency of the secure attachment of the therapy is necessary for this re-realization.

On music disks, artists have become adept at allowing the closure of one song to "lead in" to the next one. Before you know it, you are not just sensing a new sound, you are hearing a new song. In therapy this occurs when the relationship "leads in" to the work of therapy. Clients just naturally attempt to elicit from the therapist a continuance of the maladaptive pattern. Relationship-focused therapists are savvy at taking this bait. Procedurally this can be done by a studied asocial or unhooking (anti-complementary) reaction, or a metacommunication involving oscillation, a movement back and forth between aspects of the stimulus situation that are reflective of the client and the client's personal reactions to these aspects. This has been labeled *decentering* (Safran & Segal, 1990). The therapist (and client) steps outside of his/her (and the client's) immediate experience, thereby changing the very nature of the experience. Just as on the disk the music has changed, so too in therapy the therapy has changed, the relationship is now producing change. As we have said so many times in this book, therapy is dance.

What is Empathy?

Empathy has an independent and causal influence on therapy outcomes (Burns & Nolen-Hocksema, 1992; Burns & Spangler, 1998). It works. Empathy has been divided into a cognitive form, a person understands what another person feels and why, and affective form, a person feels what another person is feeling either with the same emotion or a congruent one. Empathy is also probably more. At base, it causes the practitioner to conduct a better meaning analysis of the problem situation and a transformation of motivation that enables the perceiver to inhibit a retaliatory response and substitute a better one. In recent years, empathy has undergone a shift from the absolute truth-centered perspective in therapy to a relative or narrative one. Empathy now is an active process of construal. Omer (1994) noted that, although it is easy to empathize with the suffering of the client, it is not always easy to resonate with the emotional logic of the infrastructure of the client. Here the therapist has to assume a position that the problem-saturated solution is the client's best possible solution, the best way to adapt to the situation. In this way the client stands out as heroic (Hermans, 1995).

The empathic narrative is the attempt to understand/disclose the inner emotional logic of the client's behavior. Inner means that the client buys the new therapist view. PTSD, for example, is not an opponent process dynamic; rather, it is an understandable personal fear that cannot be fully understood. Omer held that this process often necessities the admission of a mistake by the therapist, acknowledging the externality of the old theory position and striving to replace it with a more acceptable one. Restoring the client to a sense of self-meaning, even if incorrect, may be important for change to occur. In the transition from the old to the new, Omer (1994) stated:

> The narrative so constructed cannot but be external. Gradually ... through the process of empathic construal, these stereotypes may be expanded and, eventually, outgrown. The empathic narrative is thus the result of the therapist's attempts at self-transcendence. It is in the very act of renouncing our initial limited descriptions that we grow as therapists and that we can best help out clients to overcome their self-limiting views. As clients grow in our minds, we help them grow in their own. (p. 21)

In effect, good empathy attempts to cure the therapy, not the patient. In this way great therapists are great storytellers: Good therapy may just be good storytelling. Ultimately therapists must accommodate their formal theories to the client's informal theory by elevating the client's perceptions and experiences above theoretical conceptualizations, thereby allowing the client's informal theory to dictate therapeutic choices. In this way, a DSM perspective can undermine therapy and confidence in the resources of clients.

An important view of empathy is provided by Egendorf (1995). He argued for an "intuitive discernment" in listening to trauma. This goes beyond any logical understanding of the victim. It is a hearing resonance, a feel that the core of trauma is never grasped by holding exclusively to unequivocal definitions or to the readily recognizable meanings of people's stories. It arises out of the intricacy that remains hidden until uncovered. The significance of personal experience can only be voiced in a way that rings true to the suffering person. People in pain are guided from "walking through" to "working through," from the initially obscure that is viscerally meaningful to some understanding, however imperfect. What is important is often void of meaning and unsayable. Egendorf (1995) wrote:

> Resonant hearing is, therefore, an altered way of knowing and being with things, events, and people. We linger with what is before us to the point of beginning to dissolve its opacity, using attention that is at least partially freed not only from habitual judgments, opinions, thought patterns, and frames of reference, but also from the very tendency to frame, judge, etc. In this way we peel ordinary objects of perception and thought, to uncover a richness that may at first be unsayable. (p. 13)

This of course is what therapy is about. With trauma victims who are older, especially if they have carried trauma issues with them, the healing dialogue invites them to feel again the trauma, but now, more than ever, with something more, the absence in their lives. As each does successfully, each chooses not to retreat from natural avoidance and to know that they are the ones who survived and can meet trauma's demand. They did not perish, "not even in the face of nothingness." Again, Egendorf (1995) wrote:

> When you truly hear people they know it. They hear that you hear them, and you hear their hearing of your hearing them, to the point that you may hear, in addition to the ordinary meanings, the resonance's, and the presence of one who lives, another order of hearing that resounds between you. (p. 21)

It is the Therapy

"It is what it is."
Yogi Berra

Increasingly research suggests that psychotherapy should concern itself more with the client's construction of what constitutes success in therapy. It involves more too than a client-directed process that only enhances the value of empirically demonstrated differential therapeutics (Greenberg, Rice, & Elliott, 1993). There is an empathy-learned task of the therapist ("I hear that") or the exploratory necessities of therapy ("Tell me more about that"). Kahn (1991) stated:

> The clinical relationship contains within it the whole story of the patient's problems, indeed the whole story of the patient's life. It is an astonishing microcosm. And it lays before the therapist a remarkable opportunity, not only for learning the secrets of the human mind, but for helping the patient as well. It was puzzling and painful to Freud that he had not found the way to extract the full potential from this opportunity. (p. 33)

Bugental (1987) expanded listening from a humanistic perspective. Overall commitment to the therapy process is more than compliance. Compliance involves adherence to treatment, specifying acts, behaviors, and reports: Commitment is the will to "experience" the treatment process. The person of the victim is "engaged." With this focus the goals of therapy are aiding the patient to experience self as larger and more potent in life than symptoms. And, *horrible dictu*, symptom reduction or problem solution may or may not serve this purpose. It also happens that the disruptive effects of symptoms and problems are markedly lessened when this position is communicated.

The subjectivity of a person is the seat of uniqueness, of individuality. According to Bugental (1987) this involves two perspectives, *concern* and *intentionality*, both only partially conscious (for the client). *Concern* is the pulse of the therapeutic health. It has four faces: pain, hope, commitment, and inwardness. It is through these filters that the person of the victim is attended to and grows: just to reduce pain is not therapy; the amount of hope is an indicator of openness; commitment is an essential monitor for change; and inwardness represents psychological mindedness, a step toward authenticity.

Intentionality, on the other hand, represents the inward monitor of humanness, a more meaningful and explanatory notion than causality. It is not an objectification process, a diagnosis or a self-as-object view of one's condition. Intentionality is the "good" therapeutic contact that guides and recognizes meaning into client's subjectivity. It represents the healthy flow of the understanding or authenticity. It starts from the unconscious and works through more intentional processes and eventually to acts. When the patient attempts to reverse that direction—to force action in the hope of evoking an inspirited fulfillment—the result is often a dull, unrewarding enactment.

Empathic relationship resides in the intentionality of the person. It monitors the inner life of the patient:

What bothers patients about themselves?
What bothers patients about others and objects?
How do patients tell about experiences, dreams, etc.?
How do they talk about therapy itself?
How do patients ask questions of the therapist?
How do they express immediate feelings?
How do they ask for help?

With PTSD the therapist has to remain patient and humanely accept the feeling that at some point anxiety will be reduced. Again, the effectiveness of any intervention is always a function of the patient's sense of safety and the view that the therapist cares. An empathic stance is not just exploration of the fear or shame: It is the recognition of the intense vulnerability related to feelings—and it is the therapy.

Empathy Never Ends

There is no therapy then without the feel of empathy. As noted above, we return regularly to an empathic focus alone when the patient becomes annoyed or angry with the therapy. It will be used all the time: it will be the only focus on many therapeutic occasions. We especially want to see that the patient feels listened to, validated, and stroked. Interpretation or some therapeutic learning may follow but only after the perturbation melts, and only in another session. This can be done in many ways, including being personal. There are many empathic roads to Rome.

Clients seem to resonate to the reasons for their actions, but only fully "appreciate" this when accompanied by the re-experience, usually as a result of the relationship. Clients now know that they do not distort their world; rather they arrive at the most plausible conclusion, given their ambiguities and history. Letting the client know that the therapist is doing the best she/he can to understand the way the situation looks to the client (empathy) and allowing this to occur in the present. This constitutes the validation of the *client's* perception and affirmation of the plausability of the client's interpretation. Gill (1991) noted that understanding is necessary for clients but never as "explanation." This must emerge from the client's re-experiencing in his/her current life. An "optimal frustration" eventually develops; clients hunger to know why they choose that one way and how they can alter that one way. It now oozes through the interpersonal actions, the relationship. All this occurs in the presence of a therapist who meets them with interest and humanity.

Greenberg, Rice, and Elliott (1993) pointed out that therapy depends on the empathic attunement of the therapist. Often this is sufficient and the problem dissolves. Often the emotional expression of the client may deepen. In this effort, the person needs to feel valued as a worthwhile person. The interpersonal experience with the therapist, then, is the central ingredient. Generally, the amount of empathic attunement is most important and predominant in the first three sessions.

Enhancing common therapy factors and building a strong alliance are not passive therapist postures. These are proactive initiatives that require a planned, focused effort to conduct psychotherapy within the context of the client's frame of reference. This is beyond the non-specific and accepting nod of the therapist and involves an active construal of the patient. This is a critical intervention (Omer, 1994). It is a continuous and creative human attack on the theories of psychology, an articulation of the inner reality of the client.

Any "abuse" of this position can cause trouble. The therapist "assesses" the client and forms a model of care. Resistance occurs when the client does not accept this model. In a sense, the client does not accept the "external narrative" of the therapist (Omer, 1997). Adler believed that this occurs when the therapist leaves the goals of the patient: The therapist is doing something that the client does not want. The therapist then always returns to the empathic stance of the therapy.

Older Folks

Older people need to be a part of the therapy. A necessary component to relationship-building with older people is socialization. This is the word used in CBT with older people. We discuss the (our) full use of CBT in Appendix D. Here we address the practical "gate" issues of CBT as well as that other therapy that is effective with older people, IPT (interpersonal psychotherapy).

Blazer (1998) said that the most effective path to communication with the older patient is to conduct an effective interview. He means validation, mixed with respect and dignity. For many older folks this starts with a "socialization" period. It requires repeating (Gallagher-Thompson & Thompson, 1996). Done well, it allows for the necessary educative and committing features that memory is a present tense view of past events—memory exists now and can be reworked. Exposure works because the client focuses on the "now" experiencing of the feared object with a trusted therapist (Wolfe, 1996): Patients do not "re"-anything (Gendlin, 1991).

Older clients enter treatment during various stages of the change process with biases, expectations, and different degrees of motivation to change. Although this effort goes on the entire therapy period, the focus of "socialization" is in the first four sessions (Gallagher-Thompson & Thompson, 1996). Educative and committing features that normalize and place a perspective on trauma are part of this process. In effect, the relationship sets the stage for the work of trauma, the necessary validation/invalidation process. The relationship then precedes the therapeutic flow.

Box 7-7
Cognitive Behavioral Principles for Older Trauma Victims

1. Socialize (positive expectations) into therapy.
2. Be collaborative/get active (ensure pleasant events).
3. Get successes (small wins).
4. Go slow/practice.
5. Be repetitive (educate and normalize)/use Socratic method.
6. Use favorite CBT techniques (e.g., ABCs) for management.
7. Assure one coping strategy learned before trauma work.
8. Monitor work/be scientific (use Beck Depression Inventory weekly).
9. Adapt style to the client.
10. Use homework.

Several elements of this socialization are important. In contrast to younger adults, CBT with older folks relies on the therapeutic relationship to establish a foundation for accomplishing its goals (Box 7-7). The therapist is requested to be practical. The rationale of CBT is addressed and clients are told that this type of treatment has been effectively used with both younger and older patients who have similar problems. CBT is time-limited, with 10 to 20 sessions being the typical course. With older adults, the dates and times for all sessions are established. Target goals for treatment are identified (usually in four sessions). The client sees the commitment and can discuss possible problems. Barriers (e.g., transportation) are discussed and corrected. Clients are advised that they will be expected to do homework between appointments and to bring that material. CBT also provides handouts that assist in the process of care. This helps to keep the therapy focused on here-and-now issues. Throughout, we use psycho-education, normalization, role clarity, and the "selling" of the model.

Finally, we note that IPT has a long tradition fostering the relationship with older folks. The relationship-based components include (a) a review symptoms of PTSD; (b) giving it a name; (c) explaining the nature of problem; (d) giving the patient a "sick role"; (e) matching symptoms with interpersonal problems; and (f) getting commitment to treatment. Defined issues of role transitions, interpersonal disputes, grief, and social skills deficits are played out in the therapy session. The key issue here is that the relationship is tended and nurtured before work is begun as well as during the therapy process itself.

Conclusion

Perhaps because of the natural runaway vigilance of the limbic system in PTSD, this second treatment factor, the working alliance between patient and therapist, takes on special purpose. In fact, to find a description of psychotherapy with the trauma victim without the heavy endorsement of a positive relationship is virtually impossible. A healing atmosphere for the management of care is created. Attention to the therapeutic relationship is, therefore, an imperative with the trauma victim, with the older trauma victim.

You might say two "trends" are essential. One involves the minimal conditions for the work of therapy. These are the non-specific care elements that keep the client open, cooperative, and non-defensive. The second highlights relationship as the centerpiece in the work of therapy. How a person acts and then what is done to those actions constitute the main ingredients of care. The relationship is both of these; it is not an epiphenomenon, it is the phenomenon (Kahn, 1991). The transference/countertranference or the interpersonal happenings are therapy.

Perhaps the curative process of the relationship is the "eternal now." The present is not simply a rearrangement of past experiences. The present is a new whole, a new event. It gives the past a new function, a new role to play. In its new role, the past is 'sliced' differently. Not only is it interpreted differently, rather it functions differently in the new present, even if the individual is unaware that there has been a change. To say it poignantly, present changes the past. It discovers a new way in which it can be the past for the present.

As a whole, older clients, trauma victims, resonate strongly to therapy issues that arise from the relationship. These include not just the positive transference so important with old age, but the "extra mile" issues of house calls, telephone contact, being an advocate, and providing concrete help. Older people need to feel a sense of moratorium and hope, so that the process of self-repair, so natural to this age group, can unfold.

☐ Stage 3: Balance

*"... man is an animal suspended in webs that of significance that
he has spun."*
Max Weber

In Tai Chi, balance is important. "All things in moderation" goes another saying. Despite its obvious message, Stage 3 of the model is perhaps the most important one. If older people can practice a healthy life style both internally and externally, then the dis-ease process will be less intense, occur less frequently or wane. About PTSD, we know that many psychiatric processes become functionally autonomous. Given enough of this in the context of trauma, individuals organize their lives around avoidance of triggers of trauma and often have downwardly adapted. Multiple triggers of traumatic intrusions have given way to helplessness, withdrawal, low-grade suspicion, cynicism, and interpersonal problems. When this is the case, the primary attention needs to be paid to the "stabilization of the social realm." Even when this has not occurred, the issue of balance is important.

Stage 3 of this model, then, is to attend to necessary developmental and life factors that subserve treatment and reasonable living. The issue here is to assure that life is being lived well (adequately) in the broad sense. Sometimes this can be easy. In a study by Foa, Hearst, and Riggs (1995) education alone or normalization of reactions had therapeutic benefit. Only three or four sessions were necessary—education regarding post-trauma reactions, relaxation, recounting of the trauma, and cognitive restructuring. These were of great benefit in averting chronic PTSD and depression compared with an assessment control. These interventions were specific to the trauma situation alone. We are talking more broadly.

Issues pertaining to Stage 3 should be assessed and addressed early in treatment. Deficiencies are prosecuted and followed as they may cause problems. Simply assessing the person's day-to-day activities, with a special focus on coping and social supports, is often all that is required. Implied is an active stance toward life, where social skills are required. These must be applied continuously and are best done with a coping repertoire of great latitude (Hobfoll et al., 1991). If stress management techniques prove to be equally effective as exposure-based methods, then intervening with less invasive treatment is appropriate.

"The Balance"

For some time PTSD treatment has involved stress management techniques—anger management, grief resolution, meditation, relaxation, biofeedback, relapse prevention, education, spirituality, fitness, and leisure groups. They have been applied in inpatient (and outpatient) settings for trauma care of Vietnam veterans. As cure became impossible, better living was. These ideas come from old places: The physician William Osler said that, if stuck feelings do not have a valve for expression, then other organs will weep. The word is out that diet and exercise help: What is not as clear is that the whole gamut of psychological interventions (social support, relationships, etc.) are equally important.

Plenty of lesions result from writings on wellness. The most important one is a perspective on living. A continuum of "treatment" can be arranged from surgery to meditation. The left side of the scale is the rational tertiary care practiced in big hospitals. Managed care surgery is a good example. The right side of the scale involves being, not doing. Paradoxical healing is one phrase used for the less rational side of care. Gershon and Straub (1987) identified seven sources of personal power: commitment, discipline, system support, inner guidance, non-rigid beliefs, love, and finding one's inner truth. People who have a remission in cancer, for example, shift from dependency to autonomy, change the quality of interpersonal relationships, express inner feelings, use a sound diet, confront disease, are less anxious and depressed, change their attitude in life, and have a spiritual focus. In effect, people in or out of trouble can feel in control of their lives—doing things, being a certain way, and acting with power in relationships. They accept self as is, perhaps the secret to health.

The connection between brain centers and the immune system is unmistakable. We know that, if you have a physical problem (like a heart attack) and become depressed, the likelihood of dying is considerably greater. When people repress any one emotion, they tend to do so with others; when they live less in one place, they live less in time and quality generally. People do better when they know that living is a journey, that life is filled with losses, that they are not special but are human beings, and that they must experience life's losses, objects, goals, mind, friends, and so on.

People who manage their upsetting emotions indulge in a form of disease prevention. Patients can benefit measurably when psychological needs are attended to (along with physical ones). We need to teach emotion management at times of crisis. The task of getting what you want cannot start from "I do not want it" position. It must be washed in the reason and feel of possibility. Attributions matter.

Practical Methods

We discuss three practical methods. First, the literature on CBT has assisted us here. The key idea of CBT as it applies to older people is to provide a behavioral armamentarium of skills and activities that increase positive behavior (Box 7-8). The application of these is straightforward and can be seen in CBT references (see Gallagher & Thompson, 1995). A loose rule of thumb is that the greater the level of dysfunction, the greater the proportion of behavioral to cognitive interventions needed (see Gallagher & Thompson, 1994). It has been helpful not to rely solely on cognitive techniques in therapy but to integrate behavioral methods and to use a variety of behavioral techniques with distressed older adults.

The Older Person's Pleasant Event Schedule, for example, can be used (Gallagher et al., 1981). This is a scale that identifies pleasant activities and attempts to maximize their occurrence. Simple tasks like being active and dealing with life's problems by being assertive and appropriate, have an impact on day-to-day living. These have been described by Lewinsohn, Biglan, and Zeiss (1979), Lewinsohn, Munoz, Youngren, and Zeiss (1978), Dick and Gallagher-Thompson (1995), Emery (1981), Thompson, Davies, Gallagher, and Krantz (1986), Thompson et al. (1991), and Zeiss and Lewinsohn (1986). Each of these interventions is actually simple in practice but require dedication, application, some repetition, and some monitoring.

Box 7-8
Behavioral Interventions

Pleasant Events Schedule
Activity Scheduling
Mastery Training
Social Skills Training
Assertiveness Training
Bibliotherapy
Relaxation Training
Scaling

Second, we also seek the practice of behavioral health principles for living altered life styles, an application of developmental health psychology. Most diseases have age distributions that are unique (see Siegler, 1994). Behavioral risk factors tend to increase with age and practically all have Age × Sex interactions. Even though age increases risk for all, those individuals who abuse these areas the most, have a greater number and amount of problems (Kannel & Vokonas, 1986). The behavioral risk factors (Box 7-9) most amenable to change are smoking, alcohol use, obesity, cholesterol level, Type A behavior pattern, job strain, psychosocial stress, and sexual behavior. Modification of risk factors are worth the effort. For cardiovascular diseases alone, Foreyt and Poston (1996) emphasized psychosocial factors (including hostility, Type D personality, depression, stress, and adherence to treatment).

Similarly, the major factors that reduce risk include sound preventive behaviors (Box 7-10). Practice of these represent an integration of the theoretical perspectives of developmental psychology (Baltes, 1987) and behavioral medicine. These apply to a daily regimen of care. In fact, the therapist can apply almost any outlined and clear

---

Box 7-9
Behavioral Risk Factors

1. Smoking → Bone loss, osteoporosis, CHD, myocardial infarction, CA of lung, bladder, mouth, and larynx, COPD.
2. Alcohol → CA of the stomach, breast, and falls.
3. Obesity and high lipids → HTN, diabetes mellitus, CHD.
4. High fat/low fiber → CA of colon, rectum, breast, and prostate.
5. HTN and diabetes → CHD.
6. Type A behavior, hostility, and job strain → CHD.
7. Sexual behavior → AIDS, cervical CA.

Box 7-10
Preventive Behaviors

1. Vitamin D and Calcium → Reduce bone loss.
2. Exercise → Reduce bone loss and heart disease mortality.
3. Aspirin → Reduce heart disease.
4. Fat reduction → Reduce heart disease.
5. Social support → Reduce mortality.
6. Internal control → Increase self care.
7. Good health habits and regular medical care → Overall health and vigor.

---

program involving exercise, diet, and behavioral habits. About these practices, Siegler (1994) writes:

> It is not sufficient to consider the older person who comes to the developmental health psychologist for assistance from only one perspective. If one does so, important variables may be ignored. (p. 137)

To this, Weil adds breathing deeply, balance in eating and drinking, a varied diet and water, exercise (45 min./day), spiritual health, meaningful relationships, and the assemblage of a medical team. Viscott (1996) adds positive interests; vacations, relaxation, meditation, entertainment, hobbies, sex, sharing, friends, love, work, mentors, and belief in self. Whatever combination of health factors promulgated by the therapist, they need to be committed to, regulated, and rewarded. And last, centenarians, those who live to 100+ years, perform most of these behaviors and do it with a sense of control (Poon, 1999).

Third, although we have addressed this before, social support deserves special mention. This task is, of course, multidimensional, a construct that entails the social skills of both the recipient and a significant other (sometimes a caretaker). Blazer (1998) stated that social support is the provision of feedback from the social environment that enables that person to negotiate intermittent or continual environmental stressors. With older folks it is often measured by roles and available attachments, the frequency of social attachments, perceived social support, and instrumental support. As the culture is the playground for the social environment, a friendly one for older people is always beneficial.

How people perceive social support is related to their own identity and social view of self (Whitbourne, 1985). In regards to trauma, if the trauma is intense and if the social support (and coping mechanisms) is inadequate following the trauma, the risk of pathological adjustment is high. We know of course that trauma events disrupt social networks (Solomon, 1986). Freedy, Shaw, Jarrell, and Masters (1992) assessed the "total" resources of victims (social roles, possessions, self- and world-views, and energy) and found that resource loss was directly related to psychological distress. Therefore, an evaluation of the quality and quantity of social support after the trauma, as well as tending to clinical interventions in these areas, are important. Interestingly, it might be argued that success of post-trauma processing of social support is related most to the degree of discrepancy between the client and others' perception of the trauma—who believes it to be more serious. If the client feels that others believe the trauma is less consequential, social support is lacking. This has applicability to older people in general.

Conclusion

So, this is what we are interested in: To alter lifestyle habits. If wanting, the application of educational or behavioral techniques for change is provided. Normalization and education are modal interventions. Suffused though the above tables are the tasks of having social support, being able to cope daily, and use of social skills on a bed of treatment expectation and acceptance. A not insignificant portion of change is attainable by explaining the reasons for treatment compliance, as well as for social supports, coping, and skill building.

Therapeutically, the older person needs two things for compliance. First, they require cognitive/behavioral beliefs that are committed to care of self. This requires many cognitive and behavioral forms and readings regarding these issues. It is a whole person commitment. Second, they should have sufficient internal (coping and social skills, as well as treatment compliance) and external (social supports) "power" to undertake and appreciate the therapy. Again, this is the province of the therapist. There are many "teachable moments" in the care of the older person here.

☐ Conclusion

Older people come in all varieties, those that are in trouble due to trauma, those who thrive, and those who do well but relapse by reworking the original trauma at developmental stages. Although this is not popular, many older patients use therapy for immediate results and for emotional refueling. Our task as health care professionals is to read each and help as individuals. We do this because we know that the difference in success with people is often simple: Given problems, those who are optimistic, who have hope, and who commit to act, do better.

In this chapter we have addressed the first parts of our treatment model. In this beginning effort we are managers and human caregivers, more than anything. This requires a friendly and listening ear. The "protective belt" that metaphorically surrounds later troubled listening of the older client is outlined in these three stages of the model. In many cases it is comprised of prescriptive and proscriptive rules. These are actually simple "do" and "don't" rules for action that are sufficient in and of themselves, or set the stage for the latter model parts.

The target here is to keep people committed and curious, encourage experimentation, and set the stage for other world views. This is important because we not only need narrative redress (Models 5 and 6), but behavioral ones as well (both sayings and doings). In order for these narrative components of care to be effective, the self management components must be in place. The clinician must be assured that the lifestyle is reasonably healthy and not interfering with life or (later) narrative repair. Healthy living is also its own reward. Interestingly, early purveyors of therapy of older people, those outlined by Tobin, Erikson, or Maslow, noted that treatment goals are related to control and empowerment (Walters & Goodman, 1990). Of course the trend in retirement living is total living, viewing the person as an active producer in self care.

In the grand scheme of things the treatment of the older person is human care. The task is just to get the person back to where we are, active and thriving. This applies at later life more than with any other age group. Often the psychotherapist is dealing with human problems. Unfortunately psychotherapists may be good at issues of therapy but not as good with problems of life. For good care, this status must alter at later life. This applies equally well to the person in the throes of trauma, and the one who remits.

The PTSD literature tells us that to be efficacious in treatment of trauma, two processes (exposure and assimilation) are involved. These are distinctly absent in these three model parts. This treatment requires a stage that provides more than validation by the therapist. Therapists in these stages are more than just apostles of permissiveness and self-tolerance. We need more: we turn to the more.

Finally, we note that there is overlap between Chapter 6 and Chapter 7. This is intended. The reader can go back and forth between Chapter 6 and all the stages of the model. Again, this is intended.

8

CHAPTER

Personality

Our contemporary understanding of personality structure is a fabulous ac-
complishment by any criteria, given the complexity and centrality of per-
sonality and human affairs. It is, I believe, the equal of the so-called Grand
Symposis in physics or Table of Elements in chemistry. Knowledge is power,
and I believe that self-knowledge is the ultimate power. It underwrites wise
decisions and intelligent choices of life, and psychology can contribute pro-
foundly to people's self-knowledge, empowering them to successfully navi-
gate this strange passage. We also have much to contribute to making people
healthier and happier.
Frank Farley (1996, p. 775)

A course in abnormal psychology usually ends with the chapter devoted to personality. It is that which is left over. In fact, one can argue that the reason that personality
is such a poor stepchild to the Axis I Disorders (like vice presidents to presidents) is
that they are derivatives: They are considered clones. However in the last decade and
a half personality has received considerably more respect.

Probably at its simplest level, personality represents traits that somehow maintain
consistency and pervade most facets of the person's actions. When personality crosses
some arbitrary threshold, it becomes a problem, a personality disorder (PD). It tends
to perpetrate itself, to foster vicious circles, and to cause an adaptive inflexibility
(Millon, 1984). What started out as a vehicle to provide order and organization in an
integrated system becomes itself a passive resistant creature that perpetuates a "bad"
status quo.

If personality is anything, it provides order, often an understandable "madness."
In this way, if knowledge of personality assists the clinician, it provides theory/
cohesion/treatment rules and information. This is a vision of the person on prototypes of action. These are personality styles. Personality then is the infrastructure for
the expression of problems. In this way symptoms have a functional value for the personality. And in this way too, clinician and client become participants and observers
in the processes that, if used properly, assist integrated treatment.

Personality is also about treatment in an integrated way. An integrated approach
respects both reason and emotion. The person needs to know and respect the biologi-

cal dimension and how these states created problems as well as how mind–brain interactions have ensued with a concatination of "givens." Personality (via temperament and overlearning) obeys few social contexts. To ignore the truth of this is tantamount to telling people to hide their nature. Kimble (1989) noted that behavior is an increasing function of independent underlying factors: Relatively enduring "potentials" of action and relatively more temporary "instigations" of action. We can change people by changing the habits (potentials) or by changing drives (instigations). Durable changes only occur with (long-lasting) potentials. This is personality. The "feel-good" therapies occur because they address the transient instigation: emotion, motivation, and inhibition.

For PTSD, personality is important because it is the construct that provides an understanding for the management of the victim. It is also helpful because for "usual PTSD therapy" the therapist needs help.

In this chapter we discuss Stage 4 of the model. We approach personality as a construct, and how the information of aging and trauma is transduced by personality. Just as mind and body are not separate but share a single information system, so too personality operates as a shared commitment to the needs of the person. We then borrow a theory to assist us: one can translate testable constructs into the implications of etiology and link these to interventions. Millon's biopsychosocial model assists in the knowing and caring for clients with trauma problems. Our goal is not the reconstruction of character, although possible, but to provide strategies and tactics for treatment that prevent protracted problems, or an excessive reliance on medication, or worse, nihilism. Supportive psychotherapy, the modal treatment effort to return the patient to baseline, is one that can serve as a needed backdrop for change (van Denberg & Choca, 1997).

This stage of the model then is about the background management of the victim. Personality is the one area where a careful study of individuals shows a congruency of attributes, a coherence and stability of functioning. It is a multioperational construct where there is an internal logic for care.

☐ Stage 4: Personality

"Life is managed: it is not cured. Learn to take charge of your life."
Phillip McGraw

What exactly is a personality? (See Box 8-1) There are several answers. As we march through the person from inside to outside, personality represents complex emergent processes of the brain. No one neural pathway, lobe, or hemisphere is the "site" of any complex personality function, such as impulsivity, obsessiveness, or hysterical regression. This is despite efforts of Eysenck (1981), Gray (1991), and Damasio, Tranel, and Damasio (1991), who have provided biological bases for personality. They have affixed names in the cerebrum that subserve behavior. Translated into psychological thinking, Oldham and Morris (1990) have ascribed a particular self-image and a particular style to each of the DSM disorders. The obsessive-compulsive patient, for example, sees him/herself as "conscientious" and develops a style of "correctness." Inner script and core conflicts become crucial issues, organizing principles of the unfolding personality. They "determine" whether the person evolves along normal lines or abnormal ones. Presumably these are titrated to "brain" functions.

To the perveyor of the construct personality, the essence of structure is covariation. Conceptually, personality structure is best viewed as hierarchical in nature; specific

---

Box 8-1
General Facts of Personality

Personality is a covariance structure of "understandable" components.

Personality is a category (PD) or a dimension (trait), a type and amount of several traits.

Personality influences symptom formation of Axis I disorders.

For each personality, selected domains are more "core" than others (proto-typical).

A portion of personality is based on a hard-wired component (of personality) labeled temperament.

There are several models of personality. The predisposition model suggests that the personality directs the expression of symptoms.

Personality has measurement problems.

Personality is both a moderator and mediator of other variables.

Personality causes problems (see below) in treatment. The treatment of personality involves integration: Selected PDs probably react more poorly to treatment outcome (e.g., borderline) and other PDs (dependent) are more amenable to care. Severe PDs cause special problems (i.e., schizotypal, borderline, and paranoid).

---

covarying behaviors give rise to narrowband constructs, such as pervasiveness; then mid-level constructs evolve, such as dominance; then higher order constructs, such as extroversion. Personality, of course, is loaded with constructs: locus of control, self-efficacy, optimism, resilience, to name a few. Although the constructs are different, they have in common the feature of being trait-like and they are positioned in such a way as to be useable. They can be easily translated into personality traits. They are, in effect, a middle level that represents the science of factor analysis and the practicality of the diagnostic system (Millon & Davis, 1996). It is at this meso-level that the researcher and clinician alike can take some comfort in the "explainability and usability" of the construct. Watson, Clark, and Harkness (1994) noted:

> There is remarkable conceptual overlap and empirical agreement among the various systems, and researchers of normal-range personality. Personality has reached a broad consensus on its structure. (p. 216)

Personality is then a covariance structure of the salient domains of the person. Personality measures person parts both visible and invisible as part of the validation process. Each personality possesses a set of necessary "constraints." To the extent that the personality of the person approximates the prototype, then understanding is complete. Personality also is structurally integrated. If the clinician sees trait feature A, it implies B. If one or a few components are absent, that is not a problem. Of course this rarely occurs and the idiographic features of the person are present. It is both science and the person that makes for the understanding.

Personality can be considered as either a category (personality disorder; PD) or a dimension (trait). The border between personality and a PD is conceptually unclear. Traits are especially fascinating because they account for more of the variance in predicting psychopathology and outcomes in general (Millon & Davis, 1996; Widiger, 1991). It is probable that a PD is an extreme of normal personality (Strack, Lorr, & Campbell, 1992), a prototype. The DSM-IV holds that a PD (categories) markedly deviates from the norm and manifests a pattern that is both fixed and affects the person's life in multiple and clear ways, having been with the person for long periods of time. You might say that each personality has a domain of success in which they have no problem. Core beliefs are likely to have "zones of safety" until attacked by stress. It is when the person moves outside this comfort zone that problems arise. Then they are activated. Then the personality becomes rigid and creates problems. The purpose of treatment of PDs is to relax the constraints of the domains. That is, the professional tries to provide the person with more flexibility.

A person is then both a type and amount of several traits related to personality. As such, the person can be categorized and have a varying amount of that category. The person in effect has a profile of traits. Interest is both on the degree of pathology or threshold above which a person has a problem, as well as the type of person with a unique profile.

That said, some personality features are more "core" than others. This implies two things. First, there are selected personality domains that are protypical representations of the construct. For an avoidant personality, the issue of cognitive mistrust is central, for example. We will discuss this below.

The second issue involves "modifiable and non-modifiable" components of personality, basic tendencies and characteristic adaptations (Harkness & Libenfield, 1997), ones that are changeable and ones that are not. Paris (1997) believed that 40% of the variance between individuals is due to heredity. This probably represents traits and not PDs. Consensus has it that temperamental (non-modifiable) variables determine the form taken by the personality pathology but are insufficient to determine the presence of a PD itself. This points out that heredity and early learnings pose as risk factors in the development of a PD and are not themselves causative.

This is relevant because in treatment one's biology is not about limits but about the perimeters of comfort. Temperament is primarily biological and instinctive and secondarily learned, influenced by thoughts and interpretations. In this way emotions or moods, the temperament side of personality, is biological and less a product of early learning. Therapies that ignore temperament run into problems because they try to change something that is hard to change. Personality then is about many things and one of them is temperament (Magnusson, 1999).

The model that best "explains" the interaction of personality (Axis II) and symptom disorder (Axis I), between trait and state is also important. Every psychological test evaluates both states and traits. Nature cannot be carved well at its joints here. Perhaps this explains in part the fact that there are several comorbid models of personality (Hyer, Brandasma, & Boyd 1997; Starcevic, 1992). For our purposes, these can be reduced to predisposition or interaction models versus complication models. For the former, personality dictates the adjustment of the individual; for the latter, the situational stressor alters the complexion of the personality causing it to be more dysfunctional, even blending with the Axis I disorder. With the onset of PTSD then, personality traits may both alter and be altered by an Axis I problem. In a way the predisposition model organizes the pathology but remains affected after an Axis I disorder. The personality both dictates and remembers. It even creates more trauma.

In addition, several possible relationships can exist between PDs (or traits) and Axis I (or Axis III) disorders. Clinical syndromes and PDs can co-occur; people with Axis I have a PD; not all Axis I patients have a PD; the relationship between the two is one of degree; and both are distinct categories of psychopathology that can co-occur.

Several measuring problems of personality are also present, internal or external to the construct—comorbidity (McCrae, 1987), poor reliability (Mellsop, Vargese, Joshua, & Hicks, 1982), and diagnostic validity (Widiger & Sanderson, 1995), to name a few. In addition, personality is also messy because it seems to moderate and mediate many other variables. That is, personality dictates "when" certain events will hold (moderator) and will predict the outcome of other variables (mediator). A PD at later life, for example, moderates the expression of bereavement. An understanding of these provides more precision for the clinician. So, although the construct personality is "alive" with possibilities and thereby a problem, it has several things to offer.

In sum, personality may be viewed as "set in plaster," as William James (1902) held. It provides trait consistency and is amenable to understanding and change. Perhaps the best take of this construct is that it represents an enduring profile of a person's traits. With stress, the personality style suggests a way to adapt for the person that is persuasive. It often directs the expression of symptoms. PTSD is one result. The clinician can use a double-think attitude on both personality and symptoms. Progress (or lack there of) can occur on both fronts.

Treatment

We treat PTSD clients with PDs differently because they are different. As a rule, such clients do not comply in therapy, have chronic problems, are often unaware of their impact on others, are often in crises, and do not change. Typically, therapists become frustrated, are often more directive, provide a lengthier therapy, place a greater emphasis on historical data, and question their ability to perform therapy ("Am I helping this patient? It is my responsibility to ..."). What a way to make a living!

But the construct provides important information for treatment. Magnavita (1997) wrote:

> I believe that the challenge for the next century is to further refine and develop these integrated short term treatment models so that they offer help for the personality disordered individual. The task is to increase the treatment potency and also shorten the length of treatment. In order to accomplish this we need to determine which combination of approaches will be effective with which patient. We need to develop multimodal treatment formats that are sequentially applied and based on in-depth assessment of personality structure. We need to reconsider the assumption that personality is set and alterable only after many years of extensive psychotherapy." (p. 94)

It is only in recent years that the perspective of personology has been useful in treatment. This has involved the integration of care emphasizing Axis II (Clarkin, Francis, & Perry, 1992). Several are worth noting. Beutler (Beutler, 1991; Beutler & Clarkin, 1990) emphasized the clinical complexity of presenting problems and argued for personality-based components to treat people, paying less attention to diagnostic titles and more to reactance levels, coping styles, and motivational arousal (personality factors). In this way, treatment-matching should focus on a more theory-driven conceptualization of a case before forming a treatment plan. This group boldly asks whether a knowledge of Axis I really assists the clinician in treatment. Blatt and Schrichman (1983) and Beck (1976), among others, developed bivariate typologies of treatment (as well as measures) based on personality. Both have become rather popular.

Of course patients with Axis II problems worsen treatment outcomes or the course of treatment (Hyer, Brandasma, & Boyd, 1997). Several studies address the influence of

PDs on the symptomatology, severity, relapse, and treatment response of psychiatric disorders, especially anxiety and affective disorders (Garyfallos et al., 1994; Millon & Davis, 1995; Ruegg & Francis, 1995; Sperry, 1999). In a summary paper, Ruegg and Frances (1995) briefly discussed 30 studies (50 when eating disorders and substance abuse are included) between 1992 and 1995 that reflect the relationship between Axis 1 problems and PDs. The message was that different PDs influence the expression of symptoms. Also, this group identified 16 studies that had a relationship between PDs and medical conditions, especially pain and HIV. Ruegg and Francis also showed that the presence of PDs worsened the psychiatric outcome of 10 of 13 studies. These authors noted that the time has come to assess more judiciously the etiology, pathogenesis, treatment response, and cost of PDs.

There are several methods developed that highlight the relevance of personality, the therapeutic need to restructure affective, cognitive, and defensive styles, and to integrate moments in therapy (e.g., Laylen, Newman, Freeman, & Moore, 1993). There are at least 16 established case management systems that argue for the influence of interpersonal patterns (Eells, 1998). Several therapists view personality as a tiered system, a graduated problematized taxonomy of PDs. Stone (1993) mentions three: (a) high amenability, which includes the dependent, histrionic, obsessive-compulsive, avoidant, and depressive personality disorders; (b) intermediate amenability, which includes narcissistic, borderline, and schizotypal personality disorders; and (c) low amenability, which includes paranoid, passive-aggressive, schizoid, and antisocial personality disorders. The problem-maintenance structure that serves as the substrate for each disorder is different, the prognosis perhaps depending on the degree to which traits of the disorders in the third category are present. The role of personality is clear but the form is cloudy.

Retzlaff (1995) outlined six possible options for the treatment of a client with a comorbid Axis I and Axis II disorder (Box 8-2). The first option is the most typical used in clinical practice. Clinicians treat Axis I disorders only. It is the fourth (aware/treat), fifth (aware/treat), and sixth (use to help/treat) that are most typical of personological therapists, however. They involve the treatment of the Axis I disorder in the service of the Axis II problem. The therapist can make an informed decision to care for the client with an awareness of both problem states. At the least both disorders should be in therapeutic awareness.

Box 8-2
Psychotherapy Decisions with Axis I and Axis II Comorbidity

Clinical Syndrome	Personality Disorder
Treat	Unaware
Unaware	Treat
Treat	Aware
Aware	Treat
Treat	Use to help
Use to help	Treat

☐ PTSD and Personality

"Personality traits play an important role in the nature and treatment of the human stress response. This is not to say, however, that formal psychotherapy needs to be an integral aspect of all stress treatment/stress management paradigms. Processes such as relaxation training, biofeedback, and even health education practices are clearly capable of altering dysfunctional practices. Yet, there are instances where chronic stress-related diseases are a direct function of personologic disturbances such as dysfunctional self-esteem, persistent cognitive distortions, irrational assumptions, inappropriate expectations of self and others, and so on. In such cases, some concerted psychotherapeutic effort would clearly be indicated. The most effective "mix" of therapeutic technologies (e.g., relaxation training, psychotherapy, hypnosis) remains to be determined by the therapist on a case-by-case basis."
George Everly (1989, pp. 117–118)

PTSD has been treated for years without a recognition of the workings of personality. Maybe this should not be the case. In a recent publication, Keane and Wolfe (1990) provided an endorsement for a better understanding of personality in the formation of PTSD by "enhancing the sophistication of these (personality) assessment methods." Hyer and Associates (1994; Hyer, Brandsma, & Boyd, 1997) have identified over 50 studies in this area. A common finding is the one found by Weisaeth (1984). He followed victims of a Norwegian fire over time. Results showed that the prevalence of acute PTSD was related mostly to the initial intensity of the exposure, but after 4 years, pre-accident psychological functioning was a more important determinant of PTSD. The variables found to contribute consistently to predisposition adjustment models in other studies of chronic war trauma PTSD are drug abuse or dependence before the military, being raised in a family that had a hard time making ends meet, having had symptoms of an affective disorder before going to war (Vietnam), and exhibiting problem behaviors in childhood (Kulka et al., 1990). van der Kolk (1999) has noted that the combination of early abuse, chronic dissociation, physical problems for which no medical cause can be found and a lack of adequate self-regulatory processes is likely to have profound effects on personality development. These may include disturbances of self, such as the sense of separateness and disturbances of body image, view of one's self as helpless and damaged, difficulty in trust and intimacy, and self-assertion among others.

Prospective studies on the influence of PTSD have also been attempted. Using early grade school (Card, 1983) or premorbid college data (Schnurr, Friedman, & Rosenberg, 1991), early "personality problems" were noted with (Vietnam combat) victims with a lifetime prevalence of PTSD symptoms greater than those who had no symptoms. Two additional studies (Foy, Osato, Houskamp, & Neumann, 1992; McCranie, Hyer, Boudewyns, & Woods, 1991) have confirmed the person–event interaction or threshold model of PTSD etiology. In addition, the psychodynamic literature (e.g., Emery & Emery, 1989; Emery, Emery, Shama, Quiana, & Jassani, 1991; Hendin, 1983; Hendin, Pollinger, Singer, & Ulman, 1981; Horowitz, 1986; McFarlane, 1990; Wilson, 1988) and a handful of studies addressing traditional diagnostic (DSM) personality problems (Hyer & Boudewyns, 1985), especially antisocial (Lipkin, Scurfield, & Blank, 1983; Wilson & Zigelbaum, 1983) and borderline traits (Berman, Price, & Gusman, 1982), have been supportive. Most notable among this grouping is the work of Horowitz et al. (1984), who developed a method of treatment for PTSD based on the information processing of the stressors and character structure of the person.

It is not surprising too that several authors have developed a model of PTSD in which personality factors received considerable attention. Joseph, Williams, and Yule (1995) disaggregated personality factors according to attributional style, a relatively stable personality characteristic, locus of control and interdependent constructs based on generalized expenditures of reinforcement and attitudes and beliefs, where dysfunctional individuals have negative assumptions that predispose to anxiety or depression. These authors believe that ideation is influenced by personality appraisals and reappraisals. Joseph, Williams, and Yule (1995) stated:

> What is likely … is that personality attributes help shape the specific cognitions about the trauma which in turn determine the nature and intensity of emotional states, such as fear, rage, guilt or shame, which in turn influences the choice of coping and level of crisis support received. It would seem useful in helping to explain the individual differences in the severity and chronicity of symptoms to take into account the role of stimulus appraisal and personality factors. (p. 537)

The research literature is in agreement that PTSD is strongly influenced by the intensity of the trauma and that personality factors can influence one's susceptibility to experiencing the traumatic event and the severity of the symptoms, once the event has occurred (Lauterbach & Vrana, 1996). Helzer, Robins, and McEvoy (1987) noted that, even after accounting for the variance due to the level of trauma exposure, personality variables continued to make a significant contribution to the prediction of trauma severity. There is also evidence in support of the hypothesis that trauma exposure elevates the "exposure personality traits" (Resnick, Foa, Donahoe, & Miller, 1989). Thus, there may be a reciprocal relationship between personality traits and trauma exposure. Elevated levels of these personality traits may increase the probability of experiencing a trauma event, which in turn increases the level of the personality variables.

In the extant literature, a handful of studies now exist too that have used a personality scale—the MCMI (Millon Clinical Multiaxial Inventory)—in the evaluation of PTSD (combat-related). The Passive-Aggressive/Avoidant code (8-2 or 2-8) has been "universally" found on this scale to represent the personological effects of trauma (Hyer, Davis, Woods, Albrecht, & Boudewyns, 1992; Hyer, Woods, & Boudewyns, 1991; McDermott, 1986; Robert et al., 1985; Sherwood, Funari, & Piekorski, 1990) and for the MCMI-II (Hyer et al., 1994; Munley, Bains, Bloem, Busby, & Pendziszewski, 1997). Bryer, Nelson, Miller, and Krol (1987) replicated this pattern also in sexually abused women. In all these studies the borderline personality was in evidence also, suggesting the intense nature and increased pathogenesis of problems (Southwick, Yehuda, & Giller, 1993). This profile was also noted among elder veterans of Korea and WWII (Boyd, Hyer, & Summers, 1996).

The presence of a PD is so prevalent among this population that different attempts to define this chronic form of PTSD have led to personologic speculation; labels such as *complicated or reactivated trauma* (Catherall, 1991; Hiley-Young, 1992), *abusive personality* (Dutton, 1994), one characteristic of abusers, as well as our own *traumatic personality* (Hyer et al., 1994). Personality may become "complex." Complex PTSD represents an alteration in regulation of affect and impulses, manifest by problems in the modulation of anger and aggression; alterations in attention and consciousness, manifest by the amnesia, transient dissociative episodes, and depersonalization; alterations in self-perception, manifest by feelings of helplessness; alterations in perception of the perpetrator, manifest by feelings of vengeance; alterations in relationships, manifest by isolation; alterations in somatization, manifest in chronic pain or sexual symptoms; and alterations in systems of meaning, manifest by feelings of despair (van der Kolk, 1999).

In the context of PTSD, then, symptoms "do" something to personality or vice versa. Or maybe a diathesis applies. Personality may mediate the influence on outcomes. Ford et al. (1997) noted that successful treatment of PTSD involves a fundamental skill in containing and modulating intense emotion and arousal, in effect, better object-relational skills. Additional analyses suggested that the object-relations measure may serve as a good mediator variable, which accounts for the modifying affect of personality disorder status on treatment outcome. Interestingly, Perry, Lavori, Pagano, Hoke, and O'Donnell (1992) used a "mini" longitudinal design and showed that the pathogenicity of interpersonal events was not by itself related to problems, but rather to the type of personality psychopathology. Evidence, then, exists that "vulnerable" victims respond poorly after the trauma (e.g., Benedek, 1985; Black, 1982).

Unfortunately, few studies exist on which patient characteristics interact positively or negatively with exposure treatment of PTSD (Hyer, McCranie, Boudewyns, & Sperr, 1996). Also, there are few data that provide information on the effect of acute and short-term trauma on personality and vice versa. Nonetheless, we believe that treatment problems and probably the treatment symptoms (the actual trauma memory) are best *managed* by an awareness and use of personality. Again, the clinician is requested to "double think," person(ality) and trauma interpersonal styles (Horowitz et al., 1984; Hyer et al., 1994; McAdams, 1990; Ulman & Spiegel, 1994). In the context of trauma, the initial phase includes a careful understanding of the meaning of the trauma and other symptoms—their functional value (secondary gain) for the person. A personality assessment and a developmental history (life-style) then can be introduced. Core interpersonal/cognitive/emotional/behavioral domains are isolated and addressed (see Millon & Davis, 1995).

☐ Aging and Personality

"If we understand how people change as they age, we will be in a much better position to interpret the course of an individual's life."
Paul Costa (1994)

Personality, as it applies to older folks, is an issue about which there is little agreement. Personality has been touted as both stable and changing. Reacting to Freud, Erikson, the theoritian of the elderly, told us that a stage theory applied delineating developmental tasks that occur throughout the lifespan. Or, maybe traits influence a person only when the situation is relevant or matches the trait sensitivity. We would hope that whichever model applies, that assessment of this approach would be broad enough to allow for the expression of the aging trait. How would an older extrovert look, for example?

In recent years, research on personality and aging has witnessed two shifts: one away from the use of categorical types toward an analysis of personality traits and psychological dimensions; the other away from psychoanalytic models toward cognitive and behavioral paradigms. Mostly, however, writings have been interested in the phenonemon of aging and its influence on personality. This has taken the form of research addressing the constructs at later life most related to personality.

In this section we address the several issues of personality related to older folks; history, change (and the special case for dementia), PDs at later life and assessment problems, stress at later life, the interaction of personality and the narrative, and, at the end, the special case of dementia.

History

From an aging perspective, the history of personality is fascinating. After the guiding theories of Erikson and Jung came early data sets and speculation, much of it in search of new theoretical perspectives (Block, 1971; Butler, 1963; Lowenthal, Thuner, & Chiriboga, 1975; Maas & Kuypers, 1974; Neugarten, 1979; Reichard, Livison, & Peterson, 1962). In the late 1970s a new generation of theories of adult development appeared (Gould, 1978; Livenson, 1978; Vaillant, 1977). Despite an absence of scientific rigor, Gail Sheehy's (1976) *Passages* was a bestseller. In the 1970s also came a series of longitudinal studies of adults (see Baltes, Reese, & Lipsitt, 1980). These data provided a way to test many of the theories and to describe the course of personality in adulthood.

On the heels of this also was born clinician-thinking (Gould, 1978) or life transition-thinking (Levinson et al., 1978) postulates relevant to the lifespan. These were men who intensively studied small samples. They were built on Erikson's model. It was an easy transition for psychobiography and life narratives to appear on the scene (Levinson, 1990; McAdams, 1990). In the background were "the" aging theories of the time, which affected this thinking, including disengagement theory (Cummings & Henry, 1961) and activity theory (Maddox, 1976).

In the last decade, several theorists highlighted personality variables as they relate to age. Whitbourne deserves special mention. Noting that loss is part of life, Susan Whitbourne (Whitbourne & Collins, 1999) noted that the concept of identity serves the clinician well in the aging process. This involves a person's sense of self over time, including physical functioning, cognition, social relationships, and experiences of the world. Whitbourne saw identity as the organizing principal through which the world is interpreted. Physically this is most relevant to older people as they watch for a "threshold" over which they may roam and in so doing see themselves as aging or in some trouble. This probably begins in midlife.

Assimilation/accommodation, identity assimilation, and identity accommodation, to be precise, are the constructs of importance here (Whitbourne & Collins, 1999). The former allows us to get away with the slights of aging ("This is not that important") and the latter reminds us excessively that there are problems ("I am over the hill"). The ideal is a dynamic equilibrium or balance in which the individual holds a stable sense of self but is able to make changes. In one study, Whitbourne and Collins (1999) identified thresholds of appearance, competence, and cognitive functioning reached at middle age. Where appearance is concerned, a threshold is reached early; with competence, it occurs at age 65 or greater. Competence is more important at these ages than looks.

Other personality theorists too have been concerned about the processes of aging and personality. Baumeister (1991) believed that people add up changes favorably regardless of the insult; Emmons (1986) asserted that people hold personal strivings that are based on a personal goal system, allowing them to feel positive; Cantor (Cantor & Kihlstrom, 1987) developed a life theory in development (we are content depending only on the life tasks we identify with and accomplish). More recently, the life narrative has become popular: Memories are markers of adult development and maturity (Kotre, 1995). Although it is probable that memories are influenced more by personality than the other way around, the interesting point is that we do not have an age-sensitive personality focus.

Personality Change

Botwinick (1984) presented three views of personality development: personality does not change, personality changes are due to generational impact and not aging, and personality changes because of age with a maturational or biologic basis. This is a strange mix in which, on the one hand, personality is reasonably stable and, on the other hand, adult development is an ongoing dynamic process. We believe that change occurs against a background of stability. Developmental change impacts on the stability of personality at later life. This can occur for the better or for the worse.

For starters, most data suggest that older people seem to think that they are doing well relative to younger ages. As one example of this, older folks believe that they stayed "pretty much the same" (51%) or had changed "a little" (35%). Not surprisingly, the direction of change was positive: 69% felt they were now lower in neuroticism, 78% more "curious, open-minded, and imaginative," and 73% felt they were more "helpful, sympathetic, and trusting." Older adults see themselves as less impulsive or driven by anxiety (Gynther, 1979) and more emotionally complex, with more complex reactions to events (Schulz, 1982), and more complete experience of and ability to control emotional states (Labouvie Vief et al., 1989). Zweig and Hillman (1999) argued for the development of a greater range of emotions and greater experience of the transformation of emotions as likely outcome of increased experience throughout life. If this is continual throughout life, the implication is that with increasing years, there is at least the potential for greater self-knowledge and the development of a more complex self.

Most evidence suggests that the process of personality change is a normative, maturational phenomenon that does not alter much after age 30 (Costa, 1994). After all, both Freud and James said so. Studies looking at longitudinal comparisons of personality traits at later life found general stability (Costa & McCrae, 1978; Schaie & Parkham, 1976; Siegler, George, & Okun, 1979). In a review of these studies, Botwinick (1984) felt that the preponderance of evidence leans toward stability of traits across time and within respective cohorts, with change occurring only in scattered traits.

Currently, the most accepted taxonomy of personality traits (that have documented trait stability across time) rests on the five-factor model (see Costa & Widiger, 1994; McCrae & Costa, 1985b, 1987). Those familiar with this model of personality know of the work of Costa and McCrae (1992). These authors point out that five comprehensive, universal, and heritable traits have been consistently derived from multiple studies: neuroticism, extroversion, openness to experience, agreeableness, and conscientiousness. With respect to these specific traits over time, studies have found decreased extroversion (Costa, McCrea, Zonderman, Barbano, Lebowitz, & Larson, 1986), increased introversion (Eysenck, 1957; Gutman, 1966; Heron & Chown, 1967), and stability in neuroticism (Costa & McCrae, 1984; McCrae, 1987) defined as the "tendency to experience negative emotions such as fear, anger, and guilt" (Costa & McCrae, 1988, p. 259). Studies on related traits have found a decrease in activity and impulsivity (Douglas & Arenberg, 1978; Eysenck, Pearson, Easting, & Allsopp, 1985), increased depression as measured by the MMPI (Britton & Savage, 1966), increased hypochondriasis (Botwinick, 1984), low levels of clinically significant anxiety (Schulz, 1985) with a linear decline across time (Schaie & Geiwitz, 1982), and stability of subjective well-being (Larson, 1978; Costa et al., 1987), with no increase in negative emotions (Malatesta & Kalnok, 1984; Schulz, 1985).

Costa (1994) stated:

> These findings are of great importance in understanding the course of normal aging. Age is only weakly related to personality traits; attempts to describe periods of life in terms of characteristic dispositions are therefore unlikely to succeed. Stereotypes that depict older men and women as depressed, withdrawn, rigid, and cranky are without empirical foundation. Adults of all ages show a wide range of individual differences, and these differences are likely to be more important in predicting well-being, coping, and interpersonal relations than is age.

Analyses then from many personality scales support the conclusion that there is little or no change in the mean levels of traits in any of the five domains of personality in adulthood (Costa, 1994). This applies to tests that assess different domains of personality also. Given variation both within and across studies in the stability coefficients for different scales, "there is no doubt that there is substantial stability in individual rank-order for adults" (Costa, 1994). Interestingly, some groups have found women to be more flexible in their organization of personality across the lifespan than men (Haan, Millsap, & Harka, 1987). Interesting too, this group concluded that in spite of considerable stability across many transitions, the organization of personality in late life was much different from that of childhood.

In sum, there is some consensus then that change is best represented by a negatively accelerating slope with a positive gradient for most traits. Of course, it is also clear that the nature of a trait may alter across time: an extroverted youth may present as a different extrovert at later life. This especially applies to emotions (see below), and whatever pattern is applicable for the person, this can be altered to some degree when trauma or some major precipitating event occurs. Pervin (1983) quite correctly noted that any change across the lifespan is determined by the definition of change, the time period measured, and the method of measurement. In a refinement of this, Kendrick and Funder (1988) noted ways in which persons and situations interact: Traits influence behavior only when the situation is relevant and that traits are more easily expressed in some situations than others. And, Mischel and Shoda (1999) holds that the situation is the role determinant of a person's activity. Age is tied more to the situation than the personality.

PDs in Later Life

The literature on PDs in late life is sparse, given the history of uncertainty about whether the DSM Axis II even represents an appropriate nosology for the elderly (Fogel & Westlake, 1990). Various authors have suggested a lower prevalence of PDs in older than younger adults in clinical and epidemiological samples (Casey, 1988; Kroessler, 1990), suggested no differences between elderly men and women (13% prevalence rates; Ames & Molinari, 1994), and have found fewer personality disorders represented overall particularly in Cluster B (Abrams, Rosendahl, Card, & Alexopoulos, 1994; Kunik et al., 1994). Among older inpatients, prevalence studies of personality disorders found a high incidence of dependent and avoidant personality disorders and traits (Abrams et al., 1987; Casey & Schrodt, 1989). Prevalence rates for PDs among these and other studies (in hospital-based psychiatric settings) found figures ranging from 1% to 56%.

In perhaps the best overview of this area, Abrams and Horowitz (1999) used a meta-analytic approach to review the literature for trends concerning the frequency and distribution of PD symptomatology in older adults and to consider implications for future investigating. Eleven articles published from 1980 through 1994 met study criteria, including a focus on older adults (age 50 and above) and an assessment of PDs that included the full spectrum of disorders. Overall, the prevalence of PDs in this age group was 10%. The frequency of PDs in the individual studies included in the analysis ranged from 6% in a sample of geriatric patients treated for depression to 33% in a separate sample of recovered elderly depressives. It appears too that older people with a PD are at increased risk for other Axis I disorders.

In an update (in a meta-analysis between 1987 and 1997) Abrams and Horowitz (1999) again assessed 16 articles on PD and older people. Among older patients with affective disorders the prevalence of a PD is between 6% and 72%. Cluster C is the most common. The prevalence rate was 20% with paranoid, self-defeating, and schizoid being the most prevalent. This would of course argue against an age effect on PD. PD does not burn out with age.

Several other authors, Abrams included (e.g., Kunik et al., 1993), have commented on the relatively high proportion of personality disorder, Not Otherwise Specified (NOS), in their samples, suggesting that personality dysfunction may be more frequent in this age group than would be indicated by the number of subjects meeting full criteria for specific disorders. For this reason, the use of assessment instruments that provide dimensional as well as categorical data, such as the Personality Disorder Examination (Loranger et al., 1987), can be helpful in capturing the contributions of personality dysfunction to the overall clinical picture presented by older patients. Further, older individuals with a PD may be more vulnerable to the selected Axis I disorders, as major depression (Abrams, Alexopoulos, & Young, 1987), or, when a PD is present, the first episode of depression may occur earlier in life (Abrams et al., 1994; Kunik et al., 1993).

For example, Devanand et al. (2000) assessed PDs in the elderly and found that they were associated with an earlier age at onset of a depressive illness, a greater life time history of comorbid Axis I disorders, a greater severity of depressive symptoms, and a lower socioeconomic status.

Clustering PDs may be a better way to capture the essence of aging and the effects of personality on behavior. There is at least more agreement on these areas than the specifity of the Axis II pathology with advanced ages. Perhaps old ideas of a global personality (e.g., mature and immature), are sufficient to explain the effects.

Assessment of PDs

The study of PDs and personality in general in the elderly has been clouded by conceptual and methodological difficulties. As implied above, the state of this literature may lead some to underestimate the clinical importance of PDs in the aging population. Criteria for the various PDs are probably age-biased.

Personality patterns may "naturally" reformulate to accommodate to the needs of later life. Solomon (1981) distinguished between labile disorders, characterized by affective and behavioral lability and including Borderline, Narcissistic, Dependent, Histrionic, and Antisocial disorders, and stable disorders, characterized by overcontrol of affect and impulses, including paranoid, schizoid, schizotypal, and compulsive disorders. He proposed that labile types decrease in symptom intensity with aging, with less impulsivity and violent crime, but with depression and hypochondriasis serving as common endpoints. Synder, Pitts, and Gustin (1983) believed that it is uncommon to find a borderline diagnosis after the age of 40. In terms of dramatic cluster disorders, narcissistic and histrionic personality disorders are thought to show gradual improvement (Solomon, 1981; Vaillant & Perry, 1990). Alternatively, individuals with narcissistic or histrionic personality disorders may be especially devastated by losses in physical function and attractiveness, occupational opportunities, self-esteem and self-identity, along with increased dependence on others (Goldstein, 1992). Epidemiological studies have found a decreased prevalence of antisocial personality disorder with age (Zweig & Hillman, 1999). Individuals with anxious cluster disorders may be particularly vulnerable to many of the age-specific stressors cited by Sadavoy (1987) and Solomon (1981). Stable types, on the other hand, remain so or become more rigid. Symptoms of compulsive and passive-aggressive disorders may be exacerbated at later life, being especially vulnerable to depression (Solomon, 1981).

Similarly several aspects of previously maladaptive behaviors become more adaptive in later life. The detached and dependent personalities especially may alter. Avoidant and schizoid individuals may value the enhanced social isolation brought about by limited mobility and resources. Schizoid individuals may better tolerate social losses. Dependent individuals may welcome newly available health and social services, and value having fewer social and occupational responsibilities that require decisions (Gurland, 1984). Solomon believed too that schizoid and schizotypal individuals become more eccentric, withdrawn, and anxious, and often develop secondary psychopathology. In addition, behavioral changes due to age-associated stresses, such as the appearance of dependent or avoidant behaviors, may meet criteria for a personality disorder without a previous history of maladaptive behaviors on the presence of other pervasive criteria. The presentation may represent the re-emergence of previously maladaptive behaviors, brought out by the stresses of aging, without a clear or available history of similar behaviors.

Kagan (1980) labeled the "face change" of a variable across time as *heterotypic continuity*. This refers to the way a variable alters as a result of age. Attachment, for example, means one thing to a 6-year-old and another to a 70-year-old. *Functional equivalence* refers to the unique behaviors that emerge from a latent construct at various ages. The child who kicks when young, hits other adolescents when older, and is verbally tactless when old is an example. Functional equivalence then is the primary feature of heterotypic continuity. This raises many possible problems with measurement of personality: Is it the context that causes the difference or is their something in the "equivalence" (in the person): Is their something in the interaction of the person and the situation (and age): What are the best ways to assess this and the best ways to analyze this? Lest we become nihilists, we say again that people are reasonably consistent in regards to personality across time.

Stress in the Context of the Older Personality

Results of longitudinal data sets suggest that trauma can influence personality stability but only mildly. Several personality models have addressed the issue of loss or stress in their formulations, but the experience of stress does bring on problems. Stress can be both internal and external. Referencing older people, Sadavoy (1987; Sadavoy & Fogel, 1992) proposed three major pathways of symptom expression: (a) aberrant interactional patterns with social contracts, such as clinging, depressive, panic, or angry entitlement; (b) hypochondriasis, where the body is used as a form of communication; and (c) depressive withdrawal, sometimes culminating in suicide. Solomon (1981) also supported the view that aging provides unique stresses, often simultaneously, which can sometimes overwhelm psychic defenses and coping styles. In response to overwhelming stress, PDs may first manifest in later life because maladaptive behaviors become exaggerated, social networks are insufficient to absorb stress, or major psychiatric illnesses, such as depression or dementia, intervene.

A diminished sense of mastery over one's environment can start a chain reaction leading to helplessness, fear, or anger. Jacobowitz and Newton's (1990) model of psychopathology in late life focuses on the importance of stress, but from the perspective of premorbid character structure. Individuals who are prone to late life psychopathology, such as those with an underlying PD, enter adulthood with impairment due to unresolved interpersonal or intrapsychic conflicts and injuries. Being less able to draw on earlier relationships, positive values, and other sources of self-esteem to build internal psychological strength, personality problems develop. Griffin and Grunes (1990) believed that late life development is characterized by the adaptive construction of a highly stable sense of self, and that psychopathology can present for the first time when internal or external stresses threaten this sense of self-continuity. There may be, then, an age-related tendency away from unfamiliar, less differentiated and complex depiction of self and others to more constricted, familiar ones.

Finally, two "semi-personological" problems influence the expression of personality, organicity, and narcissism. Brain pathology expresses itself through the organic insult itself, the meaning of the cognitive decline and the way of defending against this onslaught. Whereas brain pathology accentuates or exaggerates personality patterns, the latter two reflect long-standing personality trends. Addressing this, Friedman (1993) wrote:

> It is not an either/or question of organic or functional but rather a both/and situation; organic disorders extenuate personality structure and the perception and personal significance of organic impairment are altered through the personality. (p. 170)

Additionally, all of us have vested interests in our thriving. Narcissistically injured older people use narcissistic defenses to externalize the disruption of their self-esteem. The most typical personality change in response to cognitive compromise is not a personality change, but rigidity and intensification of the prior personality structure (Breslau, 1980). A prescription for care with an older compromised person often involves a clarification of any organic components, the establishment of a narcissistic alliance, involving an understanding of the patient's self-esteem and the nature of the threats to it. A "narcissistic alliance," then, seems logical, if not therapeutic, in treatment, a sense of recognizing, respecting, and supporting the sources of the patient's self-esteem (Mehlman, 1977). From this concept too comes the formation of a coherent narrative, one that is narcissistically contrived.

Addressing the narcissistic PD, Silver (1992) noted that the increasing loss of control over social and economic resources that often accompany aging is compensated by the use of defense mechanisms and emotional states that help restructure the balance between social demands and emotional needs. This restructuring is facilitated by the weakening of superego demands and the lessening pressures for social conformity. The importance of personality in this context is that aging individuals become more "pure" personality types. This might be influenced by cerebral change or organic damage (Abrams & Horowitz, 1999). Thus the narcissistic elder becomes more easily wounded. In effect, the older person uses defense mechanisms to secure a sense of authority or control that fits the personality style.

In later life then stress can be external or internal. At a conceptual level personality moderates and is changed by life changes. PDs moderate the effect, for example, of caregiving and bereavement and recovery for heart disease, and PDs are influenced by life transitions and organic insult as with dementia. Trauma also is altered and alters personality.

Personality/Narrative

Personality really is but a stable constellation of styles in the form of domains (see below) with which an individual faces new stresses or challenges. A personality is a process construct but is also a content, suffused with personal meanings and a personal identity. Personality then has both a form and content. We have addressed mostly form, as personologists study the form (of personality). We have implied that as age occurs, content becomes important. The content is concerned with the wishes, fears, expectations, and meanings with which the person faces the world. The content reflects and is reflected by the ongoing narrative of the person. Little work has been done to operationalize the content of personality in a way that would allow experimental verification of its stability or instability with aging.

Where the personologist is concerned, any intervention on personality involves the identification of the ego syntonic mode of making sense of the world: Where the PTSD therapist is concerned, the exposition of how the patient integrates life, the narrative, is critical. Both are important and play off each other. We might say too that, to a significant degree, distress arises when one's life experiences do not fit with one's personality style. This necessitates a narrative review, some type of rewriting or reworking. Hopefully too, the narrative is provided by the person him/herself and not imposed by the mental health professssionals.

Remember we live a life-span. For the elderly, the personality/narrative dynamic serves to reflect the person's past, especially past sources of self-esteem, and direct the present. In this way, we all are continually writing and rewriting the story of our life, both at a conscious and co-conscious level, including how age and illness fit into our narrative. Such narratives not only express the experience of illness and suffering but create it and potentially can alleviate it (Brody, 1987; Kleinman, 1988). In a sense, consistency and loss play out with a depleted self-esteem and sometimes cognitive decline. The central purpose of personality structure, especially in old age when self-esteem is under assault by progressive losses, is to compensate and hold the line. This it does in a largely consistent way. The narrative both assists in this process and is influenced by it. With trauma, this may take the form of normal disruptions, such as safety or self-esteem, or a disrupted narcissistic equilibrium, such as entitlement, jealousy, grandiosity, an illusion of self-sufficiency, hoarding, depression, and hypochondriasis (Cath, 1965; Levin, 1977). Or, it may lead to PTSD.

Dementia: A Special Case

Finally, we note that an area where personality can have an impact is cognitive decline—and if it has merit here, it has merit anywhere. After all, personality change is one of the most distressing aspects of a dementing illness as the expression of personality traits is a defining feature of one's personhood. In fact, in recent years there has been a spate of papers on the insight and concern of dementia patients. This has included dementia patients in groups that have a heavy verbal presence, dementia patients demonstrating insight (even with low Mini-Mental State Exams scores), and the relevance of personality measures, both premorbid and after the disease has occurred.

A small but influential literature has evolved (Abrams et al., 1998). Most of the studies can be grouped into three: personality assessment on extant scales of dementia, as with the Blessed Dementia Scale; studies on patients with head injuries; and studies on more traditional personality scales as the NEO-PI (Corto & McCrae, 1990). The advantage of the traditional scales is that these correspond to more known personality entities and are stable. In the case of the NEO-PI, there is a rating scale for the significant other. But, despite no sure measure of the premorbid personality, knowledge of personality is helpful even with this population because the nature, change, and course of personality can monitor the disease itself; knowledge of personality will assist in the treatment of the person; and target symptoms become more understandable and "usable" for the use of selected interventions. Interestingly, Abrams et al. noted that there is little evidence that premorbid personality relates to changes in personality (when a dementing disorder occurs).

The work of Nelson et al. (1989) and Magai and Cohen (1998) is also noteworthy. Nelson et al. (1989) developed a scale that assesses changes in dementia, changes in personality not cognition. The NBAP (Neuropsychological and Behavioral and Affect Profile) uses five dimensions: indifference, inappropriateness, depression, mania, and pragnosia. In a comparison of normal and dementing elders, Nelson found differences in all scales but mania. Using premorbid scores, there were trends in changes for all scales. Perhaps subtle changes occur before the actual cognitive changes take place. Magai and Cohen (1998) also showed that attachment style predicts caregiver burden and reflects the expression of dementia: ambivalent patients showed more depression and anxiety than avoidant patients who had more activity disturbance and paranoid symptoms. Securely attached patients demonstrated less emotional disturbance than the other two attachment styles. At our clinics we use the PACL (Stock, 1997). Others note the premorbid traits of the probable dementing relative. Knowledge of the premorbid status and possible area where decline may be a problem has been fiercely received.

Personality then has some influence on the expression of dementia. Even here, where the mind is being lost this construct has information for the therapist.

Conclusion

A precis of the above ideas on personality appears in Box 8-3. We are absent answers on critical issues of aging and personality: What happens to the obvious consistency of a person as he/she ages? What happens to personality when changes occur at older ages? How do we explain the increased presence of, for example, interiority with age in a person with a set personality? How do we explain maturation in the context of a personality? An absence of answers to these questions should not deter us from the pursuit of reasonable clarity.

We are also absent ideas on treatment with PDs and older folks. Regarding these, Lazarus and Sadavoy (1996) stated that "age per se defines neither indications nor contraindications for therapy" (p. 819). There is not one article, for example, on the subject of CBT and personality at later life. Thomson, Davies, Gallagher, and Krantz (1986) opined that treatment of an older person with a PD necessitated a focus on warm and concerned relationship, where complaints are discussed as solvable problems, the patient is educated as to the nature of the treatment approach, and an emphasis that beliefs are considered as symptoms to be worked on. At its base,

---

Box 8-3
Summary of Aging and PDs

1. Age is only weakly related to personality.
2. There is little or no change in the mean levels of traits in domains of personality in adulthood. Longitudinal comparisons of personality traits show general stability.
3. Trait change is best represented by a negatively accelerating slope.
4. Despite alterations in the expression of a PD, the prevalence remains high.
5. Older people with a PD are at increased risk for other Axis I disorders.
6. Of the PDs, Cluster C is the most common. The prevalence rate was 20% with paranoid, self-defeating, and schizoid being the most prevalent.
7. Some manifestations of personality, such as affective control, alter with age.
8. Personality "naturally" reformulates to accommodate to the needs of later life. This has been labeled *heterotypic continuity*—functional value of construct across time.
   a. Changing relevance of symptoms
   b. Appearance or disappearance of symptoms
   c. Contextual factors influence all (place and time)
   d. Dynamic versus static variables: PD variables alter over the day and year
   e. Motivation in taking the test
9. There are no PD measures for the elderly. Most self-report scales have poor sensitivity and therefore should be used as a screen.
10. Stress can be internal (biology and narcissism) or external (trauma).
11. Trauma can influence personality stability but only mildly. The expression of problems is distorted through the interaction of age and trait.
12. Personality and the narrative interact.
13. Dementia also is influenced by personality.

---

psychotherapy on a person with a PD involves a careful identification of agreed upon targets, often interpersonal in nature, and the very careful application of consistency and collaboration.

☐ Theoretical Directions

"A man's fate is his character."
Heraclitis

Patients who have the same diagnoses do not possess the same problem. We need something more than a diagnosis. Lazarus (2000) holds that the elimination of dysfunctional patterns of behavior, sensation, imagery, cognition, interpersonal relationships, and possible biological processes is successful in direct proportion to the number of specific modalities deliberately invoked by any therapeutic system. If this is so, comprehensive therapy involves the correction of irrational beliefs, deviant behaviors, unpleasant feelings, intrusive images, stressful relationships, negative sensations, and a possible biochemical imbalance. When problem identification (diagnosis-assessment) systematically explores each of these modalities and therapy can be applied, the focus is personality. This is personological therapy. Regarding this, Beutler and Clarkin (1990) noted "the characteristics that the patient brings to the treatment experience are the single most powerful sources of influence on the benefit to be achieved by treatment" (p. 31). For this we need a theory.

Millon Model

"To uproot a personality disorder, one must wrangle with the ballast of a lifetime, a developmental disorder of the entire matrix of the person, produced and perpetuated across years. By any reasoning, the pervasiveness and entrenched tenacity of the pathology, soaks up therapeutic resources, leading inevitably to pessimism and disaffection for therapists."
Theodore Millon

The Millon system of personality posits that four components be applied: theory, taxonomy, instrumentation, and intervention (see Box 8-4). This is a personality model: The information regarding the person is based on the entire matrix of the salient domains (of that person; Millon & Davis, 1995). Personality allows the clinician to understand and treat Axis I (and Axis III) problems. It encompasses the biopsychosocial patterns of the person, is predictive of adjustment, both psychosocial and medical (Ruegg & Frances, 1995). Personality, then, influences symptoms, symptom severity, and overall adjustment of treatment-seeking patients. A comprehensive awareness of the structural integrity of this linked nexus (behaviors, thoughts, emotions, interpersonal and biological patterns) serves the clinician well (Millon & Davis, 1996). If this theory is correct (Millon & Davis, 1995), then the methods of operation of the personality provide the necessary data for an understanding of the person, the most that "science" can allow.

Box 8-4
Structure of a Clinical Science: Clinical Personology

I. Theory (Personologic Polarities)
   Explanatory system of concepts and hypotheses in a specified subject domain.
II. Taxonomy (Personality Disorders)
   Features of the subject domain; differentiated and interrelated in accord with the theory.
III. Instrumentation (Personologic Assessment)
   Data sources and measurement tools for identifying and quantifying the subject domain.
IV. Intervention (Personologic Psychotherapy)
   Techniques, goals, and strategies for effecting beneficial changes in the subject domain.

Millon's model is theory-based, anchored to the multiaxial system of the DSMs (Millon, 1969, 1981, 1984). Millon sees personality as akin to the immune system, and, as such, the key determinant in the success or failure of problems or symptoms. It is the competence of the immune system that determines the reaction of the person, not the type or extent of the stressor. Core types of personality were based on the nature of reinforcement (pain or pleasure), source of reward (self or others), and instrumental style (active/passive) (Box 8-5). Initially there were eight. Two additional Axis II disorders, sadistic and self-defeating, have been added to this model after the DSM-III–R and one (depressive personality) after the DSM-IV. Three severe personality types also exist and represent extensions or exaggerations of the basic eight personalities. These are schizotypal, borderline, and paranoid. In later writings, Millon (1990) brought evolutionary theory to bear on his reinforcement model. The clinician's task is to (a) establish the basic personality pattern(s) of a person; (b) modify this information with elevations in the severe personality styles; and (c) integrate the unique personality profile with the current clinical symptoms. We have reduced the heterogeneity among persons and isolated the dimensions most characteristic of a person. Additionally, the methodology for treating PDs is in sync with the epistemology of the personality itself. The (psycho)logic allows the clinician to address treatment. For the mechanics of this, Millon has identified two sources, polarities (Box 8-5) and the functional and structural domains of personality (Box 8-6). The former considers how one seeks reinforcement and where this reinforcement is sought. People seek reinforcement from self, others, not sure (ambiguous or discordance), or are detached, and people are active and passive in these efforts. In a strange way the person with a PD has a self-reward system that says "I do this because it feels right" and a pain system that says "My way to avoid is best." Psychopathology represents an imbalance on these polarities. The clinician's overall strategy is to balance these so that the individual has an appropriate focus of change. Millon (1969) noted:

By framing our thinking in terms of what reinforcements the individual is seeking, where he is looking to find them, and how he performs, we may see more simply and more clearly the essential strategies which guide (his life). (p. 193).

The latter involves a domain-based formulation of a PD that allows the clinician to analyze the person at a closer level. Box 8-6 presents the eight domains and the 14 personalities. It shows that there are four structural domains that are relevant to the appraisal of PDs. They are deeply embedded templates, quasi-permanent imprinted features of the person, such as memory, attitudes, and needs. These are object relations, self-image, morphological organization, and mood/temperament domains.

Four functions are also involved, as the system must adjust to perpetrate itself. Functions are an expressive mode of regulatory action. They include expressive acts, interpersonal conduct, cognitive style, and regulatory mechanisms. Each patient represents a profile of these structural and functional domains.

Domains allow the clinician to analyze more finitely aspects of the character. They build on a prototype of the personality itself. In effect, they hone in on the particular points in the system that are *especially* sensitive to change. Cognitive, behavioral, psychodynamic, and interpersonal approaches might be effective at some level with all of these interventions but there are likely to be more effective and more time-efficient at particular points. Additionally, if these salient dimensions are not directly addressed, they tend to become more resistant to change over time. The schizoid personality, for example, has behavioral acts of being impassive and unengaged; phenomenological styles of being impoverished, complacent, and meager; intrapsychic patterns of seeing self and others as meager and given to intellectualization; and biological patterns of being undifferentiated and apathetic.

Box 8-5
Continuum of Patterns to Disorders

Instrument Behavior Pattern	Sources of Reinforcement					
	Independent (Self)	Dependent (Others)	Ambivalent (Conflicted)	Discordant (Reversal)	Detached (Neither Self or Others)	Detached (Pain)
Active	Unruly ↕ Antisocial	Dramatizing ↕ Histrionic	Oppositional ↕ Negativistic	Forceful ↕ Aggressive (sadistic)	Inhibited ↕ Avoidant	— —
Passive	Egotistic ↕ Narcissistic	Submissive ↕ Dependent	Conforming ↕ Compulsive	Self-demeaning ↕ Self-defeating (masochistic)	Introversive ↕ Schizoid	Doleful ↕ Depressed

Box 8-6

Expression of Personality Disorders Across the Functional and Structural Domains of Personality—Overview

	Functional Processes					Structural Attributes		
Disorder	Expressive Acts	Interpersonal Conduct	Cognitive Style	Regulatory Mechanisms	Self-Image	Object Representations	Morphologic Organization	Mood/Temperament
Schizoid	Impassive	Unengaged	Impoverished	Intellectualization	Complacent	Meager	Undifferentiated	Apathetic
Avoidant	Fretful	Aversive	Distracted	Fantasy	Alienated	Vexatious	Fragile	Anguished
Depressive	Disconsolate	Defenseless	Pessimistic	Aceticism	Worthless	Forsaken	Depleted	Melancholic
Dependent	Incompetent	Submissive	Naive	Introjection	Inept	Immature	Inchoate	Pacific
Histrionic	Dramatic	Attention-seeking	Flighty	Dissociation	Gregarious	Shallow	Disjointed	Fickle
Narcissistic	Haughty	Exploitive	Expansive	Rationalization	Admirable	Contrived	Spurious	Insouciant
Antisocial	Impulsive	Irresponsible	Deviant	Acting out	Autonomous	Debased	Unruly	Callous
Sadistic	Precipitate	Abrasive	Dogmatic	Isolation	Combative	Pernicious	Eruptive	Hostile
Compulsive	Disciplined	Respectful	Constricted	Reaction formation	Conscientious	Concealed	Compartmentalized	Solemn
Negativistic	Resentful	Contrary	Skeptical	Displacement	Discontented	Vacillating	Divergent	Irritable
Masochistic	Abstinent	Deferential	Diffident	Exaggeration	Undeserving	Discredited	Inverted	Dysphoric
Schizotypal	Eccentric	Secretive	Autistic	Undoing	Estranged	Chaotic	Fragmented	Distraught or insentient
Borderline	Spasmodic	Paradoxical	Capricious	Regression	Uncertain	Incompatible	Split	Labile
Paranoid	Defensive	Provocative	Suspicious	Projection	Inviolable	Unalterable	Inelastic	Irascible

Treatment

What might these strategies look like? For the personologic psychotherapy that is integrative, two issues are considered: (a) Modality tactics and modifying domain dysfunction, and (b) Strategic Goals and re-establishing polarity balances. Modality tactics are initially addressed (Box 8-6). Direct therapeutic acts on the domains represent the tactics of personologic change. This is the best fit in treating the individual. For the avoidant personality, for example, the targets would be self-image and behavioral acts. The clinician would want to assist the avoidant person in the development of a better self-view and to act interpersonally with less anxiety. Of course, we are talking about prototypical components, as real patients fail to conform to any particular pattern. However a careful formulation of these structures and functional domains in the context of the personality reveals a "good enough" goodness of fit for any patient.

For overall health, strategic goals are considered (Box 8-5). Among imbalances in the passive–active polarity, efforts may be made to increase the capacity and skills for taking a less reactive and more proactive role in dealing with life affairs (decreased passive, increased active). This would be a major goal of treatment for schizoids, depressives, dependents, narcissists, masochists, and compulsives. Among the avoidants too, the therapist would suggest a lessened focus on pain and a more passive stance to obviate the need/fear axis of anxiety. The self–other polarity addresses interpersonal imbalances. Among narcissists and antisocials, a major aim of treatment is a reduction in their predominant self-focus and a corresponding augmentation of their sensitivity to the needs of others (increased other, decreased self). Among dependents and histrionics, a major objective of therapy is to stimulate greater self-interest, rather than focus on those of others. For the ambivalent personalities, conflicts that underlie the behavior of compulsives and negativists, attention is best directed at the recognition of the nature of their ambivalences and at overcoming inner disharmony. Similarly, the pain–pleasure discordance that undergirds the difficulties of sadists and masochists will require efforts to reverse these pathological inclinations.

In this context there is one other division that is worthwhile. Each personality also has both "basic tendencies" and "coping patterns," the former being hard-wired in the person and less subject to change and the latter the more learned parts of the personality (Harkness & Libenfield, 1997). In the treatment of a PD, the person is asked to know and accept the core parts of the personality that do not alter. The patient is requested to be alone with the patterns of the PD. This involves an awareness of the "dark side" of the personality. It implies that this is the best way to "know" the personality and the best way to tolerate its press. The person is instructed that the brain is only interpreting their body and now they can integrate them. Ideally, the "alone" time is experienced best when the mind and body are fully integrated. The person is experiencing action tendencies, temperament, and the mind assimilates information. The person regulates emotions according to the needs of the temperament. The complication comes when the person now must act on the triggers in real life.

In effect, we require three features for PDs: (a) awareness (acceptance of the temperament); (b) disengagement (a step back before action); and (c) action (not doing the "PD thing"). Awareness involves sensitivity to the emotional and cognitive manifestation of the PD triggers. They can be internal (a biochemical burp) or external interactions with the environment. The trick in the management of a PD is in stepping back and waiting out triggers. Action follows. For the avoidant personality, the task is to await the feeling of distrust.

On the basis of reinforcement theory and on the salient domains specific to each person, then, an understanding of the harmonic balance can be organized. Like an orchestra leader the maestro therapist understands the full piece and in this context makes an effort to find a harmonized balance of the concert. Muting some instruments and increasing others results in good tonality. In this sense treatment techniques are only tactics or strategies to achieve integrated goals. The goal is toward the improvement over imbalances of deficient polarities by techniques that are optimistically suited to modify the expression of these problems. These optimal stratagies/tactics are provided for each personality and are given in Box 8-5 and Box 8-6.

Practical Issues

As we have implied, with PTSD (or other symptoms) two phases of treatment are required. In one phase symptoms are addressed. They demand attention from the therapist, but they have a functional value for each client. In trauma work, typical methods to address symptoms include exposure techniques, stress reduction, or grief/trauma therapy, among others. These are addressed in the next chapters. Additionally, at the practical level treatment of PDs requires alterations; both a procedural adaptation including longer term sessions, and process adaptation, including detailed exploration of self-protective resistance, as well as a careful understanding of the meaning of repetitive patterns, polarities, and domains (e.g., Millon & Davis, 1995; Turkat, 1991).

In Appendix A we present our model of personality as it applies to PTSD at later life. Remember that symptoms count most at the gate or when they are loud: Attend to them at that time.

Therapy is not defined by techniques but by conceptualization. It is a model of care that has rules. This is what a personality is, a construct that has some glue to its psychological space. In fact, clients will tell the clinician this: "I know I should not do this but ..." In clients with PDs their "head" changes before their gut. So, the person must experience the "sensation of the PD" and see what is really happening. As a general rule, the clinician attacks the overall rigidity in the PD, to increase flexibility and decrease self-defeating patterns.

From Appendix B this process starts with an assessment for a vision of care. Early on we test older victims with a personality scale (MCMI-III). We use this as the template for treatment of the personality. The MCMI(s), then, provide sufficient data for care and are helpful to clients (Finn, 1996). Now that we have the necessary background, what exactly do we do?

Treatment is a loose full court press. Given our strengths, polarities, and domains (structures and functions), we believe that we can target reasonably precise points (in the system) for interventions to be maximally effective. Overall, the long-range goals of therapy, the polarities of pleasure and pain, self and other, and active and passive guide our thinking. Careful strategies around domains makes possible the creation of a personologic prototype of each of the PDs in the DSM, wherein each of the domains represents a piece of "ideal," or prototypic, characterologic structure. Clients, we believe, are "addicted" to typical patterns; Dependents, for example, are preoccupied with being abandoned, avoidants with negative evaluations.

There are two "personality features" that are highly related to PTSD. One is a backup trait for most PTSD problems after a period. Avoidance (agoraphobia in many cases), a detached stance based on fear, is pandemic and intrinsic to PTSD. Soon it develops like a personality characteristic. This feature of PTSD should be addressed in the management of the person with agoraphobia. If the issue is agoraphobic avoidance, the clinician needs to assess the readiness for exposure in vivo, discuss carefully the goals of exposure and convince the PTSD patient that success is not dependent on the reduction of anxiety but the willingness to experience anxiety, that the hierarchy must take time and reflect the feared objects, that the patient must get rid of safety features (drugs, etc.), and that the patient must monitor progress. The process of informed consent and the behavior of the patient are the treatment components.

The other is GAD (Generalized Anxiety Disorder), another trait-like component of older folks and PTSD. This Axis I "symptom" has as much stability as most of the Axis II personalities and has a comorbidity rate of 91% (Sanderson, 2000). It is highly related to PTSD after period. GAD patients are worriers, chronic worriers. The GAD victim has lost the ability to problem solve and has lost the ability to estimate probabilities. They are reluctant to give up the worry. It has "magic" qualities in the service of intrusion reduction. They of course catastrophize. Cognitive restructuring is appropriate, especially the focus on maladaptive assumptions (Leahy & Holland, 1999).

The following is a listing of possible avoidant or GAD features that we address.

Problem	Intervention
Cognitive Avoidance	Awareness Exercise
Physical Symptom of Anxiety	Relaxation
Worry	Distraction
Negative Automatic Thought Avoidance	Cognitive Restructuring Experience
Maladaptive Assumptions of Danger	Behavioral Experiments, Developmental Analysis, Skill Training
Relapse	Coping, Relapse Training

Cognitive, behavioral, psychodynamic, and interpersonal approaches then are all likely to demonstrate some level of efficacy with the personality disorders (Millon & Davis, 1996). That said, we have a cognitive bias in our rules in Appendix B. It is in this domain that action is always relevant and that the most research pertains. We believe that, all things equal, automatic thoughts are most important. These are fed by beliefs (or images). Cognitive distortions bind anxiety and other psychopathologies by constructing a secondary reality that reduces the dissonance between the inner and outer world. Secondary realities are fostered further by the many cognitive distortions.

There are many ways to unearth these beliefs but all involve an explanation of core cognitions, an identification of current situations where these are operating, and a "grounding" of the experience. Often the therapist can seek the roots in childhood through early experiences. Then the therapist can do any one of a number of interventions. They could do a Core Belief Worksheet (Beck, 1995), restructure early memories (by having the adult person talk to the younger one), do a Cognitive Conceptualization Diagram (Beck, 1998), critically examine the supporting evidence for the belief, or use any one of many techniques of Young (1990), such as express anger toward the schema, be vigilant for its presence, and confront schema avoidance.

All therapy is local. We recommend also that the clinician unpack "small" instances of the interpersonal patterns of the client. The unpacking of specific instances of the person is valuable beyond words. The clinician remains data-centered, uses emotion, is present-focused, remains developmental, applies core conflict strategies, and solicits feedback from the patient. Young (1999) labeled this complex *early maladaptive schemas*. They are comfortable, learned working strategies for life that people use in most situations. They become obvious when the person is under stress. Their presence fits like an old shoe on the feet of the besieged person. The person maintains these with carefully crafted behaviors/cognitions/emotions, avoids the wrong settings for their discomfort or challenge, and compensates when necessary to assure their presence. Their presence is most notable when there is annoying consistency, when there is dissonant behavior, and when somatization is evident in conflict.

The downward arrow too is one method that allows for a quick unearthing of core beliefs and in turn silent assumptions (Beck, 1995). The clinician identifies individual or interpersonal beliefs and attacks them with standard statements. The belief is written down and the therapist asks "And, if that were true, why would it be upsetting to you?" for individual beliefs; for interpersonal beliefs, the stock phrase "If true, what does this tell about you?" The clinician follows each phrase with "Let's write that down." There is then a (usually) 5–7 sequence of phrases of negative core issues about the person. Emotions are left out of the mix, as these are not relevant to the pursuit of the person. When done, the clinician identifies silent assumptions (e.g., " I must be loved to be worthwhile," "Others attack me," etc.). Again, as with the focus on specificity, this technique is most powerful and can lead to important information.

Using cognitions as exemplars, "the mores" apply: The more central or core the cognition is, the more difficult it will be to change and the greater the amount of resistance can be expected; the more the therapist must convince the sufferer of his/her "error," the less the client will feel empowered in a cooperative fashion with a will and a skill to challenge cognitions; the more the person understands his/her personality profile, the greater the chances of success; and the more the client understands the "rules of the game" (for treatment) and understands the maladaptive influences of their cognitions, the more he/she can choose alternative lifestyles.

Finally, we note that, as part of this personality assessment, the therapist should also assess their clients' psychological skills (e.g., problem-solving, planning, communication, rational responding, perspective-taking; O'Donohue & Krasner, 1994) in order to determine how much of the problem is personological and how much represents deficits in functioning (Trower & Dryden, 1989). With older victims this has almost always proven helpful: Social deficits are part and parcel of several personalities, especially those related to PTSD (e.g., Avoidant).

These personologic strategies are only a first step. For the treatment of trauma victims they are sufficient to facilitate consistency and perhaps for overall change. That is, a careful application of this personality model to the trauma victim allows for a more stable lifestyle, one that does not reinforce trauma-related problems. In effect, the problem maintenance structure of the person is addressed. Interdependently, the therapist can act on other psychopathic features of the person, such as the trauma memory. Greenberg, Rice, and Elliot (1993) noted that two factors are predictive of better outcome: the client's awareness of and ability to report his/her intrusive negative thoughts and the client's awareness of frustrations in his/her emotions. To the extent that these abilities are available and that the clinician can remain on task, typical CBT procedures will be successful.

Role of Clinician and Patient

We feel compelled to discuss the role of the clinician and patient. On the one hand, treatment always depends on the person of the therapist. It is no secret that most clinicians rely on countertransference reactions for a PD diagnosis and its treatment. This is especially a problem in the areas of anger, need/helplessness, and disconnected/a-relational. Personality issues come into play most when an impasse occurs. On the other hand, the patient must be on board. A working alliance must be a primary target and in place early.

This is not easy work. Beck (1997) reminded us that patients forget 75% of talk therapy; PD patients even more. For the personologist, repetition counts. With a PD, clients' negatively biased beliefs and information processing lead them consistently to misconstrue interpersonal situations (Safran & Segal, 1990). These patterns must be recognized and even embraced. In Benjamin's model (1993) too the key role is that of establishing a collaboration, one in which empathic processes may or may not be appropriate. She stressed the importance of facilitating the patient's recognition of his/her interpersonal patterns of behavior. Equally significant is the task of "blocking maladaptive patterns," and the necessity for addressing the patient's underlying fears and wishes. New learning should be facilitated, that is, to encourage the acquisition of interpersonal behaviors that are more adaptive and more gratifying than those previously used. PD work should be done in stages or stepwise (like the building of a NASA project), and multimodes should be used. Behavior, mood, and cognitions (and biology) "move together": The wise clinician knows this midlevel dance.

This work is often hard and boring. Personality therapy is not sexy. This involves several changes in the rules of application. The overall psycho-philosophy is given in Box 8-7. This is an active stance that involves commitment of the patient. It is an "active" stance, the therapist must be willing to go back and forth between

---

Box 8-7
Personality Rules of Care

Respect primacy of personological therapy: Learn to think on two levels, symptoms and personality. Give yourself permission not to have to figure diagnosis and dynamics right away.

Establishing a polarity-oriented and domain-focused treatment strategy is fundamental to care.

Sharing personality diagnosis is necessary. Education is critical.

Educate patients about the nature of their disorder, as well as about the cognitive model of therapy.

Offer hypotheses about the personality problems taking place in the life of the patient.

Elicit feedback from patients to show that you value their input and to emphasize the importance of their active participation in treatment.

Monitoring of working alliance is always necessary.

Gauge success in terms of both the personality disorder and symptom remission.

Monitor self in the process of therapy.

personality and symptom issues, between success and failure, progress and resistance. Therapists should examine these issues not only as a client variable, but also as a function of the therapist's approach in the context of personality. Therapists may be inappropriately attached or reacting. They may be causing trouble; something not unheard of with PDs.

In personological treatment, the therapist's task consists of identifying the compulsive maladaptive patterns as these evolve in the therapeutic relationship and helping the client to understand, rather than act out problematic interpersonal scenarios. Therapeutic change is a client developing an awareness of self-defeating patterns and hopefully experiencing a different outcome within the therapeutic relationship itself. In order to achieve this type of "corrective emotional experience," the therapist is most of all a participant observer, there to point out and to participate in the client's problematic patterns. Millon has provided a method for this to occur. Hopefully the patient will be so.

☐ Conclusion

In the previous chapter we indicated that a case formulation is critical. This is the working formulation of our efforts. It is the playbook. After the identifying information, a problem list, an understanding of current precipitants, as well as the etiology of the problems, we plan treatment. We do this with a knowledge of personality. This allows us to identify the obstacles to treatment, to formulate hypotheses, and to reformulate a plan over time. Personality is the key element of our case formulation.

If the other two memory components of the model are not considered, then we stop here. Stop means that we treat and manage the person without memory interventions. We treat the person and their context: we give the person coping methods for any trauma intrusion; and we monitor progress according to issues other than memory. These are symptoms and personality. Again, this is management and good treatment.

Pioneers in the history of personality psychology envisioned a new discipline as the integrative center piece for all of psychology (see Millon, 1999). Widiger (1991) saw the reality of a PD as so important and complex that a written PD description be implemented on each patient separate from the diagnostic criteria for the DSM. This would involve a descriptive part of assessment. "Real" clients are complex mixtures of core person schemas, personality styles, and the current psychosocial and trauma symptoms. The final result is an interactive mix, organized by the person. Symptoms never just "burst forth" because of the excessive nature of the stressor, "unfree" of the person's (schema) influence. Symptoms serve the person from which they evolved. We treat trauma best after permission in knowing of the person.

A good theory not only incorporates extant knowledge but has "systemic input" (Millon & Davis, 1995). It organizes and assists in the development of new observations and new technologies. Because we have no grand theories, we must rely on reasonable micro-theories that both evolve and currently are sufficient for care. For the clinician who treats trauma victims with PDs, we know that the pattern of interacting masks a truth in a protective and defeating reality. It requires a new living. Knowledge of personality provides the data for these practical issues that cause problems.

Looking at personality as it relates to aging, Havens (1999) observed that all of us have character pathology. If one has a PD, the problems with the necessary tasks of aging are made difficult. One cannot negotiate the nodal points of development well.

In addition, the ability to tolerate existential anxiety is lost (What am I about?) and the older person cannot discover "truth" in any acceptable way. For the typical individual who approaches the end of life with an "aging mandate" to review, create, and integrate, PDs muck things up. Nietzsche noted that truth needed to be confronted with the question: "Can it be lived?" A person with a PD in later life answers this, "No." Knowledge of personality at least assists in the living.

We now switch gears. As the science of the person has evolved, the concept of the narrative or story developed also. While there is an arguable distinction, there is also a seamless connection. We do and say; act and store. In the next chapters we look at this connection, addressing the memory—but the personality is not far behind.

CHAPTER

9

Core Memory:
The "Good" Memory

"Positive memory traces actually encourage behavior that strengthens the bonds between you. Encouraging affirming thoughts in yourself—in other words, by recalling your partner's caress, how he or she was helpful to you this week, a look or a gesture that was particularly touching—will tune you into a positive feeling, which in turn will dispose you to act lovingly"
Daniel Amen (1998, p. 76)

Knight (1986) pointed out: "All psychotherapy involves some elements of life review" (pp. 127–128). Lieberman and Tobin (1983) saw as an essential task of old age the preservation of coherent, consistent self in the face of loss and the threat of loss. They suggested that, because human resources are so scant and the task is so pressing, life-review primarily is used to create an image intended to be believed, a myth to achieve a feeling of stability, justifying the narrator's life. For them, typically, the older person becomes the protagonist in a drama that is worth telling or having lived for. Fact and fantasy can mingle in life-review (Lewis, 1973). This is narrative truth. It requires that a new self-view be considered. Partializing the world in acceptable ways has always been reasonably adequate for change in therapy.

At its simplest and with some current consensus in the literature, a trauma memory represents rogue events that do not fit into prior schemas and are not narrativized. The therapeutic task is to bring this implicit memory (easily triggered by emotional states, interpersonal contexts, external stimuli, and language cues) into explicit consciousness and have it experienced in language that subserves the overall narrative. Ultimately, for change to occur, the narrative of one's life must be made coherent and understandable. For a trauma victim this means encompassing the trauma experience (Antonovsky, 1987). It has been argued that this is the only road to salvation. The trauma memory must be integrated or excised. It is also been suggested that transformation occurs only when the client's own interpretation of the good coming from negative events is realigned and incorporated into positive/balanced life narratives (Tedeschi & Calhoun, 1995).

But maybe there is another reality. The trauma memory is virulent or irrelevant to the person. They become numb. This may apply to many older people who have no ability to react to the memory psychologically. For them, therapy is an extension of the physician, where they wait for the curative medication. They do not want to tinker. They just want peace now. They come for emotional refueling. This seductive element of a discomfort anxiety is like gravity and the usual feel of avoidance can be rather appealing. For those who give way to this penchant or for those with chronic and unrelenting PTSD, a just-sufficient reduction of symptoms may be the only goal. They are satisficers, who embrace Erickson's view of foreclosure. McCullough (2000) views many of these patients as chronically depressed, beset with unremitting depression and a deterioration of cognitive-emotional functioning.

It may apply too to people beset with chronic PTSD (or chronicity of some form). For them, an alternative therapy is requisite. For them, therapy has been unfriendly. Recall of positive memories may be important.

The reasons for this are unclear. We have learned that reminiscence seems to have a positive influence in terms of increased self-esteem, reduced agitation, and higher ego-integrity (Chaudhury, 1999)—but it is not just because it is something that is done at later life. Recollections of a specific positive kind actually facilitate mastering of the trauma. Just as the active and controlled remembrance of a trauma event is a prerequisite for successful recovery of the trauma, life review processes are direct and structured and a developmental task that can change the total context of memories. The individual assesses past strengths to achieve better understanding of self and to determine one's life meaning. Often it is to solve present problems and cope with losses in the current situation (Sherman, 1991). In effect, if the client cannot undo the trouble, this person may benefit from a positive repetition of events.

In this chapter we address memories that are not trauma-based. Our purpose is to show that stories other than trauma memories can be helpful in the adjustment of clients. These are the "good" memories that are self-representational. The task here is to identify and build on the "better" stories. They are core representations of the self, complete with goals. These episodes in the person's life can be strung together to form a script or personality. In therapy they can assist in the balance of life and can generalize to current life situations. In therapy (or life) too these memories can be used to understand personal meaning and assist in present demands.

First, we re-consider memory as it relates to older people. We are interested in core memories that are not trauma-based. We discuss two features of trauma that apply most to trauma and older persons, reminiscence and reflexiveness. We also allude to the work of Rybarzyck and Bellg (1997). Finally, we provide ten tenets of care.

☐ Narrative Perspective

Narrative is central to the mental health of the person. It can also be the cornerstone of psychopathology. As we portrayed, narrative is encapsulated in memory. We continue to bundle information in an effort to understand the multiplicity of our experience. We reify separate entities that are important in the designation of "memories." In time, we experience our experienced lives. What has been has become the foundation of who we are. As we become aware of this, as in aging, making meaning of this experience of our experience.

Constructivist and narrative approaches are methods of such thinking, the so-called "fourth wave" of psychotherapy. It is the technology for the enhancement of core memories or the change of bad memories. People are victims of their own constructions. Listening to the life stories has an effect on patients' understanding of their illnesses and their context. Storytelling is the creation of personal meaning, identity, and relationship. It is a way of representing reality, the storyteller's understanding of his or her place in that reality, and the role others play in it. Cohler defined the personal narrative as "the most internally consistent interpretation of presently understood past, experienced present, and anticipated future" (p. 207). There is a bonus: the positive experience of storytelling establishes empathy, rapport, and understanding between the client and therapist.

Story repair or story enhancement is based on a few basic assumptions: (a) that development of identity involves the construction of a life story; (b) that psychopathology is caused by or the result of life stories gone awry; (c) that psychotherapy is primarily an exercise in "repairing stories" (Howard, 1991). Other, even more therapeutically appealing, assumptions also are evidenced in the work of therapy: (d) that the belief that social reality is co-created; (e) that small changes are all that are necessary; (f) that victims have the resources to solve problems; and (g) that the therapist does not need to know all the story or stories to solve a client's problems. In fact, as psychotherapy seeks both to simplify (in the form of manuals, self-help books, and standard prescriptions), these approaches reveal to us that human existence is connected to our memories. We are what we remember ourselves to be.

We are meaning-making beings, striving to punctuate, organize and anticipate the interactions with the world. This constructivism allows us to be as a person. People construe meaning, organized around a core set of assumptions, which both govern the perception of life events and organize behavior in relation to these (Neimeier & Stewart, 1996; Roberts & Holmes, 1999). Individual differences "determine" whether trauma is really trauma and, if so, how reality is consequently formed and apperceived. We are in effect cognitive creatures. These are almost "choiceless events" in a choosing environment. Therefore, account making, the telling and knowing of our stories, allows us to know again our own issues and obtain social validation. Thomas Moore (1994a) noted: "Storytelling is an excellent way of caring for the soul. It helps us see the themes that circle in our lives, the deep themes that tell the myths we live. It would take only a slight shift in therapy to focus on the storytelling itself rather than on its interpretation."

One more thing: In this new culture we may have a problem with the narrative. There may be a blurring of the life course as later life becomes more "modern" in its approach to life. In effect, the new aged are de-contexualized with a new consumerism, such as retirement communities, preventing the continued development of the person. Under these circumstances, the re-authoring of the person becomes a special challenge as the person is given to the moment. The past here becomes a servant of the present. Memory is a grab bag from which the material of a new narrative fits the current circumstances rather than an dig for messages of life that was lived. The person is reinvented. We think that this is okay.

☐ Assessment of Memory

Not to Treat

The first task of the therapist is to do no harm. With the exposition of trauma this may be a problem. Garland (1994) held that for some people there may be negative outcomes. Evidence exists that treatment exposure can have a negative impact with trauma victims (Litz & Keane, 1989) or some older persons (Brink, 1978; Shapiro, 1995). With some exceptions (Fry, 1983), treatment can easily stall, especially regarding clinical depression. Because the overall goal in the treatment of PTSD involves the emotional processing of the trauma memory (Foa, 1996), this issue can be a problem.

War trauma clients especially have up to five decades of poor adaptation and inadequate coping styles (e.g., internal, global, and stable). Incessant searching for meaning is associated with less adaptive functioning (Silver, Boon, & Stones, 1983). Unfortunately, many victims do not elect to address this concern. In our research we reported that 42% of Vietnam veterans choose not to allow access to trauma memories (Hyer et al., 1994).

Matsekas (1992) provided cautions with the psychotherapy with traumatized persons. Recollections of the trauma may be a sub-optimal goal. Some individuals may not want to remember the past. For them, the choice is easy: Let them be. For them, it is important not to increase stress levels, to postpone looking at the past, to consider other forms of therapy before tackling the trauma, and to assure that a safe and controlled environment is required before any therapeutic action. In a general way, therapy is best spent away from the trauma. The overall goal is containment and management (Stages 1–4).

Additionally, focusing solely on trauma memories can be its own problem. Victimization can become an over-inclusive and uncomfortable self-examination (Shiraldi, 2000). Therapists who apply a stock trauma treatment to trauma victims run the danger of minimizing the profound personal, social, and biological disruption caused by the trauma (van der Kolk & McFarlane, 1996). The goal of more flexible treatment is to give a presence to other person factors, finessing a meaningful private ending.

Addressing specific issues of older people, Lazarus and DeLongis (1983) noted that life review should not be used with older people if guilt is a primary issue. Sparacino (1978–1979) noted further that older people should not be forced to examine in detail all their past traumas, failures, losses, or misdirected efforts. For many elders, denial and repression have been effective coping mechanisms that have helped them function relatively well for years after the original trauma. Opening up these extremely negative past events can run counter to one of the major purposes of life review, to blend trauma with good memories, shifting the balance sheet of life. For these individuals a foreclosure on the life review process is appealing and must be respected. Auerhahn et al. (1993) held:

> Remembering in and of itself is not healing. Survivors are not automatically relieved of memories by expressing them. On the contrary, expression may make it more difficult to protect the self from previously warded off material. Forced recall of disavowed material constitutes a monologue that leaves the survivor angry and injured. (p. 436).

Some events then cannot be repaired so easily, no matter how much life review. Here depression, guilt, anger, panic, and obsessional rumination may ensue. For some, the distance is too great. *Symptoms and the psychopathology of everyday life (e.g., traumatic memories) correspond to the state-dependent recollections of an earlier time.* Looking back before the trauma, some older victims say "Was that even me?" Here management may be the goal.

Guidelines

Without some ability to address and treat the trauma memories, no specialized PTSD treatment is available. McCann and Pearlman (1990) believed that the clinician must evaluate and know two psychological systems of the person: schemas and self/ego resources. The schema is the core issue of the memory itself. When the individual possesses sufficient self and ego capacities (McCann & Pearlman, 1990), the clinician can facilitate access to the memory more directly, using several approach techniques highlighting exposure. If, on the other hand, traumatic memories are largely fragmented, partially or completely unconscious with a weak ability to tolerate access, then memories will be only representations of the trauma. Where an excessive level of intrusions or a reduced capacity/willingness to retrieve trauma is present, a supportive procedure is appropriate.

For McCann and Pearlman (1990), the ability to reprocess this "fear of memory" in the present was the key. Can the older victim wrestle with trauma dialogue—What are you feeling now? Where in your body? What are you afraid may happen? Can you stand back from this experience and relate it to the whole you? and What power do you have over the trauma (or it over you)? The processing of these questions as well as an understanding of the person is important in the contextualization of the processing of the trauma memory. In addition to more severe considerations (e.g., psychotic level thinking, cognitive decline), the therapist needs to know further the quality of the trauma memory, and the willingness of the client to work. Assessment in this area is not a fine art. It is intended to provide enough data for a decision about trauma work. Often the only way to be sure is to try trauma work.

Assessment and treatment processes are co-occurring events. Assessing the client's inner dialogue, his/her ability to tolerate pain and affect, ego skills, and general level of information processing constitutes a "parallel processing" with the actual uncovering of traumatic memories. In general, the more movement or elaboration of the trauma memory, the greater the success. The more practiced the older victim in relaxation and imagery, the better the response (often, relaxation-based techniques alone have a desirable effect). Alternatively, the less skilled client may respond best to a more active therapeutic stance (partializing memories, reframing negative stories, using alternative coping, and challenging or changing stories). The more the client remains in the "now" and is able to experience the feared object or memory, the more change occurs. Preparing the older person for trauma work is perhaps the most important part of therapy as trauma victims do not access autobiographical memories easily or well (McNally, Larko, Macklin, & Pitman, 1995).

By and large telling the trauma story gives rich information on whether to pursue trauma work. We have pilot tested many ways of repairing traumatic life narratives: active reminiscence (Sherman, 1991), renarration (Hermans & Hermans-Jansen, 1995), biographical grids (Neimeyer & Stewart, 1996), time lines (Stewart, 1995), active therapeutic alteration of the story (Bornat, 1994), narrative organization (Foa et al., 1995), newer forms of exposure (e.g., Ochberg, 1996), isolated targets of self-repair (Wolfe, 1995), and transformation (Tedeschi & Calhoun, 1995), among others. However the client must be ready. It is when the client is having trouble with many of these criteria that the methods of this chapter apply.

Practical Issues

If the client has problems with the necessary skills (for work on the trauma memory), it is better to address positive core memories (PCM). Our rules of thumb are given in Box 9-1. If traumatic memories are largely fragmented, partially or completely unconscious with a weak ability to tolerate access, or if excessive level of intrusions are present, supportive procedures are more appropriate. Where the individual possesses sufficient psychological mindedness (self and ego capacities; Hyer et al., 1994; McCann & Pearlman, 1990), the clinician can access the memory more directly, using trauma-based methods.

A useful exercise to assist in this process is one that requests the client to become active early in the trauma memory process. The clinician requests the client to: "Close your eyes, focus on your trauma memory. After seeing and feeling this, take a view

---

Box 9-1
Client Indicators for Trauma Work

1. Trauma memory: Determine if memories are whole or fragmented.
   If fragmented, get whole or some pseudo-narrative for treatment.
   If excessive dissociation, provide supportive interventions.
2. Trauma work: Will you allow access to the trauma memory?
   Yes: If intrusive symptoms or painful responses are noted.
     If client consents to trauma work.
     If adequate ego skills are present.
   No: Stop
3. Psychologically minded clients:
   Can access thoughts (What were you thinking then?).
   Can access feelings (What were you feeling then?).
   Knows/accepts their client role (This is your job here).
   Have the ability and willingness to stay on task and struggle non-defensively.
   Collaborate—provide ongoing feedback to experience (e.g., SUDS levels).
   Possess adequate imagery and verbal skills.
   Is not excessively defensive.
4. Outside the therapy session clients can:
   Use self-skills in the environment.
   Tolerate frustration/pain.
   Avoid a self-condemning evaluation.
   Use calming self-talk.
   Can place symptoms in perspective.
   Can cope outside of therapy.
   Are able to be alone.
5. Harbingers of success:
   Reduced avoidance mechanism.
   Less anxiety/pain within/across sessions.
   Committed to the procedure.
   Future-oriented and demonstrate hope.

---

from a distance and think about what would stop you from discussing this with me? What fears do you have? What strengths do you need? What strengths do you have? What can I do to help with this? How do you prevent you from exploring the memory?"

The client's reluctance to focus on traumatic experiences does not imply resistance. Chief among the client's efforts to manage trauma symptoms are behavioral and mental avoidances, ineffective repetitive solutions, rigid patterns and rules, and unreflective dysfunctional behaviors. However the clinician should beware: "The patient has no motivation" is probably the commonest epitaph in our therapeutic cemeteries (Omer, 1994). When clients demonstrate readiness to work through post-traumatic symptoms and memories that hamper functioning, the therapist must be careful to work within the "therapeutic window" (Briere, 1994), or the "affective edge" (Cornell & Olio, 1991, 1992; Olio & Cornell, 1993). This is defined as the personal material that the client can safely work through to gain new awareness and integration without triggering a level of intensity that may flood the client with unmanageable amounts of new material.

All-too-often clinicians become scared off, avoiding a full exploration of events and fearing that the client will be adversely affected. Equally troubling is that the client has felt or experienced "bad" reactions to trauma, such as excitement at the events, at times behaviorally contributing to these events, as well as sadistic fantasies of revenge. Clients need to emotionally know up front that these events have happened but now are over. In this sense they are normal or acceptable as past events, as something that others also do and something that requires work now for integration. This value judgment is central to the therapeutic experience.

☐ The Good Memory: PCM

"... people are self-organizing, proactive, self reflecting, and self regulating,
not just reactive organisms shaped and shepherded by external events."
Albert Banderra

The positive core memory (PCM) is a form of therapy. Butler (1963) said that an understanding of the PCM allows for optimal psychosocial adjustment. Typically, this occurs in several ways: biological (offspring), parental (nurturing children), technical (teaching), and cultural (leaving something for culture, art, business, etc.). In fact, when the narration is moving well, the PCM is most important and generativity occurs.

Attempts to standardize administration of life-review are of comparatively recent origin. In most cases, a variety of approaches are used, including written or taped autobiographies, with feedback that may include self-confrontation (in a mirror), listening to tapes and picking up areas of conflict, boring and repetitive elements; pilgrimages; reunions, genealogy; scrapbooks, photo albums, old letters, and memorabilia; summation of life work; and exercise in preserving ethnic identity (Butler, 1963). Verwoerd (1988) believed that selectively amplifying early events that the client recalls with particular clarity, highlighting key phrases that are most salient in an individual life-review, challenging as vigorously as possible "if only ..." sidetracking, and working with the client on the interpretation of unresolved dreams recurring from early life deserves priority for therapy. Summers and Hyer (1994) advocated for "interpreting upward," helping a growth/positive focus.

Brink (1979) advocated an Adlerian perspective: The life review is helpful because it has reminded the patient that life is a series of crises and protracted struggles, and that the story teller has persevered in the past and triumphed. Such an interpretation of one's past serves as a powerful motivation for one to try to cope with the new demands of the present. When the therapist debriefs the client on his/her autobiography, the therapist must emphasize enthusiastically this interpretation of the patient's life.

Growth is not a unitary phenomenon. The act of reminiscence/life review is reasonably natural at later life and, we believe, curative for older trauma victims. Most older people are "programmed" to act in a positive way through their memories. Atchley (1991) believed the elderly defend themselves against a negative self-image by (a) focusing on past successes; (b) discounting messages that do not fit with their existing self-concept; (c) refusing to apply general beliefs and myths about aging to themselves; and (d) choosing to interact with people who provide an ego syntonic experience. Viney (1987) advocated a therapeutic effort to expose four types of memories for older folks; finding positive memories, confronting painful memories, empowering memories inhibited by grief, and encouraging non-narcissistic memories. Empowering memories inhibited by grief, for example, represents an attack on the refusal to reminisce on the part of those already overwhelmed by grief. Loss and grief work are essential parts of the experience of aging, and older people in general are well equipped to handle grief (Gutmann, 1980). Also, the encouragement of non-narcissistic memories allows people to find comfort in their own "good" sense of self-esteem, not in the eyes of others.

In effect, reinforcement of these memory components assists in life change. Previously, we (Summers & Hyer, 1994) advocated to (a) reinforce the reasonable positive interpretations; (b) bring into sharper focus benefits that are implicit in the context; (c) re-engage the client's hope; (d) bring in outside world-views and reframe; (e) reinforce competence, manageability, locus of control, self-efficacy, and bring the problem into the narrative in a positive way; and (f) reinforce cognitive complexity and religious coping.

There are currently no validated taxonomies of stories of adults (McAdams, 1996). Seeking PCMs does many things for us, however. It allows a balance, a perspective during the trauma process. In the exposition of these memories, positive schemas are fostered, rewarded, and at times challenged. Transformation may occur only when the client's own interpretation of the good coming from negative events is respected (Tedeschi & Calhoun, 1995). If this is so, the balance of a PCM and a trauma memory provides a salubrious mix for understanding and change. In a way the PCM provides permission to evaluate the self differently, to see the self compassionately and more realistically. As the person confronts older schemas and grieves parts of self, he/she also learns from the other voices provided by the PCM. Integrity means that the older person comes to the realization that she or he did the best she or he could. The PCM fosters this.

☐ Principles for PCM

The following principles can guide clinicians in helping trauma victims elicit and examine their PCMs (Box 9-2). There are three levels that begin with a concern for affect tolerance and the necessary building of resources. They then elicit the PCMs and apply rules. Finally, if all fails, the therapist can alter the memory. Throughout they

---

Box 9-2
Positive Core Memory

Preliminaries of PCMs
1. Affect tolerance
2. Resource building
Rules for PCMs
1. Get the story out in chronological order.
2. Be reflexive and nonreflexive.
3. Present centered/use affect.
4. Validate the stability of the self.
5. Respect cognition.
6. PCM summary and plan of action.
Last Resort
1. Change memory.

---

can deconstruct the memory to suit the needs of the situation. Remember the goal is for the person to experience the "power" of the PCM and to have a plan of action to assist in the application of the PCM and to negotiate the day-to-day workings of life. Let us start in the beginning.

Preliminaries

The second the clinician takes the history of the person, at that moment, the story begins. It is the person's interpretation of his/her life. Ordinarily as we have noted, the therapist attempts to fully expose the trauma memory by grounding the patient in the particulars of the memory. This is done in the therapy hour. Often too, the victim is encouraged to go to the trauma site and go through the details of the event. If the person cannot go to the place, photos or diaries can be used.

Normally, the process of life review is similar to gestalt therapy. The client may present a "bad" memory and in so doing presents the eye of the storm, the issue for review. The therapist then places this in the context of the person and tries to integrate this. In a sense, the therapist summarizes and evaluates the life events as they become more integrated and reach a gestalt. Each person extracts a relevant gestalt from the total context and, if the memories are unpleasant to self-esteem, they can be more meaningfully changed.

Now if the clinician had problems, that therapist would seek assistance. The help would take the form of time, varied techniques, or a focus on the blockages of the person, affect tolerance and lack of resources. In effect, there seems to be a seesaw effect for patients who have more chronic problems. They require something more than just psychotherapy. The trauma memory is stuck preventing the processing of information. Most victims with chronic PTSD have problems with affect tolerance (consequently they avoid). They also have lessened resources. The therapist needs a way to manage this—trauma, affect tolerance, and resources instillation.

Janet held that the PTSD victim became so because he/she did not have the resources to address the trauma. They were in turn overcome by "vehement emotions."

Trauma is the reaction of the person that prevents the processing of data—the person shames self (dissociates/avoids) or is overcome by the fear response. They cannot tolerate the anxiety or do not have the necessary resources for action. If it is the former, the person requires special tending to where he/she can become stronger or distance self from the pain of the trauma; if the latter, the person needs resources to overcome the rigid patterns of life. We apply this logic to the PCM. We want positive experiences. The end of the PCM is a formal coping or safety plan for dealing with life. So, our sequence of issues is (a) case formulation with an understanding of the personality; (b) access trauma memory; (c) if problems, get PCMs; (d) apply principles of PCM (below); (e) if problems: Apply affect tolerate affect or install resources?; and (f) result in a PCM statement and plan of action.

To repeat: Trauma victims who cannot bring out the PCM need assistance in affect tolerance or resources. The trick is to teach these. If the person is compromised and cannot handle day-to-day stress or trauma cues, then affect tolerance is in order. Affect tolerance involves coping with affect, containing excitement, defending against shame. It leads directly to dissociation. Resources, on the other hand, are already factory installed. So the therapy is not an "installation" so much as it is an enhancement of extant but dormant skills.

Affect Tolerance

Key Question: "Can you handle/cope with this emotion?"

An understanding of affect is perhaps the most important and understudied area of trauma. Memories are really affect scripts that become intertwined in a memory system. In effect, the memory is an affect laden script. It holds the trauma. The patient who can differentiate emotions from one another and can trust them is light years ahead of the one who cannot. If this skill is lacking, then affect will cause problems. Often they come in scripts that start with an affective reaction. Laughter percolates to humiliation; annoyance to shame.

Affective problems can come from a number of sources. There is some speculation that the right hemisphere is activated and the left suppressed in the presence of trauma memories (Knight, 1997). Many PTSD theorists (e.g., Leeds, 1999) believe that the work of "initial" therapy involves the "right" brain. If so, we are addressing emotion; in this case the ability to distance and objectify intense affect.

Another form of problems more associated with aging is ontological insecurity. This is a more global form of anxiety in which the person's sense of coherence and intactness as a functioning self is threatened. In this experience of anxiety there is an experience of threat and vulnerability to basic self-organization. When this threat to basic self-organization occurs, affect tolerance or the ongoing supportive quality of the therapeutic bond is crucial in helping the person to affirm a sense of self and internalize the therapist's support. Alternatively, the individual anticipates future negative events or catastrophic consequences of imagined action but reacts to these in the present as though they were actually occurring now. In this situation, fear is evoked in response to the catastrophic expectation and the appraised threat. Because the person realistically appraises the current situation as safe, however, the fear response can be dampened by the application of an affect tolerance technique.

Perhaps the key to emotional problems is (as we noted in Chapter 6) emotional awareness and regulation. Linehan (1993) discussed this best. She posited that emotional regulation skills are requisite for the treatment of borderline patients. She advocated the identification and labeling of emotions, the identification of obstacles to changing emotions, reducing vulnerability to an "emotional mind," increasing positive emotional events, and applying distress tolerance techniques. This is a wholistic attitude for self-care, that includes "validating," by paying attention to the experience of the feeling, developing a mindfulness of the emotions; "knowing" that the person is "bigger" than the emotion, that emotions are self-perpetuating and subject to interpretation, and easily can become complicated by this fact; and "doing," by attending to relationships, avoid avoiding, and the use of many distress tolerance techniques.

We liberally use many of these. Several involve distancing. The use of suspending the emotion, freezing the feeling, placing it in a box or safe place, are safe and effective techniques. Other techniques involve affective coping. We use a method called REAP described below.

Case 1

Mr. Jones was a 72 year old retired professor and at a local college. He has written several books and has been considered somewhat of an intellectual. For the most part he has been a loner. He is married and has a supportive family. He lives with his wife.

Six months ago he was the victim of robbery. He was beaten and robbed of $4,000.00 while in his home. He was home alone and the robbers are still at large. He remains most fearful about this.

He came to therapy at the request of his wife. She indicated that he was more quiet and depressed than his usual patterns. He seemed both scared and angry. She found herself helpless in his presence and could do nothing for him. She indicated that he seemed to cut ties from his children also.

It was clear that Mr. Jones did not expect much from the therapy. This said, he was most anxious and suffered from Criteria B, C, and D for PTSD. He refused to talk about the trauma and indicated that he did not feel safe in his environment.

The therapist decided to pursue PCMs based on his long history of accomplishment. Before this was undertaken, however, the therapist realized that Mr. Jones needed some buffering and safety interventions. Several plans were made to interact with the police to establish some clarity and to develop mastery over his situation. The affect tolerance techniques of emotional awareness, breathing, and distancing were practiced. He was skeptical at first but agreed to try these. In short order, he felt that he had more affect mastery over his day and could extend his activity. His wife was most helpful in these efforts. He was especially pleased that he could get through his day without being so "emotional"over his intrusive fears.

Resource Building

Key Question: "What do you need to make this work?"

What would happen if the therapist were to "front load" the patient with recourses, coping patterns that were absent from early learning as well as from the patterns? That is, what if the therapist were to build in resources early in the patient (as well as to apply affect tolerance techniques). We believe that this is best done by the management of personality. That is, the strategies are best developed through an understanding of the personality. An avoidant personality can be taught, for example, that the deficient trust can be overcome by recalling the time when they were able to be trustworthy and the rewards that followed.

The key here is that the therapist is giving the patient something that they already have—resources for life. The resources come from another time and place, as they are learned. The therapist can negotiate the coping strategy with the client. The choices are Now resources and Then resources.

Now resources:

1. How would the client prefer to be acting?
2. What are goals for the future?
3. What is called for now in the day-to-day functions of living?
4. What metaphors, images, symbols, stories are available to represent the resource?
5. Who is the key mentor/model of the person?
6. Can you use prayer?
7. What about music, novels, etc?
8. What about a positive goal state or future self?

Then resources:

1. Embryonic resources for change?
2. What were the damages with caretakers (parents)?
3. What are the missing resources for each personality?
4. What metaphors, images, symbols, stories are available to represent the resource?
5. What about generic issues of safety, trust, self-esteem, independence, intimacy, and power?

This method can be used at any time in therapy. Patients seem to understand that they lack something. They appreciate that this something is a resource absent in them. A resource can be imagined or practiced or both.

In sum, a key to the installation of the PCM is the ability for affect tolerance and resource building. Trauma victims have "adapted" by avoidance. This occurs with the use of positive memories also. They require a boost to allow the PCM or trauma to be accessed. This boost involves affect tolerance or resources or both.

Case 2

Mrs. Smith has been in the same town all her life. She was widowed four years ago and this caused problems. She felt "at sea" for several years. She received some counseling from her pastor and her children became more active in her life.

In fact, Mrs. Smith has been a worrier. She was concerned about her abilities and believed that she had to have everything just right to make life tolerable. Her husband was most tolerant and open to her ways. In the past year she had become used to his death.

One year ago she was in a motor vehicle accident. She was "the cause" of the tragedy totaling her car and injuring the driver of the other vehicle. She felt both scared to drive and guilty about her role in the accident.

Before she could address the accident she felt that she was "lacking" in her ability to continue with her life. The therapist applied a resource building procedure. She was asked to identify a recent problem. She indicated that she could not go to church as this was too embarrassing for her. She felt both emotional and shame.

The therapist asked her if she could "see" herself going to church. She could and she could identify what she needed to do this, courage and confidence. She was asked to provide a time in her life when she had either of these. She could not do this. But she discussed how her husband could do this. She was most detailed and admiring of his abilities of self confidence and skill. She was able to image this and to see herself "internalize" these skills. She related that it was what she most admired about her husband and she had often thought of this.

Through several sessions she could image herself being in the church and being more confident. These images were grounded in her (feel them in her heart) and she became more and more confident. She also related in this process that she was able to see the areas where she was "weak" and that this was helpful. She related also that she had these abilities in school. She felt that now she could do something about this.

In three weeks time she went to church.

Rules for PCM

Overall, once the patient becomes engaged in the process and is comfortable with being a storyteller, the interviewer need focus on only two tasks: to ask questions and to make facilitating comments that implicitly pursue process goals outlined below without hampering the storyteller's spontaneity. The interviewer must work hard to maintain rapport and acknowledge the patient's experience, and at times shifting the focus to more positive topics. When the patient fails to take cues to follow-up on pleasant experiences, the interviewer can change the topic to a positive one.

Given negative experiences, it is best to acknowledge these briefly and then redirect the interview toward something positive. The same is true if the patient becomes tearful, as happens on rare occasions. The interviewer should acknowledge the tears by offering a tissue, give the patient a moment to recover, and then, with the permission of the patient, move on to the next topic.

The most effective way to encourage reflection is to reinforce an interviewee. The interviewer can give reinforcement by showing increased interest, by nodding, or simply by asking the participant to elaborate further. Reflection can also be facilitated by questions that are provocative and stimulating.

Once the participant has gotten into the "groove" of discussing challenges successfully met, the interviewer should underscore strengths and resources that allowed the participant to meet a specific challenge. The goal is to identify, reinforce, and validate positive attributes that are already part of the participant's self-concept.

The final few minutes can be used to summarize the strengths and resources that have emerged from the life story. The objective of this part of the interview is to reinforce the positive aspects of the patient's self-concept and coping strengths that were brought out during the interview. This can be accomplished in different ways.

What are the conditions that facilitate growth through the PCM? These are the questions that drive the engines of research and therapy. We answer them here with the following principles.

Get the Story Out in Chronological Order

Key Question: Introduction

Based on Ryborzyck and Belly (1997), we introduce the care process thus: "You've lived a pretty long life, and you must have some wonderful memories. There have been many moments that you have an experience that has been so much a part of you as to be defining, perhaps where you lived and what you did, interactions with your children, or a long intimate conversation with someone. No doubt you have stepped back and thought of this. What each of these moments has in common is that they attempt to answer the question 'who am I?'"

"Reminiscing about early life gives real pleasure and puts people in a good frame of mind, which would be very helpful for somebody having difficulties. This may really help people get through problem times. I think people's lives are very interesting, and I would enjoy it if you want to go into detail about things you like to remember."

"For today with me the idea is to talk about your life and to begin, more or less, at the beginning. It seems to work better to do it chronologically, starting with the very earliest memories, and it doesn't really matter how far we get. What are some of your earliest memories?"

The therapist can make the past vivid and the story personal. In approaching the PCM, it is important to remember that memories can be changed, especially at later life, through words. The "unsaid" is something that already exists. It is not lying hidden in the unconscious or waiting, fully formed, to be noticed and described in the cybernetic structures of family interactions. Rather, it emerges and takes shape as we converse with each other. Therefore, it matters what therapists attend to as they listen. In other words, listening is not a passive activity. When we listen, we interpret, whether we want to or not.

Guided imagery can also been helpful. Several exercises may be particularly helpful for clients who have difficulty in "switching on" to life-review. The client can be asked to describe in words or any other medium of their choice themes selected to reflect individual interests, their life "as if" it were a house or a garden, and to proceed to fill the space with a vivid picture of life-experience. Gonclaves (1994) advocated the use of a "prototype narrative," which serves as a sort of root metaphor for one's life experience. Clients are actually taught to objectify and broaden this narrative with specific focus and detail. Then clients are taught to subjectify experiences and feel the inner experience. Next, narratives can be given metaphors using basic symbols. Finally, the client can be taught to project, construct, consolidate, and evaluate the new narrative.

Older clients, however, may have difficulty achieving clarity of the image. The therapist may have to suggest more detail in setting the scene than is the case with younger persons. Retaining an imagined scene may also be more difficult. Breaking the scene down into smaller parts (as was done with the sample hierarchy described in this section) may help. However just the act of retelling creates healing. After a healing atmosphere is established, a narrative foothold unfolds in the story details.

Be Reflexive

Key Question: "Tell me the story: What does this mean to you?"

Consciousness is a great unsolved problem. It is an internal narrative whose processes supply comment to thoughts. In consciousness, the here and now is flanked by the past which illuminates them, and by the anticipated future. The drama of life comes from consciousness and that makes life, life. Being reflexive allows an understanding of this.

In fact, we go back and forth between reality and the self-created version of reality we "create on our moments." We carry around a load of this superimposed reality and we drop it onto every moment and interaction. In a strange way life keeps trying to show us the real reality and we keep trying to push it away. We feel safe in our imaginary reality. Our defenses work. You might say that we are only half alive. You might also say this moment is only a moment by an awareness (of the moment). This latter task is done by reflexivity.

The narrative plays the role in the organization of the event knowledge and self. This is, of course, reflexivity, a dialectical approach helping the person examine the self from multiple perspectives. Dialectics in its most essential form is the splitting of a single whole into its contradictory parts. The polar parts, when brought into contact, interact to produce transformation. Novelty then emerges from a dialectical synthesis. The dialectic with which we are most concerned is that which constitutes consciousness—the dialectic between concept and experience, between reflexive explaining and direct being, between mediated and immediate experience (Safran & Greenberg, 1991; Guidano, 1991; Mahoney, 1991). People are continually engaged in a process of reflexively constructing reality from the dialectical synthesis of these two sources of experience. In fact, development is a transformational shift as a person moves from one system of structuring the world to another. It is not a cumulative process but a transformational one. This occurs in this reflexive process.

Foa and Meadows (1997) noted that a substantial part of the understanding of the unfolding of the treatment of trauma is discovery oriented. This is invested in observations and emerging postdictive strategies. A focus on understanding the process of task solution and building explanatory models of the processes involved in resolution may be important. This may involve a working cognitive map by the clinician of the observations.

Gendlin (1991) described this "meaning changing" process of therapy. He requested that the therapist seek a "felt sense" where the client feels the problem. An exercise that may be helpful is to imagine a troubling scene and its emotion, and "try on" the questions noted below. Usually, the "bad emotion" evolved from a more flexible, wider context to a narrow one. Trauma victims are stuck in that narrow emotion feeling. But, as these probes are considered and experienced, the context may change again. Gendlin labeled this a *shift*. Typical suggestions are: Can you get a broader sense of that feeling? Can you stop and sense the meaning of that feeling? What is that feeling? What is that "sore spot" up against? Can you get in touch with the whole issue? What say do you have over those feelings? What word/image/metaphor goes with that? What's in the way of this being okay? What is the worst of this? What are you all about? How are you stuck? Just sit quiet, clear a space, and see what else is there? Be friendly to yourself, create a space, and let your body tell you what all that feeling is about.

What occurs here is that the whole of the person is activated. This involves the body, an alteration in the present as the new textures of background unfold. The gentle acceptance of "what is" eventually feels "right" or fits, and, as it does, the victim changes.

In sum, reflexivity enables clients to have their cake and eat it too. They could use the structure of narrative to protect themselves from having to acknowledge explicitly their inner feelings. Or, through the act of telling a story a person comes to understand self more fully, although there was no necessity to configure that understanding into the story. Hence, the PCM creates a situation in which they could try on past or current positions. So, the therapist is encouraged to keep a balance between experiencing and reflecting.

Be Nonreflexive: Present Centered/Use Affect

Key Question: "Stay with that: Experience that feeling."

This, of course, is the other side of the reflexivity task. We know that the trauma victim is stuck in the past. To process the past, more than "re-experiencing past" must occur; a processing of the past in the present must occur. How does the present change the past? By the very act of making the past present, a new re-experience, a carrying forward and a new texture evolves. Often more "differents" occur: metaphors, images, feelings, new information, and so on.

Memory is present consciousness. Bring the person into the present by attending to current feeling, sensations, and thoughts. A crucial task of therapy is to facilitate experiential processing rather than conceptual processing, to enable the person to process holistic, emotionally toned experience in more effective ways. It is not insight into abstract patterns of behavior across situations, such as "rebelling against authority," or "pushing people away when they get close," that is searched for in therapy. Rather it is the re-experience of a concrete, particular instance that is sought after. Therapy needs to open people to more internal and external information and to stimulate and evoke the emotion schemes that generate the person's fundamental experience and that serve as the basis of emotional meaning. By exploring a particular situation as completely and fully as possible, people can access their fundamental, holistic models of the world, the models responsible for their experience, of self. It is these holistic models, not conceptual meanings that need reorganizing.

Another monitor of presentness is affect. Affect stimulates cognitions. With the mere identification of the emotion the therapist assists the person in the understanding and acceptance of conflict. A vivid description of the situation as well as the client's differentiation of the intersubjective experience. A vivid description facilitates emotional arousal and facilitates recollection. The patient that is present in the room and involved re-experiences and changes the past in the present.

It appears to be the full experience of a single instance of an experience that will bring forth all the elements of the actual experience from memory. So the task is to keep the patient in the present. The mindfulness of the present is necessary and maybe sufficient for change.

Validate the Stability of the Self

Key Question: "How does this reflect YOU?"

Nothing is a random event in therapy. The clinician can celebrate the positive, listen, and enjoy. This involves making vivid the notion that: "This really was you!" This is actually a pleasing and simple task: to attend to issues of the past and present that are empowering to the self. This enables the client's sense of agency in the context of the past. It is best if fresh and spontaneous. Examples of statements about strengths and resources are "You've always been a resourceful person"; "You were willing to make a lot of sacrifices to achieve your goals"; "You really stand up for yourself when you need to"; "You seem to be very good at making adjustments"; "Your family really stuck together"; "The work ethic was very important to you"; "You have been good at finding creative solutions to things"; "Your willpower got you through again"; "Your sense of humor served you well"; and "You seem to have had lots of love in your life."

Validation or invalidation of the most central expectations or schemas is a critical focal point. Broadly speaking, when validation occurs the strategies used to cope with changes are flexible and adaptive. However, when invalidation of those constructs is experienced, such strategies become rigid and self-defeating. With validation of central role expectations, then, the older victim moves easily between tight and loose construing. In other words, they move easily between stable and more varying anticipations of events, a flexibility of construing for dealing with change. With invalidation, the construing can be either too loose, sometimes resulting in confusion, or too tight, sometimes resulting in their repeated and inappropriate blaming of others. With validation of role expectations, clients are able to develop new constructs and alter old ones.

One more thing here. People have a self-ideal, parts of self that are more equal than others. Some people value honesty, competition, intelligence, loyalty, etc. They are almost "traited" in this or that area. When trauma occurs, the victim becomes sensitive to these areas. As a result, the victim may overcompensate by excessive sensitivity to honesty, competition, etc. In effect, these become hot areas. They "cause" problems, often unaware. The person now is hurt or angry because of the overly sensitive stance of a loyalty breach or competition slight. This brings on the feelings of the trauma without direct trauma stimuli. When the stability of the self is identified and reinforced, the person of the victim can be "freed" to react or not. Again knowledge is power.

Respect Cognition

Key Question: Assimilation queries include the following:

1. What evidence do you have to support this thought?
2. Is there any alternative way of looking at the situation or yourself?
3. Is there any alternative explanation?
4. How do you think I, your therapist, would view this situation? How would (valued person) think of it?
5. Are you shoulding or musting on yourself or the world?
6. What's the worse possible outcome?
7. How long will this unpleasant situation last?
8. On the grand scale of injustice or badness, how unjust or bad is it?
9. Are you confusing a remote possibility with a high probability outcome?
10. Are you overestimating the amount of control or responsibility you have for the situation?
11. Are you discounting or discrediting positive aspects of the situation or your ability to cope with it?
12. What does this problem say about who you are?

Narrative psychotherapists (e.g., Terrell & Lyddon, 1999) have accessed the change processes in the creation of a meaning event. Meaning events have been found to be particularly important in the recovery of traumatic processes. The symbolization of therapeutic intervention found in the creation of the meaning episodes formed an important component of the integrated constructed treatment for addressing issues in trauma survivors. Creation of meaning refers to the individual's need to construct an acceptable understanding of an emotionally charged experience by putting it into words. It involves the development of linguistic symbols to represent the meaning of an experience while one is feeling and perceiving the emotion generated by the experience. This means cognition, the formation of the acceptable "insurrection of knowledge."

The change in thinking regarding a memory is similar to the processes shown in cognitive therapy. Remember, here we are interested in a PCM, a positive memory. The rubrics of CBT provide a map for intervention. Making incorrect or automatic judgments represents a "deep habit" that requires awareness. Recognition of thoughts perpetuating habit is often all that is required. The client is a practical scientist who makes observations, sets up hypotheses, checks their validity, and eventually forms generalizations that will later serve as a guide for making rapid judgments of situations. This can be unearthed by the simple and persistent application of a cognitive focus. Stalemated dualities such as: husband/wife, parents/children, patient/"others," and supporters/persecutors. Ideally, the therapist should maintain the neutral stance of interpreter or commentator, instilling movement into the hardened polarities.

PCM Summary and Plan of Action

Key Question: "This is who you are and what you can do/did." "Here are some rules to assist in living"

There are two features here (Figure 9-1). They are the learnings of the PCM and coping. The summary, however, is just that—a positive, but fair representation of the salient learnings of the PCMs. The idea is to cull from the person necessary agency and self-empowered patterns and learnings that apply. This is crafted over time and over PCMs.

Summary:

_____

_____

_____

_____

_____

_____

_____

_____

_____

PCM Learnings:

_____

_____

_____

_____

_____

_____

FIGURE 9-1. Positive Core Memory

Coping (REAP):

Recognize _____

_____

Evaluate(SUDS) _____

Act(Iwill) _____

_____

_____

Prevention

Physical risk factors _____

Emotional risk factors _____

Cognitive risk factors _____

FIGURE 9-1. (*Continued*)

In addition, the learnings of the PCM are developed. This is a narration of the PCM and the core learnings. It consists of two parts then, the summary itself (a few paragraphs), and salient messages from the experience. Messages are a series of statements, like "I can handle adversity," "I can change my circumstances," "I was able to share feelings," "I was the one who initiated the change in my life," "I care for people," etc. Practical day-to-day coping strategies are also part of the process.

Regarding the PCM, we have noted that stories are the most important components in therapy. They help develop and maintain a sense of identity. Stories provide guidance by which to live lives and place order on the sometimes chaotic events. At the end of life we need closure and to provide a legacy.

Additionally, adult developmentalists argue that personality continues to grow and develop through the life cycle. At various points in life, challenges "ascend"—inner needs meet cultural demands at a particular age period. As we have argued, at later life something happens that increases tolerance and willingness to "look again" for authenticity. How does the Me of yesterday become the Me of today and the anticipated Me of the future? Transitions set off events that invalidate extant core constructs. Generativity influences this interplay in later life. The therapist can foster this with a focus on empowering choices. A generativity script of the present is initiated. People really do change by life review.

In a way the therapist helps the client organize the self as better "voiced characters." The future and possible narrative receives a "privileged status" over and against old traits. The "You did this" phrase can be most empowering. The new story now can serve as higher order discourse for purposes of the unification and integration of disparate elements into a meaningful unity. The therapist just has to ask.

Regarding coping, the goal is for the person to apply both integrating and coping features of the PCM to life. This by itself is the goal of many therapies. The idea is for the person to have a memory plan that includes growth. The person now has an improved integrated view of self. This allows for an improved sense of self-esteem.

But the plan also allows for something else: a coping profile that includes many of the features of a relapse plan. We use a plan called REAP. The person is taught to

Recognize—here it is. I can do this.
Evaluate—use of a device for scaling (SUDS).
Act—relax, think, cope, do something.
Prevent—organize environment for safety and positive events.

The risk factors include (a) physical—people, places, and things that put the person at risk; (b) emotional—feelings associated with problems; (c) cognitive—cognitions and self-talk associated with problems.

With this plan the trauma victim can apply what was learned with the PCM. The person both organizes life for integrity (PCM) and plans for problems (coping).

☐ Last Resort

Change the Memory if Necessary

Key Question: "Let's switch gears. Give me that good time you had when . . ."

If memories are virulent and negative, the therapist can become therapeutically practical during the PCM task. If the memory is negative and stuck, the therapist can change the memory.

Nichols (1991) outlined a positive recall procedure, labeled *core goals*. A core goal is the single feature of the person that is best situated to account for behavior. Satisfaction or dissatisfaction results because the core goal is or is not met. Knowing what is wanted explains what is rewarding or dissatisfying. Applied to the trauma victim, he/she is asked to identify "best moments" or positive experiences. As with PCMs, best moments are isolated. These are developed from positive memories, so they are "real" and appealing. Since they are emotional experiences, the goals often become "alive" and assume a life of their own. Again, goals have a direction setting function and are the motivation behind behavior (see Nichols, 1991).

It is of course possible to have patients who can give no positive experiences. Often the judicious use of time, as well as a therapeutic foraging in the past, is required. With some, "moral jogging" may assist (Seligman, 1998). The task here is to have the patient give to others as a way to "jump start" the moral process of non-depression (optimism). The patient may be asked to volunteer, for example.

The therapist is cautioned against the use of the PCM with recently or pathological grieving victims. (See Chapter 11.) The highly depressed patient also can be a problem. But, the therapist can usually elicit a PCM and this can serve as the sediment for change.

In sum, the restructuring reality with PCMs is both simple and sometimes complex. It is done simply with clinical interest in the new memory itself. This interest is of course one that exposes the positive epiphanic moments of the new memory. It can also be more complex as the PCM gets stuck. In such a case the client is not ready. Management is necessary, and deconstruction also always applies.

☐ Special Case: Deconstructivism

"An abnormal reaction to an abnormal situation is normal."
Frankl

There is a middle way. How else can the therapist defuse toxic memories? In the telling of the story, the therapist can also be an interested listener, one who uses constructivist interventions or storining. We repeat a theme. The patient narrates, the therapist listens and directs, even interprets. Eventually predominate stories "get the message." Perhaps there is a story synthesizer present. If psychotherapy is anything, it involves an alteration of acquired meanings. This is done by language—language allows you to "hover over" the experience.

This appears to occur in several ways. The co-construction of new meaning occurs during the ongoing dialogue of treatment. The past alters because it is spoken. Memories in this sense are a recollection of the past in terms of present meaning (Duncan, Solovey, & Rusk, 1992). There is no memory without a present context, but the message alters also because it is never the same. Because the current interactions are always changing anyway, there is never one absolute memory. It is this continuous meaning revision, the juxtaposition of past in the present context, that, we believe, is the curative agent of psychotherapy. Deconstructive therapy sees change as unfolding naturally.

Meaning-making is also about the journey of development and the creation of self—the activity of each person who is both shaping a self and shaping a coherent, meaningful life. Development is not from something absent to something present: It progresses from the simple to a new "simple," perhaps now complex. Development occurs as a person moves from one system of structuring the world to another. It is then both a cumulative process and a transformational one. With complexity of thought and self-knowledge comes an increasing capacity to achieve personal creative solutions and new forms of knowledge (Carlsen, 1988, pp. 12–13). In this process are the movements of personal knowing that can take a person into "more epistemologically powerful (inclusive, viable, integrated) ways of making sense of the world" (Lyddon & Alford, 1993, p. 32). For some, this journey constitutes a life project.

At its simplist level, deconstruction involves the therapist's accepting the client's frame as logical up to the point where it produces troublesome behaviors, thoughts, feelings, and perceptions. The therapist explores the client's situation, sometimes in great detail and at great length looking for a focal point or some puzzled moment. When one listens "deconstructively" to people's stories, listening is guided by the belief that those stories have many possible meanings. The meaning a listener makes is, more often than not, different from the meaning that the speaker has intended. Through this listening, an open space is sought for aspects of people's life narratives that haven't yet been storied. People are invited to relate to their life narratives, not as passively received facts, but as actively constructed stories. Therapy is a process in which "we are always moving toward what is not yet known" (Anderson & Goolishian, 1990, p. 159). This implies not asking questions from a position of pre-understanding (Andersen, 1991; Weingarten, 1992) and not asking questions to which we want particular answers. This may be especially important for brighter older victims.

White (1980) introduced the idea that the person is not the problem; the problem is the problem. People who suffer abuse tend to internalize the traumatizing events to which they have been subjected as inner dialogues. They stay in narrow views of self. Deconstruction questions help people unpack their stories or see them from different perspectives, so that how they have been constructed becomes apparent. Questions, for example, encourage people to situate their narratives in larger systems and through time. The idea is to broaden the scope of the landscape of now-only-seen problems.

The design adopted in our formulation of sequential meaning-making unfolds from a philosophy of care that espouses the importance of language in the social construction of meaning. Box 9-3 notes the therapeutic processes in this formation of new meaning. In this table, logical therapeutic processes involve therapist interventions that are both more passive, simply accentuating or contrasting statements, and more active with therapeutic altering and questioning. They are intended to create an atmosphere of dialogue to upset the expectancies of the patient. Eventually these may unearth or disrupt the comfort of old thinking.

This therapy is a part of all therapies. Destructuring also hypothesizes an interactive relation between experience that is construed in the isolated subsystem and experience for which constructs are never developed. Experience of the latter type would produce anxiety or confusion in the individual. This anxiety actually initiates movement within construct subsystems. Often this is sufficient for change in therapy.

We are advocating for a new voice, a new point of view; different contexts, different time frames, motivation, hopes, and goals, as well as values and beliefs, knowledge, and leanings. Once the landscape of the problem has been broadened through deconstruction questions, there are numerous vantage points from which unique outcomes or "sparkling events"—those experiences that lie outside of the problem-saturated narrative and would not be predicted by it—might be brought forth (Friedman & Coombs, 1996). Hardened stories are softened and often confess their weakness. At the least, the person is empowered with ambiguity. Waxing poetic, a healing resolution may not be a function of its absence. Rather, resolution occurs when meaning is provided or, when little is left to be learned (Epstein, 1990).

Finally, we put on a scientific/critical thinking cap. The development of the narrative is complicated, beyond this representation. Undigested dimensions include the domain of the narrative (i.e., how narratives are defined in terms of textual structure), the individual's involvement in the developmental process (i.e., the relationship between some internal and external forces and the organism's own active participation in the developmental process), the course of development (i.e., whether it is continuous or discontinuous and whether it perceives in an edited fashion or is regressive over phases, and what is the impact of transitional points), the goal of development (the implicit notion of target points that are appropriate in developmental processes), the mechanisms of development (i.e., the forces or conditions that both instigate the developmental process and keep it moving), and the methodology (where and how to look for the establishment of a developmental framework of the trauma). But, lest we be caught in the vortex of the confusion of these potential quandries, we can act with the assurance of a clinician whose one friend is clarity and knowledge, a fair exposition of the person's take on a topic with many perspectives and voices.

☐ Conclusion

Throughout life, the internal and subjective and the external and objective are negotiated. Psychological development occurs where we interpret and reinterpret our

Box 9-3
Selective Process Interventions in Constructivist Psychotherapy

Overall Positions
1. Realities are socially constructed.
2. Realities are constituted through language.
3. Realities are organized and maintained through narrative.
4. There are no essential truths.

Deconstructive Actions

Safran and Segal (1989):

Intervention	Description
Empathizing	Indwelling the client's meanings and communicating an understanding of them
Analogizing	Developing an image or metaphor to explore or capture an experience
Accentuating	Focusing the client's attention on an important feature of experience that might be overlooked
Nuancing	Highlighting in passing an aspect of the client's communication for further elaboration
Dilating	Widening the field of discussion to include broader issues or implications
Constricting	Narrowing discussion to a single focal issue
Contrasting	Exploring a sensed conflict or discrepancy in the client's experience
Structuring	Articulating or organizing diffuse material in a way that clarifies its implications for action
Ambiguating	Fostering a looser or more approximate meaning
Weaving	Overlaying or connecting strands of related material

de Shazer (1998):

1. Making exceptions into the rule.
2. Changing the location of the complaint pattern.
3. Changing who is involved in the complaint pattern.
4. Changing the order of the steps involved.
5. Adding a new element or step to the complaint pattern.
6. Increasing the duration of the pattern.
7. Introducing arbitrary starting and stopping.
8. Increasing the frequency of the pattern.
9. Changing the modality of the problematic behavior.

(continued)

Box 9-3
(Continued)

Freedman and Combs (1996):

1. Give memory a plot: Externalizes the problem and pathologizes the pathologizing pattern itself.
2. Relative influence questioning: Map the influence of the problem in their lives and relationships and then to map their influence on the life of the problem.
3. Contextual influences on the problem: What "feeds" the problem? What "starves" it? Who benefits from it? In what settings might the problematic attitude be useful? What sort of people would proudly advocate for the problem?
4. Asking for openings: "Has there ever been a time when the problem tried to get the upper hand, but you were able to resist its influence?"
5. Look for preferred experiences: "Does this interest you?" "Did that surprise you?" "Is this something that you want more of in your life?"
6. Think like a novelist or screenwriter: "What was the look on his face when you told him?" "What did he call you? "When he was saying that, did he refer to you by a special name?"
7. Characters and multiple viewpoints: Ask about other people's points of view.
8. Dual landscapes: Both with action and consciousness. The action (agentic) self is reinforced. "How did you do that?" The landscape of consciousness involves meaning question. "What does that mean to you?"
9. Hypothetical experiences: "Were there times when you've done this kind of thing before?" "Who would have predicted this event?" "What have they seen you do before that would have led them to believe you would have done this?"
10. Link the past with present: "Now that I understand its foundation in your past, do you see how this recent development in your relationship makes even more sense to me?"
11. Extend the story in future: "If we look at these events that we've been talking about as a trend in your life, what do you expect the next step will be?"

---

experiences. The integration of these reinterpretations is the primary characteristic of psychological development. This is especially important for our more central, core constructs about ourselves, housed in our memories. This focus is a "true continuation" of psychological maturation and development. Given adequate ego resources and a sustaining, supportive environment, most elderly people can do this and master the challenges of later life.

Of course there is loss. Cath (1965) characterized the middle and later years as a balance between factors that promote a person's self-esteem and sense of self (e.g., wisdom derived from lifelong experience, the attainment of a satisfying philosophical and religious world view, past accomplishments), and factors leading to emotional depletion (e.g., failing health, cognitive impairment). Trauma is also a loss, sometimes so much as to prevent the presence of anything positive.

However in this chapter we advocated for a true integrative therapy. Here we emphasize the positive. Just as the longitudinal course of PTSD is a total person response, the way out of trauma can be broad and flexible. If the process of (trauma) decline is impacted unduly at first by fearful and intrusive experiences and accommodated to by a symphony of poor adaptation, the strengths of later life are the needed ones that redress this frozen self. The wise clinician then can treat the person of trauma victim at later life with this other clinical focus. Fortunately, we believe, a simple massaging of PCMs can be all that is required.

10
CHAPTER

The Trauma Memory: The "Bad" Memory

"The exploration of personal meaning of the trauma is critical: The pursuit of the meaning of the trauma is the central goal of therapy."
Bessel van der Kolk

The alteration of the trauma memory is the work of therapy in PTSD (van der Kolk, 1996). In the previous chapter we considered the "lighter side of treatment." This is not less important. It simply considers other aspects of the person. Additionally it massages memories in an "easier" way. Also interventions related to reminiscence (expose the story, unearth obvious distortions, and provide methods for alternative beliefs) apply.

In other chapters we learned the dirty secrets of the trauma memory. In other chapters we also noted that several techniques exist that are apt for the exposure and rescripting of the trauma memory. The traumatic event is less elaborated, fixed in hierarchical assignment, isolated, unable to enter into subsets and supersets with other construed events, and therefore less likely to be related by associative or transitive propositions with the rest of the individual's conceptual structure. Consensus also exists that the more the trauma memory is organized, narrativized, and placed into explicit memory, elaborated, disclosed, validated, and retrieved as less a summary memory, the more general improvement occurs. These efforts at explanation of the personal meaning of the trauma are critical because patients cannot easily undo past grieving (van der Kolk, McFarlane, & van der Hart, 1996). Exposure techniques of any ilk, direct or otherwise, are staples but often not sufficient to effectively treat PTSD. The proper application of cognitive-behavioral assimilation techniques within the context of a supportive and collaborative therapeutic relationship also is required. Merely uncovering memories, then, is not enough. They need to be modified and transformed.

The use of CBT/AMT methods and those applied to the narrative are apt for trauma alteration of older victims. After all, trauma psychotherapy is a continual retelling of self, shifting from previous negative narratives to more positive ones (van der Kolk, McFarlane, & van der Hart, 1996). With the combination of assimilation

(CBT and narrative work) and exposure work (AMT + exposure), trauma codes can become habituated (desensitized) *and* assimilated (corrective cognitive codes). Initially, intrusions of fragmentary memories of the trauma may predominate. Here exposure and desensitization are what patients most urgently require. At a later stage of the progression of the disorder—when individuals have organized their lives around avoidance of triggers of the trauma—primary attention needs to be paid to stabilization or management, in the meaning or social realm. In general, it appears that the persistence of the intrusive recollections drives the biological and psychological components of PTSD, even if avoidance provides its virulent quality. For this victim, probably the only recourse is management of the symptoms (Stages 1–4 and 5).

It is at the end that we consider the intrusive element of the trauma, that component that is there first and last. Most victims then will not receive the methods in this chapter. The core of our treatment is AMT, the management of anxiety, and EMDR, an efficient way to process information. We also highlight two issues that are critical for success, booster sessions/relapse and the broader focus of care, the caretaker/family. We do this not because they are afterthoughts. In fact, these are built-in to the care equation from the beginning. These are, therefore, not ending issues. As we have done in many previous chapters we consider the influence of aging in this mix first.

☐ Extant Models

Treatment books of PTSD are generally in concert. We are forever iterating Freud's ideas of stimulus barrier and repetition compulsion, and later Horowitz's (1986) phase model. Today, the treatment of trauma is often discussed in phase language. Trauma occurs because the intrusion and avoidance phases are out of control, when oscillation is out of sync. Under such conditions the client's defenses are themselves bad cops, letting the wrong things occur and picking up good perpetrators.

Such models have much to offer. They outline what is necessary in care. First, develop the alliance, as the therapist gathers information from the history, both current and past trauma. Initially also, the therapist assures him/herself of the client's tolerance for treatment, especially the client's history interpersonally (Burns, 1999). Here, baseline anxiety levels must be reduced to at least tolerable levels. Soon the treatment components of encouraging action (social support, reduce avoidance, etc.) are activated. Compensatory skills are always in place before exploration. Eventually the revision of the trauma is addressed. By repeatedly redoing the trauma event, the inner and outer worlds of the client are revisited and an appreciation of cognitive and emotional meanings unfold. Eventually the person is encouraged to practice new skills, experience, and recognize the provoked emotions and thoughts, and alter these.

In actual trauma revision, the therapist proceeds with loose goals in mind; acknowledge and accept traumatized self, regain mastery, and integrate traumatic information. In trauma integration the therapist usually proceeds from the periphery to the core, with interpretations at a low ebb or at the least presented as working hypotheses. It is the re-experiencing that needs to be addressed as the mind must revise events and the body must avoid avoidance. Eventually, this intervention may give way to an activist stance, to mild confrontations. Interpretations may be useful; for example, when the client resists acknowledging any psychological distress beyond obvious symptoms (e.g., counterphobic defenses for self-protection). Stoppage points are of course red flags for therapist action. Transformation of core schemas eventually requires a working through.

In this revision process, the re-experiencing can be slowed, stopped, or fast-forwarded, as the level of tolerable dosage is found. Bad data must be processed, as trauma cannot be assimilated into existing mental schemes. Always the therapist is undoing poor responses, as in differentiating fact from fancy and encouraging an active stance for the client. The client needs to have the opportunity to initiate changes in a real way and under his/her own control. At any point anxiety may revisit the scene and the therapist response is desensitization. Success comes in many forms but always in the recognition of the traumatized self.

☐ Development and Memory

"Life can only be understood backwards"
Soren Kierkegaard

Personal narratives are not encapsulated intrapsychic constructs, which dwell in splendid isolation within the mind. They are attached to the developmental dialogue of the person and as part of other characters and storymakers (Omer, 1994). Remembering an autobiographical memory is really an active process characterized by shifting interpretations and new life situations attaching to an ongoing life narrative. In this way, delayed recall of the trauma, common in many older victims, is understandable. It exists, especially with childhood trauma. People protect their selves well even with trauma. The likelihood is that an "awakening" unfolds over time rather than after a single event and that it ascends most commonly in the context of a life's crisis or developmental milestone. People may come to psychotherapy due to recent life crises/milestones, a change in a close relationship, intrusion of memories, idiosyncratic occurrences, and abstinence of drugs and alcohol (Harvey, 1996). Trauma reminders may also serve as triggers. Over time, the active suppression of thoughts about trauma predispose individuals to stress-related illnesses (Pennebacker, 1989). At later life then developmental milestones and losses are at the ready to unleash the occult suppression of trauma.

Psychotherapy with an older adult is not simply adjustment to current problems of old age (as is often assumed in reviews of therapy with the aged). It concerns itself with working through unfinished business from earlier stages of life. While possible for someone to go through all of their life with resolved identity issues from adolescence, generativity issues from adulthood, or even autonomy issues from childhood, it is not likely. People carry baggage. PTSD people carry much baggage. Over time, the area most in need of repair (for the older person), the memory, is well protected by the PTSD-enhancing methods of operation. This includes negative interpretation as well as (un)stable patterns of interaction (personality). Older victims also have poor self-soothing skills crusted from a lifetime of experience.

However, older people also have the advantage that they can rework earlier stories, now as meta-historians, in a natural way. Later life is the time to renegotiate these choices. History and identity are both made and discovered. Priorities switch. Starratt and Peterman (1997) noted that non-egocentric events that occur to the elderly are more important than the egocentric ones because, as Erikson noted, they are more concerned with generativity than egocentric events. Frankl (1988) believed that the curative factors in existential psychotherapy with older adults involves noticing (future-oriented), actualizing (present-oriented), and re-collecting (past-oriented) events/memories, the storehouse or museum of meanings of the person. The storehouse becomes "forever real," conscious, and complete. The older client who is fully heard can assert an "aging self" and perhaps alter the lifestyle.

Viewing memory reconstruction only as necessary for resolution is, we believe, flawed. Increased access to memories is a sign that the self-structure is whole and complete. Even in a delayed state of remembering (Meiselman, 1990), the memory of trauma seems to represent the "internal wisdom" of the client. When clients express concern about not being able to remember, it is important to communicate that individuals remember their past when they are ready and that in some instances, fully functioning people do not gain complete memories of their past. As the client develops new coping skills, poor defensive postures are no longer a necessary mechanism for protecting the self.

Research data on older trauma victims are distinctly absent in these areas. The principles of getting the troubling story out and facilitating movement in the processing of the memory are paramount. The idea is to provide a perspective for a friendly review and allow the client to alter the memory. This is actually a co-creation of an acceptable myth through the story. This involves some technology also.

☐ Stage 6: The Trauma Memory

The last (and complement of the fifth) component is the "work of trauma therapy." Decondition trauma memories by the application of AMT or EMDR. Remember that we need something simple and doable for a complex problem like memory. Binder (1999) indicated that as therapists we need to make therapy part of procedural knowledge. It must exist in the therapist as a routine and natural. This seems to occur best when the therapist can teach, coach, and show. This is what is involved in the trauma memory.

We provide several pre-AMT/EMDR thoughts and then discuss the techniques themselves. For the trauma memory, preparation is everything.

Before AMT or EMDR

Initially we apply a cost benefit analysis. Then two preliminary training/education issues follow. A cost benefit analysis is a technique that allows the clinician and the patient to see the strengths and blockages for the memory intervention. Cost benefit analysis involves providing the patient with a way to isolate the factors, both primary and secondary, that can facilitate or prevent memory work. Burns (1999) espoused this as the most important technique for unearthing motivational problems. This is then an important technology.

One way to apply this is for the clinician to identify the cognition (or belief) that prevents memory work. Then a paradoxical method of the cost benefit analysis is used (Burns, 1999). This negative belief is next placed in the center of the page and the advantages and disadvantages are considered. This may take some time and each input deserves time. All are written down. At the end the "summative feel" of each is given (50–50, 60–40, etc.). A decision is then made to proceed or to work on some blocking agent.

Remember too that working through traumatic memories, including those to which the client has clear access, should not occur until the client's self-structure is relatively stable and the client can tolerate strong affect. We have addressed these issues in other chapters (Briere, 1994; McCann & Pearlman, 1990). The ability to tolerate exposure to new, painful material can be gained through assessments of the client's ability to engage in introspection, ability to manage and limit self-loathing and self-depreciation, and capacity to engage in self-soothing and calming activities, especially. Self capacities are also enhanced as a client learns concrete coping skills, including thought-stopping and stress-inoculation techniques, as well as the "dosing" of one's exposure to emotional discomfort or stressful events, and the transforming events by developing positive imagery, and taking "mental vacations" from memories just described.

The first education/training involves an explanation of the biology of trauma. Although this is given at other times in the model, it is most helpful here. Information about the world is transmitted by our senses to the thalamus, the brain's grand central station. It is efficiently sorted and assigned meaning by the cortex, and eventually ferried down the limbic system to the emotional brain, the amygdala. However in trauma, the cerebral cortex is bypassed entirely. The amygdala triggers a cascade of physiological responses from a speeded-up heart, to jacked-up blood pressure to tense muscles. The hijacking (of the amygdala) is persuasive and compelling. A subterranean pathway takes over and the new path is prepotent. Now stimuli for the trauma can be just about anything—an angry look, a feared stimuli, a critical colleague, and so on. The amygdala then makes a snap judgement on often vague evidence and a trauma reaction is under way. Often the trauma victim may not remember the reason for the stimulus, but the amygdala does. The inner trauma narrative is accessed and the rest is a script of terror or self-defeating patterns.

Naturally there is a problem if the human brain is wired in such a way that the first reaction is emotional. But there is more, especially with aging. Under extreme stress the hippocampus, the brainy friend of the amygdala, shrivels, thus preventing any logical appraisal of the event after a period. This occurs in PTSD. This occurs in aging.

What to do with people who react to others and stimuli as an animal to a conditioned fear? Can thoughts even have a chance of working in such an emotional-saturated situations? The answer is yes. The person can access thoughts easily in situations in which there is time or the amygdala can be "reasoned with" as in mild stimuli. When the cortex has a chance to flex its muscle, "thinking therapies" work. Also there is another situation. A relaxation response is possible when the client is trained to experience sympathetically and to interact with those brain states that allow for a switch to a more vulnerable state. The client must feel safe, read the signature signs of arousal, and practice their vulnerable reactions.

The second preliminary training entails coping techniques. The first is relaxation that we addressed in the previous chapter. Next, signature emotional reactions are identified. These are labeled as such. Immediately this leaves a safety feeling of understanding and perhaps control. The body is the voice of the emotions. This is the emergency brain-state that has its own profile. The moment one becomes aware of this response, the client activates the prefrontal lobes and the response can be modified. The client can be taught to practice this. The knotted stomach is a personalized reaction to the trauma. The client is then taught to "think." Initially this is a coping response. After a period this can be a full-fledged challenge to emotional reactions.

Finally, whether using AMT or EMDR, one technique that has been especially beneficial is the compartmentalization of worry, a technique applied in several CBT models. We believe that it should be routinely introduced to older PTSD clients. This technique is especially applicable to those PTSD clients with comorbid generalized anxiety disorders, ones who chronically and excessively ruminate about a variety of problems in their lives. With this procedure, clients are paradoxically directed by the therapist to worry at specific times and in specific places in an effort to get their ruminations under better stimulus control. For example, a client might be directed to think and worry about their health for an hour between 9 and 9:30 each morning while sitting in their living room and to steadfastly refuse to think about the matter at other times or in other places. Surpassingly, this is a valued technique for many older victims.

In effect, before trauma work the patient is given a safety plan. This includes a plan to activate day-to-day. It includes physical risk factors (situations, people, places), emotional risk factors (feelings, physical sensations), and cognitive risk factors (negative thinking factors, denial thoughts). These carry through and include relapse prevention.

In a previous book (Hyer et al., 1994), we argued that symptom therapy is best done with a mixture of top-down and bottom-up interventions. This involves an application of both CBT and experiential methods, used flexibility. They mix and match until success is reached. At any particular point in therapy, then, the "right mixture" of these two methods provides for the needed titration of the necessary externality/interiority of meaningful therapy. Synthesizing data from disparate sources in the integration of treatment is challenging. Used in the context of AMT or EMDR, the work of therapy is easier and straightforward. We are now ready for AMT or EMDR.

Memory Rendition

Procedurally, the sequence of memory work is straightforward. The therapist has assessed for client skills, willingness, and needed safety issues (Stage 5). At this time also, affect is not attended to but defused if necessary. At this early juncture, when emotion is present, the therapist is advised to interpret upward or to focus on reality issues. In fact, in the early stages for just a clinical rendition of the trauma, the paralyzing affect that stopped the story telling dissipates (temporally).

As with Aristotle, near enough is good enough. The therapist obtains the facts, a "clean" rendition of the events. Now is the time for information gathering. Confusion, misattribution, fears, and gaps are highlighted and gently challenged. Often new information is introduced. The objective is not an exacting account of the trauma, as there is little evidence that this helps in therapy. Rather, when a reasonable rendition of the story has been settled on, a final run at objectification (facts, sequence) is provided by the therapist. Normalization and education regarding the reasons for unearthing the memory are provided also. This is the story that will be returned to. This is not the time for aggressive treatment. The objective is not cure, but an understanding of the event and any surface construal. The time for stopping the process and teasing apart emotional accouterments is later; why this emotion, what these construals, how does the victim sees "self," and so on.

The patient needs to know some things clearly, that they are safe and that they can be fallible. Encourage fallibility. The clinician naturally will have asked about trauma events. This should not inordinately cause problems beyond the meeting (Boudewyns & Shipley, 1983). At this point clients need to know that they are "exempt" from the necessity of absolute accuracy in the representation of the memory. Routine education on the vagaries of memory are important. What is important is a reasonable accounting of the event, one that is believed in.

Many clients report that they believe that memory acts like a tape recorder that can be played back. Meichenbaum and Fitzpatrick (1991) held that the client should be told that memories are not fixed, exact replications of events. They are influenced by later events, emotions, and renderings that have followed. They can also be influenced by the suggestions of others. Briere (1992) asserted that the patient may not have to access all the traumatic events for change to occur. A core representation of events is all that is necessary. Lest we forget, trauma events also influence the poorer processing of other information.

Older clients often can be assisted by techniques involving a recounting of the incident in slow motion, at a safe distance initially, or adjusting internal sensations and thoughts that are problems. It is important for the older client to feel in control of the remembering, to process details of what comes up, and to become friendly with self in this process. At the end the therapist should not discontinue the session immediately after the imaginal exposure, allowing the client to talk about the reactions. Roberts and Holmes (1999) echoed the importance of knowing how the client feels after disclosing the trauma ("How do you feel after what you just said?"). Breathing retraining after imaginal exposure was also helpful. Issues related to new material, how the client did, and what the client was thinking were important. Again, the therapist expresses confidence.

Remember that this story is being told after several sessions have transpired, after other model sections have been addressed. Remember too that empathy and listening are always basic. Egendorf (1995) reminded therapists that in the intuitive discernment process, empathic listening—the core of trauma work—is never "the" reality of the story. The mystery remains in the intricacy that lies hidden.

Whatever technique we eventually use, the standard EMDR evaluation pre-therapy procedure for clients is recommended (Shapiro, 1994). This is an excellent and efficient method to acquire data on the target memory, its intensity, negative and positive cognitions, emotions, salient sensations, and safety cues. Again, we have a backdrop of several sessions of a relaxation training that can be eventually cued to trauma memories. This is learned at the beginning so that the client can control the anxiety associated with the traumatic event. During either procedure, an audiotape is used and the person is instructed to practice at least once daily (Hyer et al., 1994; Suinn, 1990).

AMT/EMDR: How to

A standard AMT or EMDR is used. Both appear effective and can actually be used interchangeably. (Box 10-1, Table 10-1)

AMT   In AMT, the desensitization process is applied (Suinn, 1990) with some modifications. The principle alteration is initially to have the client target a scene that is only at a moderate level of distress. As with the application of psychiatric medications for older people, start low and go slow. Always relaxation is practiced. Success must occur before more difficult issues are approached, however. Most often the target memory reduces in level of disturbance as practice unfolds. The core AMT concern is start with memories lower in SUDS levels, and apply relaxation before. Typically, the therapist does "AMT things," such as continuous feedback is received from the client; flexibility to access all target features; practice; reduction of anxiety at the end of sessions; and the allowance of sufficient time for discussion of new material for client reflection on the process. Always get success.

If little change results, several methods are used, including partializing if necessary (small wins); reframing negative stories; using alternative coping (breathing, safe

---

Box 10-1
AMT Protocol

Preliminary:	Relaxation learned
	Builds on success
	Receives constant feedback
Session 1:	T—Rationale
	T—Builds on relaxation scene
	T—Brings up old scene (SUDS = 20 − 40)
	T—Practice/relaxation for homework
Session 2:	T—SUDS at 50 and real anxiety scene
	T—Relaxation (muscle tension/easing and scene)
	T—Alternate anxiety scene and relaxation
	T—Practices relaxation
Session 3:	C—Relaxation
	T—Anxiety scene (SUDS 50) and relaxation ("Pay attention to how you experience anxiety in relaxation")
	T—Discusses "early warning signs" of anxiety
Session 4:	C—75 SUDS anxiety scene which client terminates and applies relaxation
	T—Continues to instruct on anxiety/relaxation cues
Session 5:	C—Initiates relaxation
	T—Switches on anxiety scene
	C—Continues anxiety scene or self-initiates relaxation
	T—Brings in new anxiety scene

T = Therapist Initiated; C = Client Initiated

---

places); and even challenging/changing stories. This latter intervention is only done if the story is virulent and resistant to change (see below). Other elements can also be added—cognitions, imagery, emotions, and bodily sensations. As Lazarus (1999) held, the more the merrier: The more aspects of the person accessed, the more apt the treatment. Commonly, failure results in an underresponse, where avoidance is occurring (and the clinician becomes passive in finding out and targeting the cause), or in an overresponse (where the therapist can do any number of AMT responses, usually backing up and finding a memory lower in intensity).

We have used many iterations of the following five sessions. This represents a short treatment trial and can be modified. Many older victims require more than this. Sessions are taped and used as homework.

Session 1: Session 1 involves four steps: rationale, development of a relaxation scene, relaxation training, and the assignment of homework.

After a standard rationale (Suinn, 1990) is given, the session next focuses on the development of a relaxation training and a scene. Relaxation training has already

TABLE 10-1. EMDR Procedure

Presenting Issue or Memory: "What old memory would you like to work on today?" (An old memory; avoid present referents, family members, phobias, life issues.)

Picture: "What picture represents the worst part of the incident?"

Negative Cognition (NC): "What words best go with the picture that express your belief about yourself now?" (Have client make the statement in the form of an "I" statement in present tense. Must be a presently held negative self-referencing belief.)

Positive Cognition (PC): "When you bring up that picture/incident, what would you like to believe about yourself **now**?" (Must be a present desired, self-reference belief.)

VoC: (Validity of Cognition-Measure for PC only.) "When you think of that picture/incident, how true does that (positive cognition) feel to you now on a scale of 1–7, where 1 is completely false and 7 is totally true?"

Emotions/Feelings: "When you bring up that incident and those words (*negative cognition*), what emotion(s) do you feel **now**?" (Emotion(s) client feels in the present.)

SUDs: "On a scale of 0–10, where 0 is no disturbance or neutral and 10 is the highest disturbance that you can imagine, how disturbing does it feel to you **now**?"

Location of Body Sensation: "Where do you feel it (*the disturbance*) in your body?"

Desensitize: "(I'd like you to) bring up that picture, those negative words (repeat the *negative cognition*), and notice where you are feeling it in your body—and follow my fingers."

1. Begin the eye movements slowly. Increase the speed as fast as the client can comfortably tolerate the movement.
2. Approximately every 12 saccades, or when there is an apparent change, comment to client: "That's it. Good. That's it."
3. It is helpful to comment to the client, (especially if client I abreacting): "That's it. It's old stuff. Just notice it." (Also use the speeding train metaphor.)
4. After a set of EM, instruct client to: "Blank it out" and/or "let it go and take a deep breath."
5. Ask: "What do you get **now**" or "what are you noticing **now**?"
6. After the client reports, say: "Stay with that" (without repeating the client's words/ statements). Client should be reporting a 0 or 1 on the SUDs scale before doing the installation.

Installation of Positive Cognition—linking the desired positive cognition with the original memory/incident/or picture:

1. "Do the words (repeat the *positive cognition*) still fit, or is there another positive statement you feel would be more suitable?"
2. "Think about the original incident and those words (*selected positive cognition*). From 1 (completely false) to 7 (completely true), how true do they feel?"
3. "Hold them together." Do EM. "On a scale of 1–7, how true does that (*positive statement*) feel to you **now** when you think of the original incident?"
4. **VoC:** Measure the VoC after each set. Even if client reports a 6 or 7, do EM again to strengthen and continue until it no longer strengthens. Go on to the body scan.
5. If client reports a 6 or less, check appropriateness and address blocking belief (if necessary) with additional reprocessing.

Body Scan: "Close your eyes; concentrate on the incident and the PC, and mentally scan your body. Tell me where you feel anything." If any sensation is reported, do EM. If a positive/comfortable sensation, do EM to strengthen the positive feeling. If a sensation of discomfort is reported—reprocess until discomfort subsides.

Closure/Debrief the Experience: "The processing we have done today may continue after the session. You may or may not notice new insights, thoughts, memories, or dreams. If so, just notice what you are experiencing—take a snapshot of it (what you are seeing, feeling, thinking, and the trigger), and keep a log. We can work on this new material next time. If you feel it is necessary, call me."

been given. It relies on the standard Jacobson (1938) (see Smith, 1999) deep muscle method, whereby muscle groups are first tensed, then relaxed. We use a 12–8–4–4–0 five session tense/relax procedure described in a previous chapter. Again, we do this before the scene. The relaxation scene, on the other hand, should be one that describes a real event, which is associated with feelings of relaxation or calmness. Scene details should be concrete and should attend to sensory aspects that help make the scene vivid, such as vision, sound, temperature, tactual, emotional, and other sensations. Relaxation scenes are the same as in desensitization. Once the relaxation exercise is completed, the client is instructed to "switch on" the relaxation scene and to use the scene to further increase the level of relaxation. A hand signal is used by the client to indicate when the relaxation scene is being experience. The homework assignment is to practice the tension-relaxation exercise, without the relaxation scene.

Session 2: This session involves four steps: identification of an anxiety scene, relaxation, anxiety arousal followed by relaxation, and homework. Session 2 begins with the development of an anxiety scene. This scene involves a real experience that has been associated with a moderately high level of anxiety about 50 on a scale with 100 as extreme anxiety. As with the relaxation scene, this anxiety scene must be a real event and concretely described. The scene should be a real event rather than a fantasized one to keep the client from drifting during visualization.

After the anxiety scene is identified, the therapist provides relaxation instructions, without use of the tensing component. Instead a muscle review is used, calling attention to letting each muscle group relax. This takes about 10 minutes. Slow, deep breaths are used to aid in the relaxation, followed by the relaxation scene. Hand signals continue to be the means for obtaining information—for example, when the client has achieved a comfortable level of relaxation, when the relaxation scene is clearly developed, and later, when anxiety is being experienced and when anxiety has been replaced by relaxation.

Anxiety arousal is initiated through the therapist's instruction to switch on the anxiety scene, to use the scene to re-experience the anxiety, and to signal the onset of this anxiety. The instructions include description of both scene-setting and anxiety-arousal details, as well as appropriate voice emphasis (volume, tone) to aid in anxiety arousal. After about 10–15 seconds of exposure (after the client signals anxiety), the anxiety scene is terminated, and the therapist reintroduces the relaxation scene. The client signals when he or she has retrieved a comfortable relaxation level. A brief muscle review is also conducted to further the level of relaxation.

Session 3: Two new steps, self-initiated relaxation and attention to the anxiety-arousal symptoms, are added to Session 2. The client can identify the personal signs associated with anxiety.

The first step in this session is self-initiated relaxation. Instead of the therapist giving the instructions, the client goes through the relaxation exercise on his or her own. As in the prior session, anxiety arousal is achieved through the use of the 50/60-intensity anxiety scene (new one). As before, the client signals when the scene has produced a return of anxiety.

At this point, the therapist introduces the next new instruction for attending to anxiety symptoms. The following instructions are given: "Pay attention to how you experience anxiety; perhaps it is in body signs, such as your neck muscles tensing or in some of your thoughts." Relaxation is again retrieved through the relaxation scene, with the therapist taking responsibility for switching on the scene and describing the details. This is followed by a brief muscle review for increasing the level of relaxation.

This cycle of anxiety arousal, attention to anxiety signs, and retrieval of relaxation is continued to the end of the hour—a cycle of about three to five repetitions. By training the client in becoming aware of the signs of anxiety, AMT not only teaches the person how to identify the presence of anxiety, but also makes it possible for prevention in the future. The therapist discusses these anxiety signs as "early warning signals" to tell the client in the future that tension or anxiety is building and to initiate self-controlled relaxation-coping skills.

Session 4: This session adds two new major components. First a > 75-level anxiety scene (target trauma) is identified. The session requires the client to assume more responsibility for regaining self-control after anxiety arousal. Instead of the therapist terminating the anxiety scene and reinitiating the relaxation, the client decides when to end the anxiety scene and takes responsibility for relaxation retrieval.

In summary, Session 4 repeats a general pattern, once a high level scene is constructed and the client self-initiates relaxation. The therapist instructs the client to switch on the high level scene and pay attention to the cognitive, emotional, and behavioral cues of anxiety arousal. After the client signals anxiety and when he or she is ready, he or she switches the anxiety scene off.

Session 5: This session completes the fading out of therapist control and the completion of client self-control. At the start of the session, the client self-initiates relaxation, signaling its achievement. Although the therapist switches on the anxiety scene, all activities from this point are client-controlled. Hence the client uses the anxiety scene to experience anxiety arousal, and, while still in the scene, initiates relaxation control. When relaxation is gained, the client then terminates the anxiety scene, signs its termination, and continues the relaxation until the next anxiety scene is called for by the therapist. Hand signaling is as before, with the hand raised being indicative of anxiety arousal and hand lowering indicating that relaxation has been retrieved. The latency between signals provides evidence for the progress of the client in anxiety management. Homework is the same as for Session 4.

This is a standard AMT protocol (Suinn, 1990). We of course do not get a total desensitization of the target memory. So steps 4 or 5 can be repeated. The idea is not the fixity of the protocol but the grounding of a believable procedure, a working client, and a tuned-in and clinically curious clinician. As the neural changes in trauma make the person susceptible to the possibility of further trauma, the work of AMT provides both an emotional tutorial and cognitive relearning. The client has learned if mastery is possible, anxiety signs can be identified, and that they trust the procedure.

EMDR   EMDR is an alternative. We use this method over AMT when we suspect that the client is able to handle the trauma memory more directly. In effect, they are more motivated and more psychologically minded.

In Chapter 5 we noted that this method maximizes sound psychotherapy principles, especially CBT (Hyer & Brandsma, 1997). It is fast-paced, equal to other treatments, and user friendly. It requires a set procedure, a process in which the client experiences the target at his/her own pace. EMDR uses the power of treatment expectations, accesses associative networks unique for each person, uses "clean language" (language of the client), uses traditional cognitive techniques (especially the identification of positive and negative cognitions), challenges evidence, and applies affect and necessary sensory experiencing of past targets. In EMDR also the mixture of both experiencing and meta-communication on the client-governed content is paramount: Experience, then comment on the target. This process of self-reporting on one's experiencing increases the "now" experiencing and the consolidation of this. In sum, EMDR has evolved into a sophisticated technique that blends exposure with a non-directive, free associative processing and other treatment components common to good "traditional" therapy: EMDR applies the active treatment ingredients of exposure in a patient-acceptable manner.

We also note this about EMDR: It is not a method for treating trauma alone. It is broader as it addresses blocked responses. EMDR is most of all about activation. Bilateral stimulation is an orienting response that does one thing above all else: It creates interest and action. In the trauma victim, the frontal lobes are always scanning for threat cues (witness the Stroop Test reaction to emotionally loaded words, see Litz et al., 1996), *and* the brain is also avoiding, trying to block out stimuli. EMDR addresses both, as the person scans and ciphers stimuli naturally.

Initially as with AMT, the clinician should provide the client with a positive experience with EMDR by using the safe-place exercise and teaching him/her a variety of relaxation techniques to relieve any disturbance that may arise between sessions. This is the ready-state for the work of EMDR (or AMT). When EMDR is used, this relaxation scene can be anchored with the eye movements. With EMDR too (as with AMT), the trauma memory is not the initial target. Success at the beginning is most important. We obtain mastery with practice—relaxation and more recent memory(s) at SUDS 50 or less. In fact, when the EMDR target goes to the trauma memory on its own, we return to the lower SUDS-level target. We stop there. The therapist is in control here.

In the application of *EMDR*, the patient is told: "What we will be doing is taking a physiology check. I need to know from you exactly what is going on, with as clear feedback as possible. Sometimes things will change and sometimes they won't. I may ask you if the picture changes. Sometimes it will and sometimes it won't. I'll ask you how you feel from "0" to "10"—sometimes it will change and sometimes it won't. I may ask if something else comes up—sometimes it will and sometimes it won't. There are no "supposed to's" in this process. So just give as accurate feedback as you can as to what is happening, without judging whether it should be happening or not. Just let whatever happens, happen."

In the procedure the client is asked to focus on a traumatic memory—initially a memory at SUDS 50 or less and later, if this goes well, the most traumatic point (Table 10-1). Recall that there is no need to describe the trauma exactly. The therapist then queries for the salient negative and positive cognitions related to the target memory. Words that attribute negative connotations are common (e.g., *helpless, out of control, sad, angry, shame*). The therapist asks for a rating on the believability of the positive cognition. Next, the therapist acquires the most notable feeling state from the patient. The patient is asked to concentrate on the memory, picture, and attributions, and assign a rating using the SUDS (0–10). Last before the eye movement processing, the therapist obtains information on the body sensation associated with the target memory.

Now the trauma processing begins (Shapiro, 1995). The therapist instructs the client to visualize the traumatic scene, recall the negative statement and feeling, concentrate on the physical sensations in the body, and move his/her eyes to the therapist's index finger. The finger (or some object) is moved rapidly and rhythmically back and forth across the line of vision from the extreme right to extreme left at a 12- to 14-inch distance from the client's face, two back-and-forth movements per second. The back-and-forth movement of the therapist's finger is repeated for approximately 30 seconds and will vary depending on the intensity and type of processing. After each set of these saccades, the therapist tells the patient to relax, to take a deep breath, and then describe what went on. This process is repeated as the patient "moves" the target information.

As the client processes the target trauma, cognitions, feelings, and sensations change. Sooner or later clients reveal new cognitions that begin to approximate the "desired" attribution given as the "preferred" cognition prior to beginning the desensitization procedure. When the SUDS level reaches "0" or "1," then the client's desired cognition is retrieved (and rated) and "installed." At this point the client is asked to focus on the picture along with the desired rating while more saccades are used. When a positive cognition is rated high and the SUDS is 0 or 1, the EMDR procedure can be terminated.

This is the ideal procedure. It is rarely reached quite this way. Problems occur when the target memory is "stuck" and clients cannot process the information. One example is looping. After successive sets the client remains at a high level of disturbance with repetitive negative thoughts, affect, and imagery. The client is repeating the problem state. Under these circumstances, the therapist becomes more active and applies both cognitive and experiential techniques to expose the problem, to challenge the data, or to experiment with feelings to obtain necessary movement in the treatment (Box 10-2). Often another memory or picture begins to interfere: If so, the whole procedure is repeated with the new material. At the end, the clinician has the client scan their body and summarize for him/herself the effect of the processing. The therapist says: "Close your eyes and keep in mind the trauma memory and a positive cognition. Then bring your attention to the different parts of your body, starting with your head and working downward. Any place you find any tension, tightness, or unusual sensation, tell me." Our clinical experience is that at least half the time the processing will be impeded and the clinician will have to use various additional strategies and advanced EMDR procedures to restimulate it (Shapiro, 1995).

Box 10-2 illustrates a way to think about EMDR. It outlines the basic therapeutic interventions and honors the least restrictive principle. When more assistance is required, the table specifies the needed input. Above all, the EMDR ideals of staying out of the client's way, providing choice, facilitating movement, identifying blockages, and applying the technology of the method are important.

EMDR is not a break-man test. If problems result, several procedures are available to assist in their alleviation. We use them with regularity. Use of guided imagery, grounding techniques, positive statements, breathing, and the like, with the eye movements are especially helpful. Just adding a positive statement ("It's over") can be of value. If necessary, the therapist can use a treatment hierarchy, a procedure using a graduated form of systematic desensitization (see Smith, 1991).

When the SUDS level and the negative cognition do not reach baseline, this may be due to several entrenched learnings, personal convictions, or the ecological validity of the belief. A simple query—"What prevents your SUDS score from being a zero?"—can be helpful. The question "What do you need to hold onto and what do you want to let go of?" can be most helpful also as it separates commitment from resistance. Processing of targeted information also can be blocked by the client's fear of the outcome or of the process itself. Regardless of the cause of the block, it is explored and the client's fears allayed before EMDR resumes. Once the fear is cognitively debriefed, any remnants of the fear itself can be targeted. Additionally, if the therapeutic effect has not been maintained, the fear of change may not have been adequately processed. In this case, the negative cognition associated with the fear should be explored, the present situation analyzed to identify and deal with any appropriate concerns, and the origin of the dysfunction targeted.

Box 10-2
Potential EMDR Responses

I. Narrative Attunement

Empathic Exploration: Do *not* be an active therapist but have the client listen inside and trust the process. ("Stay with that"; "Attend to that"; "Focus on that"; "Bring that up.")

Help 1. Do what is natural: Alter mode (e.g., feelings for thoughts) and get SUDS rating

Four helpers:

1. When positive or negative features of processing arise, go with negative.
2. If choice of feelings, images, or content, choose feelings.
3. Body sensations, however, are the true test of movement.
4. When there is a change: "Pay attention to tension that *remains*."

II. Doing Therapy

Help 1. Light Resistance (no change): "Where else in the past were you like this?" Become a therapist ("What prevents you from ... ?" "What would you need to have happen to move this along?" "I can't give up this memory because ...").

Three techniques are (a) query for the potential resistance, "imagine yourself" (opposite of resistance components); (b) secondary gain ("Who would you be without the problem?" "How would you like to be living?" "What would you need?" "What is preventing this?" "What would happen if ... ?"); and (c) early learnings ("Where did you learn this?" "Access early memory/event of this learning")

Help 2. Be a therapist: "What would unblock this?" "What might symbolize this cycle?" "Focus on body or feeling." Partialize events in the loop and frame-by-frame iteration of process ("Concentrate on blocking out this scene" mind and "What would allow you to feel ...?").

Help 3. Be real active: cognitive interweave, guided imagery, and relaxation

Assimilation queries

1. What evidence do you have to support this thought?
2. Is there any alternative way of looking at the situation or yourself?
3. Is there any alternative explanation?

III. Ending–Future Orientation:

Closure: See yourself in the future with this issue. Install the positive cognition.

Be a therapist: empower–"This is no worse than original trauma and you survived that"; reframe–"Something positive is happening." choice–"In the past you had no choice, now you have one."

Box 10-3
EMDR: Acute sequence

1. Obtain a narrative history of the event.
2. Target the most disturbing aspect of the memory (if necessary).
3. Target the remainder of the narrative in chronological order.
4. Have client visualize the entire sequence of the event with eyes closed and re-process it as disturbance arises. Repeat until the entire event can be visualized from start to finish without distress.
5. Have client visualize the event from start to finish with eyes open, and install positive cognition.
6. Conclude with body scan.
7. Process present stimuli, if necessary.

EMDR/Acute Trauma

EMDR also has a somewhat different procedure for an acute trauma. As trauma has not had time to consolidate, the therapeutic reaction requires a fast-line method to unearth all parts. We find that you can use the above technique. However Box 10-3 provides the standard sequence for acute trauma (we especially find 4 and 5 helpful with an acute trauma).

We have found this method helpful with older crime victims and on occasion with issues of recent loss. Caution should be used for its use with any major loss or with depressed clients. Often too clients will appear to have a new trauma. In fact, they are reexperiencing older trauma and the procedure above is in order.

Post Script: Agoraphobia   We have not considered the almost universal problem with PTSD—avoidance. We believe that it is sufficient in and of itself to warrant a separate viewing. Avoidance or agoraphobia, its DSM friend, is so pervasive that the therapist must consider it. When the agoraphobia is present then, it is addressed as a separate issue. If agoraphobia is inhibiting the person's life, a situational fear hierarchy needs to be attempted. Outside the session patients routinely are asked to perform in vivo experiments to cues in the environment that they had been avoiding. Clients are asked to monitor their fear and reactions to these situations. At times, interceptive cues may be helpful. A fear and avoidance hierarchy is established and the person is requested to start at the bottom of the list and march forward. This is done in imagination first (in the office) and later in vivo. The focus is on doing, not feeling. Also the therapist can then give anxiety exercises, to assure that the core of the anxiety is addressed. This is done for several reasons, most importantly because there is often a dysynchrony among thoughts, feelings, and behaviors.

☐ Aftercare and Relapse Prevention

PTSD does not go away. It returns. This is why the use of medication alone is not sufficient for care. A more holistic program is necessary including a relapse program. Sperry (1995) held that relapse is optimal when symptoms persist, the client remains in the precontemplation or contemplation stage (not having done anything), has a minimal social support network, non-complies with treatment in general, or has a flight into health. It can apply to compliant and remitting patients. These include patients with better relationships, a better self-concept, who trust others, have less control problems, have a good rapport with the therapist, and are willing to take risks (Salvendy & Toffe, 1991). Generally, patients who involve their family and apply psycho-education are best able to respond to aftercare well. With PTSD, these conditions are often not in evidence.

Surprisingly, the idea that the older victim can or should return for care is appealing to older people. We always schedule a booster session, usually 3 months later. This involves a booster session, made popular by CBT, but also includes a semi-formal relapse prevention discussion. We schedule it because it cements learnings of therapy and communicates commitment over time, as well as attends to the issues just raised. It continues the safety plan noted above at the beginning of therapy.

One's history of reactions to a medical illness is a good predictor of compliance of the current treatment. That said, the activation of appropriate cognitive appraisals (self-efficacy, optimism, perceived control), coping strategies (active behaviors, positive and acceptance reframing, and lack of denial), resources (social, economic, familial, and spiritual), as well as the individual's life context (stressful events, perceived stress levels, and functional level) is needed. Always the $64,000 question involves the attribution of the client at the moment that a stressor is present. This can be practiced.

This final task of psychotherapy is then an educational exchange about possible lapses and setbacks. Relapse prevention is really a method to convince the client that they can be their own therapist. The therapist works with the client to ensure that the re-experiencing of symptoms (lapses) does not lead the client back to the pretreatment level of adjustment (relapse). The client is taught ways to anticipate, accept, and cope with possible lapses and setbacks. A discussion that PTSD symptoms may re-occur when the client is stressed or under specific conditions (e.g., anniversary date) is always helpful. Now the client can exert some "authority" and "choice" over symptoms (e.g., can elect to remember or put memory aside). The therapist can highlight positive coping responses, and foster an "adaptive spiral" instead of "vicious destructive cycle." It is best to use clients descriptive metaphorical terms. Simple reconstructive ideas, like "Memories do not go away, but lose their gripping quality" or "Memories no longer are able to stop you in your tracks" are used with success. The therapist can use coping cards here.

An imaginary relapse exercise can also be of value (Lazarus, 1999). The client can imagine a relapse in as full detail as possible. The client can then predict what caused it, and imagine what he/she would learn from the lapse. The client can consider what he/she could do to prevent the lapse from escalating into a "full-blown" relapse. The client too can consider what could mitigate and prevent the relapse. He/she can be helped to view lapses (backsliding) as learning experiences. Lapses and relapses provide useful information about what and how the client is likely to respond. Lapses can be reframed as "conditioned responses to stimuli" (reminders), "fear memory structures being triggered."

Box 10-4 presents a format for relapse prevention for chronic trauma problems. The central method involves the Dysfunctional Thought Record. The patient identifies a time in the near future that he/she fails. They then outline all the negatives that apply ("My therapy was only a fluke," "This proves that I am hopeless," "Therapy does not work," etc.). These are then challenged. This exercise not only consolidates the necessity for the differentiation of therapy as "feeling better" versus "getting

---

Box 10-4
Relapse Protocol for Chronic PTSD

1. Anticipate need for continuance of care—discuss issues of a change in treatment, having temporary end, and booster sessions. Graph of progress and thoughts about termination.
2. Address relapse—a formal education of the concept of relapse as well as its place in recovery.
3. Practice skills—overlearn cognitive statements related to lapses and eventual recovery. Teach skills with wide application.
4. Aggressively address negative thoughts through the DTR. Adapt a "process view" of relapse (temporary setback). Predict automatic thoughts about setbacks. Develop a short plan (breathing, thinking, automatic thoughts that needs clarification).
5. Recognize early warning signs. Anticipate high-risk situations.
6. Have emergency plans for relapse. This includes a self-help strategy.
7. Involve significant others.
8. Use booster sessions.
9. Reinforce a relapse philosophy—"I am in this for the long haul and will make self-care a necessary part. There will be setbacks but I will take control and react well. I have lots of help and can use many skills."

---

better," but it provides a needed dialogue about the impact of this therapy, a method that does not seek cure only the best management of psychological problems.

We remind the therapist here what Linehan (1993) asked: Does the individual have the capability to engage in more adaptive responses and to construct a life worth living? If not, the clinician should ask what behavioral skills are needed. This leads to a mix-and-match consideration of skills training procedures. In addition to the typical therapy focus of skills training and distress tolerance problems, mindfulness skills are worthwhile. In effect, the client is provided with a psycho-philosophy, a way to view self that extends beyond the issues of the problem. Often issues of spirituality can be highlighted and assist in the meaning-making and better living at late life.

Finally, "good" outcomes are prepared by asking clients to describe what will be different when the problem(s) that brought them to therapy has been successfully treated (Fara, Grandi, Zielezny, Rafanelli, & Canestari, 1996; Teasdale et al., 2000). This involves the solution-focused queries (previously discussed). Of course now the query addresses the process of continuing positive behavior. This frame on life creates a good possible self, a considered plan on what life has to offer, or at the least what may be blocking change. Engaging a PTSD or depressed client in this discussion naturally reframes negative or stressful events as temporary.

☐ Necessary Treatment: Family

Aging is a journey played out in a family context. For simplicity and brevity, two trends are found regarding the effects of PTSD on family or significant others, almost always women with war trauma victims. First, gerontological research has seen a dramatic increase recently in the area of family caregiving. In fact, caregiving has even been labeled a "career" (Pearlin, 1992). Caring for a physically or mentally disabled elder has been linked to increased levels of anxiety and depression (Gallagher, Rose, Rivera, Lovett, & Thompson, 1989), a compromised immune (Kiekolt-Glaser, Dura, Speidher, Trask, & Glaser, 1991) or cardiovascular system (Haley, 1996), among other problems (see Wallsten, 1997). Many studies have examined the cognitive and affective appraisals of caregivers, including the efficacy of coping with care (McFarlane & Yehuda, 1996) and premorbid personality (Hyer, Woods, & Boudewyns, 1991), as well as the popular depression models (Zarit, 1996). In general, these studies suggest that caregivers are at risk, that social support is important for mental and physical health, that marital happiness affects outcomes for the better, that containing stress is important or it will proliferate into life and cause secondary role strain (Pearlin, Mullan, Semple, & Skaff, 1990), and that several models of caregiving are effective in the treatment of caregivers (see Zarit, 1996).

The second area involves the problems of PTSD itself, and women. There have been several treatment models related to families (Figley, 1989). Glynn et al. (1997) reported on a study in which they augmented exposure therapy with BFT (behavioral family therapy). Amid a sea of homework, these authors applied many behavioral strategies, including communication, anger management, and problem solving, among others. The results were positive.

Prevalence rates (of PTSD) are generally higher for females regardless of the stressor (Riggs, Rothbaum, & Foa, 1995) or age (Zarit, 1996). Generally, being a woman is compounded with less education, lower socioeconomic status, or being a minority (Breslau, Davis, & Andreski, 1991). Regarding older veterans' wives, those in a long-term relationship with veterans suffering from PTSD commonly experience PTSD-like symptoms themselves (Nelson & Wright, 1996). This has been labeled *secondary victimization* (Boudreau, Fitzpatrick, Resnick, Best, & Saunders, 1998), also applying to offspring (Hyer et al., 1994).

It is clear that caregiving is not a unitary process, and that caregivers are very different from each other in the ways in which they cope (or fail to cope) with the demands of their role. The multivariate nature of caregiving, interventions, and their effects are just now unfolding. At the very least, one needs to assess the adequacy of the social support network, the nature of the care-receiver's disability, previous and current coping history of the caregiver, intercurrent stressful life changes, and caregiver physical and mental health. *Subjective burden* is typically viewed as the emotional costs of the illness to family members (e.g., feelings of embarrassment, resentment, and helplessness), whereas *objective burden* is defined as the disruption to everyday family life for the ill person's relatives (e.g., financial burden, loss of free time, and conflict with neighbors or law enforcement officials). Both require therapeutic tending.

One helpful tact with older trauma victims and their families is provided by Zarit (1996). He recommended a combination of individual therapy with a primary caregiver followed by family meetings, as well as support groups. Interestingly, the presence of adult children often provides assistance in treatment, as children appear universally accepted and needed at later life (Hyer et al., 1994). The significance of the reciprocal impact of the psychiatric patient on the family cannot be understated, especially in later life. Older trauma victims play many roles; the angry distant one, the submissive and depressed one, the confused and dependent one, among others. The "social" aspect of the treatment involves fundamental changes in an individual's family and social identity, along with declines in role performance. A whole family treatment focus is requisite.

The results of one important study (Teri & Uomoto, 1991) are instructive. This study investigated the relationship between depressed mood and pleasant activities in patients with dementia and a major depressive disorder, a cause of excess disability in patients. Patients and their caregivers participated in a behavioral treatment program designed to improve patient depression. Caregivers were taught to (a) track patients' mood, duration, and frequency of pleasant activity, (b) to increase pleasant activities for the patient; and (c) decrease behavioral disturbances that interfered with engagement in these pleasant activities. Caregivers of all patients successfully increased the frequency and duration of pleasant events, and decreased the patient's depression as measured by the Beck Depression Inventory and the Hamilton Depression Rating Scale. Further, increased frequency and duration of activity was significantly associated to decreased levels of depression in each of the patients. This procedure has also been applied to just dementia patients (Uomoto & McCurry, 1997).

These tasks can be simply applied. An overall treatment plan for the caregiver is given in Box 10-5. With "healthier" couples, overall rules are provided (IV), as well as one strategy (V). The rules for couple care are the positive side of things. They are based on the work of Gottmann (1999). The focus is on three principles for implementing positive behaviors (first three); knowing each other, focusing on the positive, and interacting frequently. The foundation of care is on strengthening the friendship. The strategy is based on the negative side of things, that of handling conflict. Additionally, the therapist can be of great help by making families aware of the naturalness of trauma reactions, especially that (a) caregiver anger, frustration, and sorrow are natural reactions to serious illness; (b) the caregiver must take care of himself or herself to give the patient good care; (c) caregivers must rely on their own judgment in some family conflicts; (d) role changes require time and energy to comprehend and adjust to; and (e) many complex and difficult decisions arise when needs of various family members are in conflict (Lezak, 1978). Although we have not advocated this, use of any one of several family environment scales can facilitate the pinpointing of problems in the social milieu (e.g., Family Environment Scale; Moos & Lemke, 1980).

☐ Conclusion

A high energy paradox occurs when the trauma victim focuses on the past and observes one's trauma from a perspective of safety. This last stage of the model advocates this. At base, the client chooses either to work on and integrate the memory or to keep it: If the choice is therapy, AMT or EMDR apply: If not, renarration of the PCM (Chapter 9) is appropriate or just management (Stages 1–4). With the trauma memory, the important task of therapy is to access (target) these unique associative networks (prototypical exemplars of the person) and unblock problem processing. We have been rather matter-of-fact; attack the trauma memory indirectly and then directly. We provide the older person with what they seem to need or do best, broad-based help and support, and taking responsibility for their problems (AMT/EMDR), or renarrate direct their actions. We do this in a CBT framework.

Goleman (1995) stated that you can change a problem by doing, by thinking, or by relaxing the autonomic nervous system. Our model calls for all of these. The model we provide requests that the clinician attend to everything. This allows for more entry

---

Box 10-5
Caretaker Issues

I. Overall Concerns
   Knowledge: Know disorder and what is happening.
   Rights: Acknowledge and vent your own feelings.
   Needs: Help practically and emotionally.
II. Unhealthy Couple
   A. Treatment Factors
      Track patient's mood, duration, and frequency of pleasant activity.
      Increase pleasant activities for the patient.
      Decrease behavioral disturbances that interfered with engagement in these pleasant activities.
   B. Assure Social Support
      Assess and assist.
III. Healthy Couple
   A. Rules for Couple Care
      Know each other.
      Focus on each other's positive qualities.
      Interact frequently.
      Let your partner influence you.
      Solve solvable problems.
      Overcome gridlock.
      Create shared meaning.
      Fight fair.
      Be able to say "Stop."
      Take care of yourself.
   B. Strategy for Caretaker with Identified Patient
      Choose a time.
      State feelings.
      Listen and restate what you heard.
      Admit when you had enough.

---

points into the person with a life of trauma. A substantial part of the understanding is the unfolding of treatment in a top-down way—management of the person's life. And a substantial part of the care of a trauma victim is bottom-up, discovery-oriented. This involves observations based on extant data and strategies based on the research. The focus is on understanding the process of task solution and building explanatory models of the processes involved in resolution. From this perspective, symptoms are seen as "urgent questions, behaviorally expressed, which had somehow lost the threads that lead either to answers or to better questions" (Kelly, 1969, p. 19). As we respect this position, we can see that we keep a promised land of optimism in a sea of turmoil.

In reality, the amount of change that can occur in therapy is generally limited. In fact, Jacobson (1964) may be correct that "the individual learns to run his organism according to what he believes are its best interests." Ultimately though, this is how it should be. After all, we are constantly altering our being: Change is everywhere and at every time. The natural rhythmic dialectic of life progressively discriminates and reorders. Fortunately, the older victim does not have to experience integrity (integration of life) to make it. The older person must only be vivid to self; self-consistent, coherent, and flexible.

It may be that the world's best evangelist is the aging process, which makes painfully clear how little we can do and how short the time. Aging makes possible what therapy cannot. C. S. Lewis said:

> The world is so built, that to help us desert our own satisfactions, they desert us. War and trouble and finally old age take from us one by one all those things that Self hoped for at its starting out. Begging is our only wisdom, and what in the end makes it easier for us to be beggars."

In this book, we discussed human beings, advanced by dint of age: They are just trying to be human and to be themselves. Trauma provides for a miscalculation. We provided some ideas for a better accountant, one that is both practical and human.

Grief Work and Forgiveness in the Context of PTSD

"... old pain is best resolved by admitting as much truth as possible, taking as much responsibility as you can, and forgiving others. This is the heart of the therapeutic process."
David Viscott (p. 21)

Traditional theories of grief are wanting. Traditional views of the grief experience uncover clinical issues but do not provide clarity. There may or may not be stages of grief; there may or may not be a normalcy to more severe bereavement symptoms; there may or may not be an end to grief. Perhaps there exists a dynamic component to the process of the grief response. Freud, for example, noted that people are never willing to give up emotional attachments. We do know, however, that individually people go through a sequence of some sort in the grief process and most reach some accommodation or acceptance.

Traditional approaches to bereavement are also too restrictive. A multifactorial approach is now necessary that will include issues of trauma and vulnerability of the self (Hagman, 1996). Considering just grief in the elderly, the tasks are more straightforward. At its simplist level the task of grief is to acknowledge the pain of the loss and to get on with life, but we are not talking about just one loss, one grief. With trauma, grief becomes complicated. Everything is made worse, perhaps by the presence of risk factors, both person-based and social.

The processes of grieving in the conceptualization of trauma treatment then are woefully understated, yet critical in all stages of life (Figley, Bride, & Mozza, 1997). Loss is a very common and frequent experience in life and a large component of all trauma. But most times the elderly person does not show the deficits because the scars are internal, the process habitual. The "scars" represent the loss or damage to the person's internal organization that enables them to experience consciousness as a human, that organization being their self-theory (Epstein, 1978). Most often loss is initially conceived in terms of the effects from the death of a valued, internalized other—yet all know there are many other kinds of losses. However always self-theory damage—Thomas Moore (1994) would say a soul loss—is registered. Grieving is important in the therapy with trauma victims. It allows you to be aware of your thoughts and feelings. It allows one to be human.

In this chapter, we (first) define self-theory and set it in the context of trauma. Next, we discuss the "necessary" co-mingling of grief with other diagnostic states (i.e., PTSD and depression). We believe these states are inherent components of the trauma experience. Trauma necessarily accompanies grief. A critical component then in the treatment of trauma involves the issues of loss in the trauma re-experience. Third, we outline eight tenets for the understanding and treatment of PTSD with its grief components. This is highlighted by the hypothesis that the person is best understood in the context of the stored memories that form their identity (as mentioned, a crucial aspect of the self-theory). Treating trauma is insufficient; treating the person and their self-theory is required. Fourth, we present a model of the processes and steps involved in grief treatment. In written form this model may seem simplistic and "canned," but it does possess enough abstraction, generality, and flexibility so that respect for the person of the victim can be maintained while still providing a roadmap for treatment. We believe that the literature now points to the treatment of trauma memory by directly involving grief work. Finally, we argue that the person is potentially transformed in this experience when there is an optimum level of frustration allowing for at least some disintegration, restabilization, and growth. Within this growth-healing we posit that forgiveness processes are central for change. Forgiveness too is a complex process based on one's relationship with God, others, self, and the culture, but when begun, people can become more than they were—they can repair and redefine their self-theory, and grow on.

☐ The Self

A very important part of the self is the consistent, organized set of memories, largely autobiographical, that capture in narrative form the important aspects of person, and the rules (the often implicit assumptions, propositions, and hypotheses) that hold these together. These dictate how information is to be processed. Part of this organization is a set of core memories that reference the person, ones that both organize how and what information flows and what is the conceptual "base camp" of the person. The self-concept, you might say, is the subset of these core memories that abstracts and summarizes the person more or less adequately. This is a more generalized and abstracted icon of the total self-theory. Perhaps the self is composed of modular selves and the narrative (self) organizes information and defines the person.

Each individual has a self-theory, an amalgam of implicit or explicit assumptions, postulates, corollaries, hypotheses, laws, and concepts implied or enacted in their cognitions, behaviors, and affects that organize in schemas to process experiences and initiate action. Some important schemas are body image, sources of esteem, the nature of the world, important other people (introjects), the assumption of predictability, self-efficacy boundaries, the summary self-concept, as well as a host of just world and safety concepts among others. Other components of the self have also been identified—trust, individuation, object relations, reality experience, fullness of experience, coping mechanisms, integrative capacity, and self-analytic functions (Lingiardi, Madeddu, Fossati, & Maffei, 1994). Trauma disrupts these: Key schemas of the self are disorganized and new information becomes impossible to assimilate. One's self system thus breaks down in the midst of great psychic pain.

As a result of trauma the person suffers a self loss, a wound to one's identity, damage to parts of their self-theory. With age this can include many things, internal and external. Life-cycle stressors imposed by aging may be conceptualized as forms of loss: loss of significant others; loss of social role; loss of health, function, or both parts; loss of omniportence, control, and effectiveness; and ultimately loss of life. Sadavoy (1987; Sadavoy & Fogel, 1992) addressed eight critical, age-specific stressors: interpersonal loss, physical disability, loss of external manifestations of the self (e.g., strength, beauty), loss of role, loss of defensive outlets, forced reliance on caretakers, confrontation with death, and conflict over the wish to live versus the wish to die. Although several of these stressors occur across the life-span, their concentration and impact in later life is unique. Aged individuals do not always have the time, resources, or physical abilities to cope adequately with such losses. In addition, they have a restricted range of behavioral expressions for pathological states. Interestingly, trauma victims (or individuals with personality disorders) have an even more restricted range of coping mechanisms, making them particularly vulnerable to being overwhelmed by stress, and often requiring psychiatric intervention. The longer one survives, the more ineluctable is the march of cumulative losses and the need for repetitive or partial grieving (Berezin, 1972). Perhaps "successful" aging is marked by a process of mourning without loss of self-esteem.

These are all losses of the self in some way. The self organizes past, present, and future, and, with trauma, has been wounded and requires "therapy." The self is the intention-driven actor who foremost tries to comply with its natural tendencies to heal. Rorty (1976a,b) opined that "an individual transcends and resists what is binding and oppressive, and does so from an original natural position."

From an information processing perspective, we (Bagge & Brandsma, 1994) have argued that when trauma occurs, information is not assimilated into the historical memory; it is stuck in the immediate memory. As we have stated along with others (e.g., van der Kolk, 1995), people with PTSD initially hold traumatic experiences as sensations or feeling states that are not immediately transcribed into the self, the personal narrative. It is this failure to encode information in symbolic form that constitutes the core of PTSD pathology. We believe that this is especially a problem with loss (a grief process), where time does not heal the victim's blocked grief. The appreciation of one's vulnerability, a new philosophy of self, or a new meaning is not achieved. If psychotherapy of PTSD means anything, it implies the integration of the fragments of the self, its cohesion in explicit memory. This process may be more needed or insistent in these growing elderly.

Trauma must eventually be integrated into the narrative of the person's life. Guided imagery can be used to revise and then revisit the trauma memory. This dialogue of grief allows for completion of unfinished business, the expression of affect and affection, forgiveness, and finally the goodbye. The last step of mourning involves opening up to a new future, the new remembered future, by allowing for a safe old past (cf. Melges, 1982). Grieving is essential to growth. As Erikson (Sherman, 1991) noted, there is no other task in the philosophy of life (especially when under stress) than to remember the self.

This might seem an obvious conclusion to many clinicians: A person in trauma must deal on a basic organizational level with the assumptions, postulates, and guiding hypotheses of their current self theory (i.e., Who am I in the world?). This is what is required to organize the data of experience, to balance the pleasure/pain dynamic, and to maintain self-esteem (cf. Epstein, 1973). For true healing, the path must go through this affective state. Grief has a special role, one that impacts on core memories and alters the rules of their integrity. This involves the therapies that require a coherent autobiography of self, ones of trauma. In addition to providing meaning to the old and the new, therapy also requires a necessary dialogue within the body and soul, a dialogue about the loss.

This has been addressed. Hyer (Hyer et al., 1994) noted the relationship between the necessary abuse criterion (of PTSD) and schemas of the self. Several authors (e.g., Herman, 1992; Tedeschi & Calhoun, 1995) also noted the inherent pain in the trauma process. The most poignant psychic pain is experienced when the person's self-theory has been found to be inadequate, unable to assimilate the overwhelming meaning shifts or disintegration(s) that occur in trauma.

Trauma then devastates the self, the self theory: It has a critical role in deforming the context that then usurps all set points; it affects the typical internal structures of the self most tellingly. It devastates the explicit memories that are self-defining, as these cannot accommodate to the degree of stress (Hyer et al., 1994). What is critical here is that the self (a key subset of core memories and rules) shapes the trauma response, the specific cognitions and affects. Always the problem is one of loss, self-loss. When symptoms occur, the self has not been able to assimilate or accommodate the trauma. The remembrance of the trauma, then, is suffused with the ineffable process of self-pain regarding loss. This is grief.

☐ Grief Constructs

Whether grief should have a separate diagnosis in the DSM continues to be debated (Simpson, 1997). If grief is a universal reaction to loss, many stressors are probably beyond the scope of earlier DSM's in diagnosing PTSD (Horowitz, Bonanno, & Holen, 1993). Even though the DSM-IV has been more liberal with the stressor in the diagnosis of PTSD, the psychological space for grief is unclear. In fact, many diagnostic overlays seem possible. Grief shares features of other diagnoses, especially the anxiety disorders, including PTSD and depression as well as psychosomatic problems (Cook & Dworkin, 1992). Our interest here is in the similarities and differences between grief and PTSD, as well as anxiety and depression.

The Process of Grief in Trauma

Rando (1999) noted that there is a difference between grief and mourning. Grief is always acute, is awash in anxiety, and is PTSD-like. Grief is the beginning of mourning. It is feelings and the protest that results. Mourning refers to the conscious and unconscious processes and courses of action that promote three sets of actions: (a) gradually undo the psychosocial bonds that tied the loved one to the mourned; (b) help the mourner adapt to the loss; and (c) refocus on the new world. Healthy mourning involves grief resolution and accommodation to the loss. This occurs in most people.

Whatever the process of relearning after loss is called, the critical test of therapy is whether the person is moving on in life in a healthy way (adapting to the loss). This means that there is not excessive denial or excessive "holding on," excessive pain in the process. So, although mourning may involve the longer term process of therapy, the real concern for therapy is complicated mourning, better known as complicated grief. This is a process where the person tries to either deny the problem or to hold onto the lost loved one (or self-object). The former is often the result of a conflictual relationship. The factors that subserve the problem reaction include the suddenness of the death, loss of a child, overly lengthy illness, death that was preventable, an ambivalent relationship, prior losses, loss of support, or mental illness of the mourner.

The latter form of complicated grief is a special problem, excessive holding on to the loss. This is really complicated or, if a trauma is involved, traumatic grief. We, of course, are most concerned with this. Traumatic grief is like separation anxiety. This happens between the separation and the understanding of the permanence of the loss. Separation indicates a search. It is an anxious undertaking. After the search, however, depression unfolds. This feeling remits when the loss is accepted as real. On the way to depression, however, something else becomes manifest, PTSD (or ASD).

Few empirical studies of grief reactions with PTSD victims exist (e.g., Villereal, 1991), but the two are connected. When the grief reaction is simple, individuals face problems soon into the reaction; those with more complicated reactions avoid and are delayed (Cook & Dworkin, 1992). This avoidance may be a "part of PTSD" as individuals who show traumatic grief also show many signs of PTSD. Regardless, available literature suggests that grief reactions are an abnormal rather than a normal variant when a reaction is delayed or intense (Worden, 1982). In addition, available clinical data suggest that PTSD and loss go hand in glove, whether simple or complex. Also, the affective transition is from the "emotion" of anxiety-based reactions to depression-based reactions.

Grief as Necessary for PTSD

The concept of grief has been applied to PTSD in one form or other since the inception of the construct (Cook & Dworkin, 1992; Villereal, 1991; Widdison & Salisbury, 1990; Worden, 1982). In fact, grief and its complications are universal in trauma (Garb, Bliech, & Lerer, 1987)—the issue is "how much?" At the one extreme, grief may just be a part of the disorder and "responsible" for subclinical pain and sadness, often experienced years after the trauma event. At the other, grief may be the primary explanatory variable in the acquisition of PTSD. In this latter sense it is a universal reaction in trauma victims, especially those who were victims of personal loss. As a component of PTSD, Shay (1994) and Lifton (1992) for example, posited that rage is a key byproduct (of grief); Hence these authors outline the need for personal and communal grief rituals. It is no surprise that several models of PTSD have implicated grief (Hyer et al., 1994).

Many terms have been used to address the complications of grief in the bereavement process as it relates to PTSD: delayed, abnormal, pathological, and complicated. States of grief and PTSD are descriptively and conceptually close, sharing many common features (cf. Bagge' & Brandsma, 1994). We have used traumatic grief as the phrase used to straddle the two diagnostic domains of pathological grief and PTSD (van der Hart, Brown, & Turco, 1990). This is the complicated grief noted above in the context of trauma. It represents the complicated side of loss in PTSD, a state reflective of the "biphasic symptom-swings from symptoms of arousal, intrusive traumatic imagery, and anxiety, to defensive numbing and avoidance" (p. 264).

Rando (1999) held that in traumatic grief, there are three levels of severity. First, there is acute grief with minimal traumatic stress symptomotology. This is the easy case where the grief risk factors are minimal. Second, there is more than the usual amount of traumatic stress symptomatology secondary to the presence of the high-risk factors. This makes therapy more extended. Third, there is a PTSD reaction, whether the Criterion A is met or not. The person has most of the symptoms of PTSD and indeed suffers from this state. This is often the face of PTSD that is seen at later life.

Loss is then a necessary element in the etiology of PTSD. We believe that the grief response is virtually universal in PTSD, often later fueled by clinical depression and sometimes not. We underline that this is *self-theory loss*, a loss or disruption of one's autobiographical memory, issues core to self-definition and continuity. In fact, just as meaning in the process of dying is enhanced by a self-struggle, so too trauma survivors must genuinely make inner contact with the pain of loss (grief) for growth to occur (Hyer et al., 1994).

Then Depression

We know that, as far as PTSD goes, that clinical depression asserts a differential influence on the treatment of trauma response (Foa, Molnar, & Cashman, 1995), especially in the elderly. However the relationship between depression and grief is another way to understand grief as a problematic state. Research shows that these are interdependent but different terms. Depressive symptoms can occur as part of a grief reaction and result in a clinical depression. Often, when the clinical depression remits, the grief reaction and need for grief work are still present.

Another way of coming at it is that depression can be complicated by a grief reaction, as well as anxiety. Kim and Jacobs (see Nader, 1997) examined the relationship between complicated grief, depression, and anxiety disorders in 25 bereaved individuals. Significant relationships were found between complicated grief and the anxiety disorders. Relationships were not as high in the depressed group. The authors concluded that these disorders share some common features but are not "isomorphic." More recently, Prigerson et al. (1995) assessed widowed people and found that grief is indeed different from depression and anxiety. Symptoms such as preoccupation with the dead, denial, yearning, and searching correlate with grief but not depression. With depression, there is more of a poorer sense of self. Grieving people suffer from the pangs of loss and are preoccupied with this. Also in grief there is often an open display of affect. The symptoms are up-front and present, unlike depression. And, although depression is an enduring syndrome, grief tends to be greater than one episode with distinct features, sadness, pangs of loneliness, and transient depressive features.

Perhaps what clinicians are seeing in this traumatic grief process, then, is that the person's self-theory is being altered, and the prepotent emotion is a function of the meaning of the trauma event. In this way the grief and depression of PTSD affect the information processing of the person. Depression does this in general, leading to a hypersensitive focus on self and to an overall negative or general recollection of memories. Depression predisposes the person to respond in a determined way to emotional states (state dependence), to biased cognitions, to develop avoidant coping strategies, and eventually to become numb. Depression can also form as a comorbid affective state (Boudewyns, Woods, Hyer, & Albrecht, 1990). If it does not, residual depression states are visible, often impacting on traumatic grief. This altered information processing, we believe, constitutes an important deficiency and provides for maintenance of the traumatic grief response. There is indeed a "soul death." A schema that represents the process of traumatic grief is presented in Figure 11-1.

In sum, in the context of grief, what initially starts as anxiety and pangs of fear, transits to PTSD quickly, and over time to depression. Always this process is based on damage to the self theory of the person. Rogue emotions, anxiety, and later depression and other PTSD affects, are not assimilated and act as "free radicals"

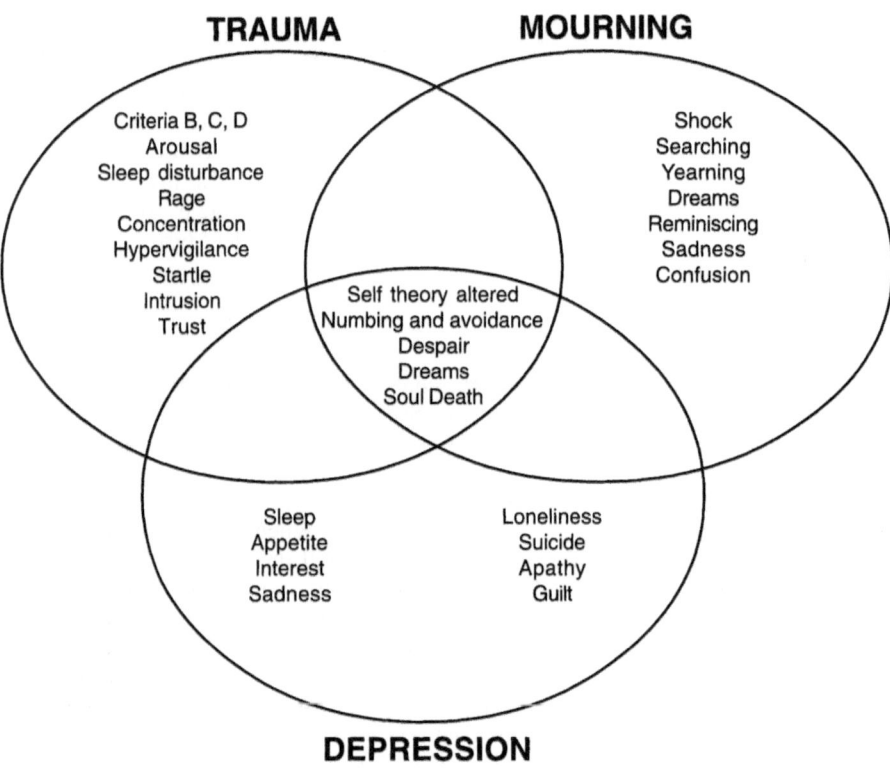

FIGURE 11-1.

roaming the thalamic region of the brain unabated until a place can be found for them in the explicit memory (van der Kolk, 1999). Over time then, depression appears to accompany PTSD modally. We believe then that "PTSD depression" is present and has had its start in grief, traumatic grief. Most emotions disrupt the internal stability of the person, but the depressive features require "grief-healing." As regards the influence of depression in the treatment of trauma, Spiegel (1993) noted:

> The working-through process is the overall therapeutic growth in which an initial trauma is recalled, abreacted, processed, and incorporated to the ongoing mental models and narrative of the patient's life. The working-through process invariably involves grieving as the advent of new knowledge destroys an often idealized sense of a significant other or of the self. Depression also commonly accompanies this grief. (p. 118)

Finally, we note that the fact that grief lies behind many of the functional problems related to PTSD and is present in nonclinical trauma populations. This is more important than finding its "correct place" in the nosology. If the clinician considers struggle against the loss of meaning in the face of at least a partial disintegration of the person's basic schemas as part of the process of PTSD, then grief becomes a part of treatment. In that treament, the clinician can focus on the excessive intensity of any grief response seen in this context (Worden, 1991).

☐ **Growth in Grief**

Among the core issues of PTSD treatment are the transformational processes found in grieving. Grief is the motivational pain that is both specific ("I lost this") and human ("I survived and must find meaning here"). Several principles underline the importance of this relationship and its potential for healing, especially in the elderly. Some of these apply to the victim, some to the therapy process. These tenets relate to the issues that we have been discussing in the book regarding the nature of the self and trauma. In this section they apply to grief and loss. They set the stage and provide the basis for the grief process in trauma treatment.

Tenet 1. People often do not merely cope with trauma, they can be transformed in their struggle with it. One result of assimilating trauma is that individuals extend developmentally where they could not go had the trauma not occurred. Positive reactions to trauma have been noted in the research literature (Lopata, 1973; Malinak et al., 1979). Affleck, Tennen, and Gershman (1985) noted that after trauma integration, most people had improved their perspective on life. Tedeschi and Calhoun (1995) more than others noted that an important sense of self reliance is learned through the struggle; surviving trauma not only leads to an enhanced sense of one's vulnerability, but sensitivity and emotional strength as well. In another study these authors (Calhoun & Tedeschi, 1989–1990) found that 83% of a bereavement group realized that they could depend on their family and could now better express emotions (i.e., their interpersonal experiences were enhanced). As another result people who suffer from trauma are more likely later to be supportive of others (Tedeschi & Calhoun, 1995).

It is our belief that a kind of phylogenetic principle applies here: A transmutation of information occurs moving from a dysfunctional to functional form, from diffuse to specific, and from negative to positive. This can occur because the vulnerability of the grief reaction in trauma is unlocked over time. A self-healing of the person unfolds as the state specific material of the obvious or subtle grief components are integrated into the core narrative of the person. Eventually the self-theory and person are actually better for this experience.

Tenet 2. Significant growth occurs only when schemas are challenged and changed by (traumatic) events: Tedeschi and Calhoun (1995) noted that change is possible only because schemas are disrupted. If you manage the event well and do it with ease, little change in the schemas occurred, but if you are rocked to the core, schemas are disrupted. Now the conditions appropriate for self-change are available and necessary.

We believe that one's theory of self provides a "platform" or perspective from which to view and initiate the information flow. Whatever the central metaphors of their living, the person attempts to match the necessities of their personal needs with life's events in their own way. This is most notable when one ages. Here the recognition and reconstruction of the self in the course of life review is an inherently satisfying component. In senescing life takes on a reauthoring process as the person attempts to separate self from specific problems. Epstein (1973) held that the dialectic import here is that one's self-theory is preserved and that the flow of information unfolds naturally without breaks in the continuity of the narrative.

Each person reconstructs memories, especially self-defining memories, to preserve identity (Singer & Salovey, 1993). As we have noted, usually a core of self memories that are representative of the person become involved. It is these memories that provide the meaning and the consistency for the self. One central part involves the drive toward sense-making by the individual. Meaning implies that one has internal patterns to guide our actions and behavior, and to regulate emotions (Baumeister, 1991; Janoff-Bulman, 1989).

In the grief process of trauma the person attempts to find meaning also but is unable to complete the process because of some self-damage. It is the job of the therapist to expose this process and to allow the affect(s) to be assimilated. This is only done when core aspects of self (theory) are challenged. Frankl (Sherman, 1991) noted that people find meaning in the suffering and struggle of their existence within the transitoriness and frailty of life. This occurs through self-pain, the survival-guilt pain of grief. Adversity does introduce a person to self.

Tenet 3. Memory is created in a present context and oriented by affect: We have addressed this before. This is a distinctly therapeutic tenet that is critical for an understanding of the change process. The emphasis here is on "now" experiencing and the process of meaning changing. Two personal experiences guarantee ongoing experiencing, affect and sensations. Singer and Salovey (1993) believed that affect is the phenomenon that provides the ordering for and association to multiple memories. Meaningful reprocessing of memories occurs in the present. When past and present commingle, what happens is that on-line expressions necessary for restructuring occur. The vehicle of change is most often affect (Safran & Greenberg, 1991).

In therapy sensations also are accessed to cement the experiential component. Bacon noted that sensations do not lie, giving a "true snapshot" of the situation (Guidano, 1991). For Shapiro (1995), sensations are the true governor of the change process. Whyte and Epston (1990) too noted that the real entrance to change is the body itself, the passage way out when thinking stops.

This is not to eschew the past; To do so is costly (Hyer et al., 1994). It is only to endorse the fact that treatment gains are optimal when the past is alive in the present. Both past memories and present affect attract the therapist's interest when they are in conjunction (Fleming & Robinson, 1990). Survivors of traumatic grief benefit from talk and exposure to the past event in the "doing" of the present. Exposure may be done in a gradual (Bagge & Brandsma, 1994), even nonsystematic way. We noted in a previous chapter that the change process never involves a "re-"experiencing of anything (Gendlin, 1991). Rather, it entails the present experiencing of the past event; present tense processing is the curative component in the change process, not the past reintegration. Reorganization is a byproduct.

Tenet 4. The narrative of one's life must be made coherent and understandable, encompassing the trauma experience: Over time salient positive and negative events form the memories of the person. As noted above, core memories are organized and form our autobiographical self. Memories are summarizations of experiences; they are at the vestigial core of development. In effect, we are our (selected) memories. A "need" to organize the biographical self to maintain continuity of meaning is paramount for optimal functioning in our species.

From the perspective that we have been developing, information about the self is organized in stories (memories) dictated by the theory of the self. It is an attempt to capture who we are at a level of abstraction that allows for historical continuity. This organization is critical because how one organizes information and scripts the story determines the adaptation process.

Importantly, trauma events must be taken in by their narrative. Strong negative events especially have difficulty becoming integrated into the self and require rescripting for change and assimilation to occur. When the self-theory becomes disorganized, the balancing processor of information is dyfunctional. Information does not move freely and core experiences become damaged or stuck.

Rescripting is the treatment. We are arguing here that these negative events must be incorporated into the ongoing self to be completed and processed. Because they cannot be exorcised, they must be exercised. The person comes to know that she/he is greater than the pathology: The self is the director of and responsible for the change.

Tenet 5. There is a need for a degree of consistency and continuity in the theory of self: That is to say, there is a need to bind time, to have a connection of coherence with what happened then, is happening now, and what will happen in the future. No superior new self is warranted; The person must be as she/he was but with the incorporation of the new data. The aim is not a new rendering of the whole self-theory; It is to make the person aware again of postulate breakdowns, to bring back the past as it was but alive and immediate and needing of attention for present and future. The person moves on to the next "viable you," not to a superior self (Neimeyer, 1995).

The simple point here is that change occurs with genuine inner contact. This leads to evolutionary change, a sense of acceptance and renewal, not revolutionary, discontinuous recreation. This is the consistency side of the change balance. The self is remarkably consistent, even in its own distortions. In reminiscence the "earlier person" is made vivid to self. As this occurs the self becomes more coherent, consistent, and intelligent. This process starts in childhood, has new intensity in adolescence, and builds across the life span, but is "my" identity always (McAdams, 1990). The natural iterative process of finetuning past, present, and future is ever unfolding.

Tenet 6. The person has to confront older schemas, grieve parts of self and certain experiences to grow: Organisms that ignore their own natural feedback do not adapt well. This involves giving up, for example, old assumptions of invulnerability and power, sometimes the harsh judgements of others. Also a commitment to live life better and to be generative toward others is often in order. In the search of the examined life the person becomes more what they intended to be (Jung, 1971). This is an unfreezing of the past, but not just nostalgia, it is a true generative process. If sufficiently close to the self-theory, the balance of pleasure/pain and esteem for one's self is incorporated. It is narrative truth, with acceptance for the only self that could have been at the time.

The self-narrative that denies truth to make events more pleasant or to "get by" runs counter to the possibility of change. One can "foreclose" in the Eriksonian sense, but this is a faulty compromise that allows for minimal satisfaction only. People must "come to terms" with their problems and feelings, and accept life's events. This is why treating trauma is insufficient: Treating the person and their self-theory are required.

Tenet 7. Transformation occurs when the client's own interpretation of the good coming from negative events is respected: Again this applies to the therapy protocol. Reflection and unconditional positive regard are only rarely overused. Then a gentle learning procedure, a dosed exposure that encourages change by facilitating choice and mastery over state-specific information is always efficacious.

Two issues are important here (Tedeschi & Calhoun, 1995): (a) Being respectful of the individual's processes of coping and (b) letting the client do the work. In allowing the person to feel validated while listening to the narrative they create, respecting their pace and their self-protective ways, the therapist creates the holding environment for the healing work of therapy. Clients learn that fear does not kill and that anger does not have to be all-consuming. They unlearn maladaptive responses "naturally." Once old schemas and the inherent tensions are re-experienced, they become relieved, and new meanings emerge. Revised schemas generate new behaviors and reactions.

Second, the client does the work. McCoulough (2000) noted that the biggest problem in CBT is that the therapist takes over for the client. The trauma victim is requested to "just talk" from self. As the dialectic process with the inner self continues, presumably an old problem can create new meaning. The client becomes a witness to the rigid and chaotic musings of their inner dialogue. The therapist first helps by explicating the target memory and next commenting on the processing style.

Everybody has their own way to struggle with trauma. Some act out more than others; some immerse themselves in the emotions and struggles; others in more rational processes. Clearly if the crisis is continuing or intense, the struggle will be more difficult and take a longer time. A balance must be struck between passive acceptance of the problem with denial/distortion of the event versus the problem-solving that is required for change—between what must be and what can be.

The essence of the grief process in trauma is a transformation of fear/depression into a new contact with self that allows for change. As the memory is changed, the person's self-theory is altered, self-concept and self-efficacy are touched for the better (Shapiro, 1995). One message is that, although loss is important, it is not the only thing. Grief can even enhance growth in the family system. Brabant, Forsyth, and McFarlain (1997) suggested that recovery is an individual process, involving common factors. These include Frankl's three tasks–doing a deed, experiencing a value, and suffering. These provide meaning in life, which is essential for life. Good comes from bad.

Tenet 8: The treatment of trauma may never be complete; most often the reason is grief-related (i.e., the refusal to mourn and forgive): The life span of the grief reaction in the PTSD survivor appears to be set during the first few months—and the story often becomes "bad start, bad finish" (Brandsma & Hyer, in press). Probably as a "result" of the early (mal-)adjustment to trauma, the pathological types of complicated grief take form (Parks & Weiss, 1983).

However something more important is implied. Marcel (Sherman, 1991) noted that life is a mystery to be lived, not a problem to be solved. The grief in the trauma process is the "natural suffering" of life. It is a key aspect of life. It should not be removed fully—in fact, it cannot be. This is the reason that the narrative of one's life must be "understood" (stood under), as the person "becomes" and encompasses the wisdom of the processes that undergrid life.

Of course, people must come to terms with their problems and how they cope with daily events. This is only to say that life goes on, and that practical issues must be attended to. Most therapists know that the amount of change that can occur in therapy is limited: "Real" change occurs in the life lived. It is probably folly to think of a person as an authentic self; Rather, people become realized selves in the sense that they are dealing with the realities of life and human nature itself. Hopefully in response to self-damage, the person comes to know that the only life that could have been lived, was. With trauma, this occurs in the feeling and acceptance of the pain, then the grief and the hard tasks of forgiveness. We elaborate below.

Each tenet implies meaning-making. Mason (1996) noted that change at later life involves an inner climb that starts with commitment, an act of will. It involves facing the edges of one's fear (fear of failure, fear of success, fear of the unknown, fear of engulfment). It continues with a crucial choice at some point. The person must act in some way that says "goodbye" to a shared dream. This is a restructuring of a life, a transformation to live, a commitment based on caring. Then, it is just a question of enduring, with the establishment of life anchors, social supports, and a covenant to live.

In this process too, loss is deconstructed. This involves questions of self:

1. What is the experience of loss for you?
2. How are you active in the construction of loss?
3. What are the limits of your particular conception of loss?
4. How can you obtain a more holistic view of the loss?
5. How is your world forever transformed by the loss? (It cannot be returned to premorbid status.)
6. How is grief played out in the larger family context?

☐ Treatment Model

We expand here on the grief therapy model that we previously outlined (Brandsma & Hyer, in press). As we noted before, many grief therapies exist (e.g., Worden, 1982), sometimes outlined by the focus of the therapy, like psychodynamic (e.g., Horowitz et al., 1984) or cognitive-behavioral (e.g., Fleming & Robinson, 1990), sometimes by components of the grief process (e.g., Melges, 1982), sometimes by stages (Parks, 1970), and sometimes by tasks (e.g., Worden, 1982). When PTSD is chronic and unrelenting, however, these methods have only loose application clinically. After all, grieving in PTSD is "traumatic," resulting in an alteration of basic physiological responses (Hyer et al., 1994), as well as enduring dysfunction in basic character structure (self-theory; Herman, 1992). In working with the sick soul—the chronic PTSD client—that the healing of the human being may extend, we believe, beyond that required by the curing of the patient's symptoms.

Stages in Grief Work

Six identifiable stages in traumatic grief work were identified (Brandsma & Hyer, 1995). These stages overlap with the tenets just noted. In this process the therapist recognizes that he/she cannot take away the pain, that the "presence" of the therapist is seen as therapeutic, that the therapist reach out to the person, that caring is the order of the day, that personal needs determine the experience of the bereaved, that loss cannot be explained away in religious ways, that the situation cannot be minimized, that seeds of hope are planted, that the processes of mourning be encouraged, and that the expectation of hope is fostered. Of course in any "real" sense the process of the grief reaction is not step-wise and clear. It is muddled and non-linear. Often it falls short of acceptance.

Verbalization of the Loss—Some stated recognition that a sense of loss was or (preferably) is being experienced. Here the therapist's task is twofold; to get the "grief story" out and to create a healing atmosphere. Merleau-Ponty (1964) noted that "man expresses self to discover what he means to himself." The client articulates the trauma, and the therapist validates it.

One form of validation is the universal sense that something deep in the soul was involved. In the pursuit of a narrative understanding the therapist attunes to the client and makes the past vivid (validation). There is an increased saliency regarding the interiority of the person ("What happened inside?") that leads to a need to talk through what are important core self issues. In addition, the therapist must create a healing atmosphere, she/he must listen and understand.

There is a critical element here in the two classic motives of human striving, agency (striving for self-enhancement) and communion (the need for contact with others). The grief side of loss requires expression for the self and to others. Direct queries into loss are helpful: What does this mean/take away from you? Comparing you now to before the event, what do you notice?, and so on. In some cases even repressed subselves reflective of the loss may be exhumed so that a balance can be seen (e.g., the quiet self as contrasted to the active one).

At the risk of over simplification regarding the trauma response, a chronic grief reaction is individually driven but tends to follow the two "classic" paths (often both) of PTSD, numbing and intrusion. That is to say, the person experiencing the grief tends either to get stuck in a pain barrier, in the intensity of the experience (trying unsuccessfully to avoid), or severely suppressing or inhibiting the response(s), often becoming numb to feelings and given to acting out (Fleming & Robinson, 1990). While these may be the "final common pathways" of the grief/trauma response, when the therapist accepts and truly validates the experience, information is forced to confess itself again, and an epiphany can unfold, often a reorganization of the core schema.

Psycho-education of the Grief Process—The tasks of healthy forms of grieving can be "taught." There are of course many informative pieces of data about grief, many myths too (Worden, 1982). The issues that are important (among others) involve experiencing the loss, the identification of its components, its sequence, and predictable responses, among others. These are as important in the treatment of grief as they are in the treatment of PTSD. Information titrates expectations and builds an appropriate compliance pattern in the service of realistic goals. Clients who have had a lifetime of opportunity to deal with grief in various pragmatic ways can still be only vaguely aware of their problem and the course to change in treatment. They need to become aware of their habitual ways and learn some new approaches.

We mean more too. The therapist who truly believes that stories (memories) are habituations and that these memories are important can use this model to treat with confidence. The therapist who knows that memory exists in present consciousness can be free to validate the pain and parse out its components. The therapist can make issues vivid that allow for an understanding of the grief process.

Tedeschi and Calhoun (1995) noted that the therapist can facilitate the psychoeducational process in several ways, including positive framings on the struggle, generic benefits accrued by the person in that context, a re-engagement of hope, new perspectives on possible growth, as well as a selective reinforcement of competence, manageability, locus of control, and efficacy (i.e., those personality variables noted above). The therapist can also assist in integrating the problem into the larger life narrative.

Talk through, Then Work through a Loss ("Once More with Feeling")—Exposing the positive and negative aspects of loss, always guided by affect. The therapist's task is to foster any movement of information, to allow the story to unfold and to keep it moving. The therapist is to keep statements simple with affective involvement high, and thus allow the natural healing (integration) of the therapy. If the client remains stuck, the therapist task is to keep data moving. The intent is to keep the client processing in present time to allow the natural healing processes of assimilation and accommodation. Worked properly, new information is accessed.

As in most dynamic therapies the therapist has one key rule—to keep information moving. Hopefully this involves a mix of expressive and instrumental tasks for the client. The therapist moves back and forth, being reflexive ("What does that say about you as a person?") and nonreflexive interventions ("Stay with that"). Other tasks are to bring the focus into the present; to access other modalities, especially sensations, to allow for "genuine inner contact," to appreciate the primacy of affect, to tag (label) emotions, to keep the client experiencing in the present ("Feel it now"), to support the tolerance of unacceptable feelings ("It's okay"), to tighten poorly integrated concepts ("Tell me more about that"), and to loosen deviant cognitions ("When were you not that way?"). Eventually the therapist more actively facilitates change ("What prevents you from . . .?"). This leads to the next stage.

Guided Imagery—Resolution unfolds in imagination with an awareness of several blocks to the affective flow. The therapist's task again is to keep the information flowing and to tag problem areas. Melges (1982) argued for the use of imagery in this process: He used present-time guided imagery, which optimizes the imagery skills usually already present in these individuals. Melges advocated that imagery be used at two times in grief work, believing that in pathological bereavement feelings of loss and grief are components of the psychopathology of PTSD. The first step is to identify the losses that the individual has experienced and the blocks that have become obstacles to resolution. A list of obstacles found frequently in grief work has previously been provided (Bagge' & Brandsma, 1994). For example, an individual who gives evidence of persistent yearning for the deceased may keep the clothing of the deceased in closets long after the loss. A key step is to help the individual to remove the obstacles by revising scenes through the use of present-tense imagery. This helps to reactivate the grieving process in a controlled manner.

In Box 11-1, it can be seen that guided imagery is the key to the whole grief process. Revision of the scene through talk or creation of new imagery is then planned with the client to allow opportunity for completion of unfinished business. It begins with

---

Box 11-1
Grief-Resolution Therapy

Techniques for Removing Obstacles	Process
1. Decision to regrieve	1. Decrease of defensive avoidance
2. Guided imagery	2. Controlled detachment
Relive, revise, revisit scenes of the loss	
Last positive exchange	
News of the loss	
The viewing	
Funeral ceremony	
Burial	
3. Future-oriented identity reconstruction	3. Building new images and plans

a decision to regrieve the losses. The patient is asked to relive the scene(s) of the loss in their imagination as it happened at that time. The more traumatic and foreign the experience, the greater the difficulty with this stage. This reliving often helps to identify blocks to the grieving process (e.g., things not done or done and regretted).

For an individual with traumatic grief, this process can be initiated with some ease as the client has already had intrusive images usually related to the loss.

"Saying Goodbye"—This somewhat ritualized component can be a powerful closure to a traumatic memory. This is the logical extension of the previous stage. The person's blocks are negotiated to enable the saying of the needed "goodbye." In conjunction with the previous stage one woman was unable to express a goodbye to her deceased son because of the presence at the funeral of her husband's former wife. In the revision, the scene could be reconstructed without the offending individual, thus facilitating the expression of unfinished business. This then is effected in a controlled environment by revisiting the scene and allowing opportunities for "dialogues with the dead." Affective exchanges (both love and anger), confrontation of conflicts, expressions of guilt, and finally (but empathically not of least importance) the giving and receiving of forgiveness, are important elements. When carefully done, this allows for a controlled detachment from the deceased. These sessions are often intensely emotional, which supports Bowlby's (1980) contention that weeping and anger appear to be necessary components in helping the patient recognize and accept that the loss is final, the bond is broken.

We add to this one technique that has been beneficial for the more resistant client, those who resist change in their position of grief. The lost person is most often seen in a distant and absent way. Often intrusions occur. The grieving person cannot experience the lost person with good feeling, or if so, the rush of grief is so great that the effort is aborted. So the therapist can assess how the lost person is experienced: What is the "felt presence" of the diseased? We do this in a positive way: "You are having trouble with the sadness of the lost person. This is not what you miss. What you miss is the good memories, love, and comforting presence of the person. Recall a time when you and _____ were in a valued place and time. Recall the love and the comfort." This feeling is then anchored in the person, perhaps by a word or image. This will be a template to be recalled when the person desires. This is the image that the client will re-associate with the person. The person must feel the presence as positive and empowering. It is practiced. The client will often cry but see the benefits.

Future Orientation—Imagery is used to help the individual construct a future in terms that recognize the finality of the loss and the need to continue in life. The therapist's task is to focus toward the future and to empower, give choice, and if needed, reframe. Again, imagery is used to help. The therapist allows for a series of feasible steps in which the client creates a new future and then anchors it. Often the client can be asked what a full life would be like in the recent future.

Withdrawing cathexes from the past allows the renewal of a present–future focus. Using guided imagery, the individual can look to the future (as well as to the past). This can be done shortly after the completion of the guided imagery phase of grief-resolution therapy. The patient is asked to imagine that he is visiting a place once cherished by himself and the deceased together, a place of safety and warmth (Melges, 1982, p. 207). Then the individual can look toward the future and perhaps can look back on the present. The elderly with religous faith may look forward to meeting loved ones once again. This ability to flexibly distance (observing ego) is a good test of the efficacy of the grief work; it shows the new flexibility of the healed self-theory.

☐ Forgiveness: The Special Ingredient of Grief Therapy

"Haven't you forgiven yourself yet?" is the common sense reaction by many to the extended grief reaction. Grief is a process that humans go through to mourn (process) their many possible losses. We believe that losses in traumatic grief are for the most part shame-based. Shame and guilt are bookends that are often confused. Guilt refers to specific acts that one is sorry for, whereas "the experience of shame is directly about the self, which is the focus of evaluation" (Tangney, 1995). For example, if one would list the losses related to guilt and shame with regard to combat, on the guilt side of the equation we would find such events as taking life, not saving friends, illegal and immoral acts. The shame side of the equation is much longer and more insidious and pervasive. There is the loss of the ability to work, to behave appropriately and consistently, the capacity to love, the sense of a niche in humanity and community, missing body parts or functions, control, integration of self, potency, innocence, vitality—all with their negative impact on the summary self image (self theory). These shame-based losses have an important impact on the theory of self because they are directed at the self, not at specific behaviors. Shame-based losses abuse the central valuations of the person, and they strike at the core of the person's belief system, the self-theory. In effect, the self-narrative is damaged, and the only way back is through self-healing. The Russain poet Yevgeny Yevtushenko held that shame is a most powerful motivator.

Interestingly, more recent therapies for shame and guilt have involved cognitive (Kubany, 1994) or spiritual (Hebl & Enright, 1993) interventions. For change to occur, forgiveness must play a crucial part. Forgiveness is central to all aspects of mental health. Forgiveness mainly deals with the insults and losses to one's theory of self. Mourning and forgiveness are intimately linked. They both represent processes that progress toward a more realistic acceptance of the self and world as it currently is.

In the last decade forgiveness as a therapeutic concept has blossomed. Conceptual clarification has made great strides, and this has led to operational definitions and interventions useful both scientifically and clinically. A brief historical and philosophical analysis of this term has been presented by Hebl and Enright (1993) and provides an excellent conceptual foundation for interpersonal forgiveness. For our purposes, forgiveness is defined as overcoming of negative thoughts, feelings, and behaviors *not* by some form of denying the offense or the right to be hurt/angry, but by viewing the offender at least with acceptance so that the forgiver can be healed. At a simple level, it is the realization that one does not condone the transgressed act nor absolve one of responsibility, but it releases resentment. It is a change in perception—a recognition that this is emotionally over. Forgiveness, then, is not forgetting. At a deeper level it is an act of self-interest and self-love. When one forgives, one must own the pain that was experienced in the situation. Once it is owned, the pain of the past looks to the future.

Once again we refer to our tenets: To begin the process of forgiveness, the client must be stabilized enough to feel that she/he is safe and in a relationship with a therapist that will be as supportive as necessary. The client must know that the

---

Box 11-2
Ego Skills Necessary for Forgiveness

1. The ability to empathize and give up one's egocentric position. This involves a discovery of likeness or similarity, and respect for the personhood of the other.
2. Appreciation for the self and growth of the self-theory apart from the other person in a relationship (autonomy).
3. A differentiated theory of motives.
4. Ability to discriminate boundaries between parties.
5. Understanding of vulnerabilities in all parties.
6. Ability to tolerate and clarify emotional contradictions (i.e., ambivalence, confusion, logical contradiction).
7. The acceptance of limitations in self and other.

---

therapist understands his/her predicament. As therapy proceeds, however, forgiveness depends on several higher level cognitive processes. Many of these are listed in Box 11-2 (cf. Brandsma, 1998).

The growth of these ego skills requires a relationship, insight, and time for effective working through. Particularly important is the operation of empathy and altruism as processes that underlie forgiveness.

These are often hard to attain with trauma victims until a conceptual shift is experienced, from competition to cooperation, and eventually compassion. This is a true reformulation of one's valuations, one that then has less reason to grieve.

From the therapist side of the equation, McCullough and Worthington (1994) added five elements that must be provided by the therapist (Box 11-3). These underlie the key therapeutic interventions with regard to forgiveness.

Most therapists trained in secular institutions do not think in terms of forgiveness or understand its various possibilities in technique. Thus clinical questions abound with the primary one being how explicitly a therapist should encourage forgiveness and, if so, in what forms and at what points in time? There are now available psycho-educational, time-limited programs for teaching people the processes of forgiveness

---

Box 11-3
Key Therapeutic Interventions for Forgivness

1. Unconditional positive regard to explore feelings.
2. Refocusing attention away from negative emotions by reframing or viewing from a larger context or different perspective.
3. Enable empathy for the offender.
4. Discuss reconciliation if possible.
5. Focus attention on forgiveness of the self.

---

that address these issues by plowing through them. However there are many pitfalls and pseudo-forms of forgiveness interacting with personality diagnosis and level of moral development that limit effectiveness (Hebl & Enright, 1993).

Viscott (1997) held that forgiveness is necessary or emotional debt follows. Emotional debt leads to *toxic nostalgia*, the emotional script that is unfinished and unfriendly. It is the emotional newsclip of life that is superimposed on the present. It is the source of unmourned losses in life, the key method where the unresolved past attempts to define the present. Unforgiven events serve as determinants in life everywhere, and can lead to self destructive grudges, lower self-esteem, prevent the understanding of present feelings, and result in excessive hypersensitivity, just to name a few. Worse, symptoms of "emotional stuckness" are everywhere. They sneak around denial to remind the person that peace is an illusion, make the person excessively defensive, cause old feelings to rush in all at once (often unannounced), download guilt when unnecessary, and establish that old pain is unresolved and not going away. Positive feelings are defeated also. Both pleasure and pain are the puppets of unforgiveness.

We propose that an engagement with the issues of forgiveness in some explicit form is very useful in the resolution of traumatic grief and PTSD. It is often the missing piece in the therapeutic puzzle that prevents movement toward a new gestalt or schema. We note that although the processes of therapy surrounding forgiveness have been clarified greatly in recent years, especially where it involves other people, it is forgiveness of self that remains a more difficult conceptual conundrum. This is the ultimate act of humanity, perhaps what makes a person, a person. It is often a silent personal war within a war; it is the essence of the human struggle. It involves a high degree of ego-splitting and skill. It is compassion for self, a friendly view of self, and it is the part of the PTSD response that applies to grief.

☐ A Caution

At its simplist level reasonable structural strategies of the therapy apply, the correct balance in the experiencing of the pain of the loss, approach and avoidance techniques. For grief work in the therapy, the client should have as a minimum the ability of the three Ps—pacification (calm self down), partition (distance self from loss), and perspective (see context of life). They should be able to care for themselves (as we noted above).

However this is often not sufficient. With many grieving people, especially older victims, the penchant for an attachment for behaviors that do not work is monumental. People repeatedly use methods of self-care that do not work. Often a questioning of the person's position is an act of futility. Many grieving clients possess restraining forces that are so prepotent as to require coping and management, just as with trauma. For these clients just fostering stable psychosocial adjustment may be preferable, a form of supportive therapy.

We know that most psychotherapy outcomes covary inversely with chronicity in PTSD. Many clients with chronic PTSD will not benefit equally even with the practice of our musings. In other chapters we address the assessment of the trauma victim and the readiness for treatment of the trauma memory. Over time, many simply do not have the "object relations abilities" to struggle with these issues; that is, they do not possess sufficient cognitive complexity, a flexible capacity for emotional investment and detachment, an understanding of social causality, or enough affect tone in relationships (Ford, 1995). For them we manage and encourage the practical necessities of life, simple balance, activity, and support.

As a way of "quick" assessment, we have found two questions have been helpful in an understanding of this tact by a patient: (a) "Does this view of the lost object really work for you?" and (b) "Are you headed in a direction that you would like to go?" The patient can see more clearly that the traumatic grief is present and asserts a cost.

☐ Conclusion

By way of recapitulation, a better understanding of the treatment of PTSD results by looking at grieving processes. PTSD and grief cohabitate, initially by anxiety and later in the form of the depression. In fact, these can be independent "symptoms." We argue that issues of loss necessarily influence the formation of PTSD. We provided eight tenets that reflect the PTSD grief process and its treatment. Central to this understanding is that the person of the trauma victim is affected and, as such, both is influenced by and influences the loss response, the grief reaction in PTSD. In addition, we outlined a treatment model useful in the therapist's response to grief in the context of PTSD. We have ended with forgiveness, usually an ongoing task in one's life, as a necessary component in the care of grief in PTSD.

Grieving is a choiceless event that accelerates the decisions of the victim. Time may stand still for the phenomenology of the person, but it speeds up where life choices are concerned. Hundreds of choices including whether to absorb the caring and loss of the loved one or distribute it to others present themselves. At base too, grieving (like PTSD) involves a dual process, a vacillation between engaging versus avoiding. A choice allows for a relearning of the world disrupted by the loss as well as a relearning of self.

At a basic level also the inability to accommodate to the trauma is due to the severity of the event and the internal resources of the person at the time of the trauma. In the past decade we have come to know that treating trauma memories alone is insufficient. After all, the traumatic memory is only a descriptive summary for events that are experienced under high levels of arousal. Loss is there. Forgiveness, the essence of which is a personal reframe on one's theory of self, is part of this grief care equation also, as it addresses both loss and PTSD. The existence of loss in this reaction is no less important than any PTSD symptom. To turn a phrase the "care of the PTSD soul" demands this hearing (in treatment). To do less compromises the treatment of PTSD and certainly is not the treatment of traumatic grief.

12

CHAPTER

Using Assessment Data to Inform the Treatment Plan

"... the evaluator can rarely determine exactly which symptoms or difficulties in an adult survivor of abuse are in fact directly related to a given instance of abuse. Furthermore, it will almost never be true that psychological testing "alone" can serve as an absolute litmus test for whether abuse has occurred in a given individual ... instead such data should be combined with all other available information to provide hypothesis about what may be abuse affects in someone who has reported abuse."
Briere (1997, p. 49)

"Every man is in certain respects (a) like all other men, (b) like some other men, (c) like no other man" (Kluckhorn & Murray, 1953). A person is ultimately unique. The more you know, the less you know. The longitudinal course of PTSD is a total person response, a process of decline impacted unduly at first by fearful and intrusive experiences and later accommodated to by a symphony of poor adaptation. In time, the symptom numbing comes of age. Regarding older people, this is a story of a smorgasbord of these vulnerability factors but also resilience and of a disorder that has many parts. Information about PTSD will follow from this understanding.

In this way too the clinician's role in the assessment of PTSD in older persons is, we believe, important. The practicing clinician begins in a professional setting, addresses a problem of significance to the client who presents it, and is faced with a need to respond to that problem in a humane and effective manner. If scientific knowledge is sufficient to the task, the situation is an easy one and desirable behavior for the clinician is readily apparent. Science meets taxon. In such a situation the professional can apply easy-to-use or validated techniques, but professionals also must be prepared to deal with those problems that do not clearly lend themselves to scientifically verified approaches. In fact, it rarely is the case that scientific knowledge is sufficient to the task. Science only presents at best a partial solution. Critical judgment becomes crucial.

Most clinicians are aware of the gap between the global nature of research findings and the usual specific nature of clinical dilemmas. Good clinicians want to know

257

both, the how and why. The goal is to reconstruct a circle—from rich idiographic individuality, to nomothetic commonalties, to nomothetic individuality. In a sort of strange way clinicians must give up the person to ultimately get him/her back (Millon & Davis, 1995).

In this chapter we discuss the importance of assessment. We start with overall considerations and suggest a format for evaluation. Next, we consider the idiographic formulation, its problems and necessities. We then address the "players," types of measures that we and others use. We end with a discussion of the other necessary components in the trauma response of the older person. These include depression, coping, health, dissociation, and therapy.

☐ Overall Considerations

"A theory of evaluation is as much a theory of political interaction as it is a
theory of how to determine facts."
Cronbach and associates (1980)

At the least, assessment should inform treatment. The clinician looks to the assessment data for help in informing his/her interventions. A victim's assessment always starts with a history. In some corners this constitutes 80% of the diagnostic picture. With PTSD victims, these "context components" of treatment are indeed important. Previous trauma history, previous psychiatric history, and the illusion of invulnerability (an almost universal belief) especially are important premorbid factors. The type of trauma, especially war or sexual trauma, fear of injury and actual injury, are some negative stressor-related variables. Excessive levels of stress, lack of social support, negative cognitive appraisals, and causal attributions that reflect learned helplessness and negative safety beliefs are some variables that affect the course of care for trauma victims.

Given these concerns, assessment (for us) involves several areas (Box 12-1). Briere (1997), for example, believed that seven areas are necessary for evaluation: pretrauma functioning, trauma exposure, social supports, comorbidity, malingering or secondary gain, and PTSD. The first issue addresses the target trauma. We have discussed this. Second, we measure intervening trauma (both current and past). This may be as or more important than the trauma itself. The assessment of trauma across the life span with an older person assumes the form of a life review. Third is comorbidity. Information on comorbidity and the influence of current stressors should be examined and treated immediately. The clinician should be especially concerned about depression and dissociation.

The fourth issue involves assessing how the person has "aged" since the trauma. How is the lifespan affecting (affected by) the trauma experience? What are coping and social support resources? What is the person's physical health status? What are the person's expectations? "It is part of the cure to expect to be cured" (Seneca). This issue also involves the "rest of the story" that comprises the life context surrounding the person's trauma history. These are age-related issues, as well as coping, health, and resources. We consider this also in other sections of the book.

The fifth issue involves skills necessary for the dialogue of the target trauma itself. These involve sufficient self and ego capacities, whether traumatic memories are largely fragmented, partially or completely unconscious with a weak ability to tolerate access, and the level of intrusions. Again as discussed in Chapter 9, we are interested in whether the person is able to handle the stress of therapy with the trauma memory.

Box 12-1
Context Knowledge for Treating Trauma in Older People

Issue 1: Assessment of PTSD
        Severity/type/frequency of trauma
        Can the person tell a story?
        Does the person want to do this?
Issue 2: Intervening trauma
        What additional trauma occurred/is occurring?
        When did PTSD first show itself?
        Trajectory of trauma?
Issue 3: Complications
        Comorbidity (including dissociation)
Issue 4: Developmental issues
        Age-related issues
        When did trauma first show itself?
Issue 5: Self and ego skills
        Can access thoughts (What were you thinking then?)
        Can access feelings (What were you feeling then?)
        Knows/accepts their client role (This is your job here)
        Has the ability and willingness to stay on task and struggle non-
            defensively?
        Collaborate; provide ongoing feedback to experience (e.g., SUDS
            levels)
        Possess adequate imagery and verbal skills
        Is not excessively defensive
        Use self-skills in the environment
        Tolerate frustration/pain
        Avoid a self-condemning evaluation
        Use calming self-talk
        Can place symptoms in perspective
        Can cope outside of therapy
        Is able to be alone
Issue 6: Personality
        Methods of operation of the person
        Strategies and tactics of everyday life
Issue 7: Related issues
        Social support
        Coping, health, and resources
        Interview significant others
Issue 8: Positive Core Memories (PCMs)
        Other stories
        Who is the person?
Issue 9: What is the best form of treatment?
        Has anything helped?
        Likelihood that a particular intervention will achieve goals
        Will the patient be able to partake and understand in treatment?
        What if they resolve this problem?

The sixth issue involves a knowledge of the client's personality processes. There may be no other variable in the clinician's armamentarium as important as data that address the ingrained patterns of thinking, feeling, interacting, and behaving. This information assists in the application of tactics and strategies of care. We address this also in other chapters.

The seventh concern involves the other issues of trauma. They include social support, health concerns, and coping, as well as an interview with a significant other. These are the deceptively simple and important components of care that the research suggests influence everything. They do.

Eighth is the narrative. We are interested in the PCM (positive core memory), discussed in Chapter 9. In standard case formulation of an older person, the intent of the clinician is to rule in problems. This issue enlarges the field of view to encompass a broad range of factors. What are the core defining memories, PCMs, that the person uses to characterize his/her sense of self? The clinician requests core, self-defining memories from the client and uses these to renarrate better current self-views. We discussed this also in Chapter 9.

Finally, the treatment itself is relevant: What is the likelihood that a particular intervention will achieve its goals with this patient? Here the interest is whether the patient is able to partake and understand in treatment and the implications of this.

It is stressed that these issues relate to our overall assessment of the trauma and the context. It does not specify tests or ratings. The clinician should be open and flexible with our "hard and fast" positions. We need a map, a largely conscious strategy for achieving psychological goals. To the extent that this is not so, the assessment and

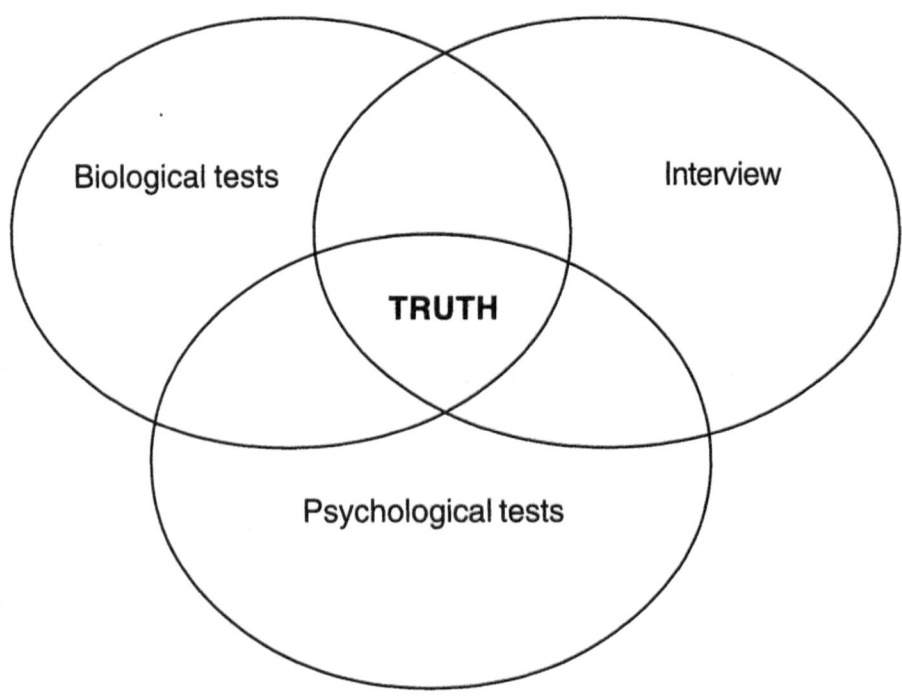

FIGURE 12-1.

plan require alteration. In another sense the clinician needs to re-evaluate his/her own epistemological model and establish better bridges between logical and practical matters.

Also, we note this. The Venn diagram in Figure 12-1 indicates that assessment is a complete process. The three legs of clinical interview, psychological tests, and biological tests often constitute the playing field for the assessment. To this could be added conferences with significant others and peer consultation at least. Regardless, the center represents the convergence of data, wisdom.

☐ Idiographic Formulation

We do not know all problems that prevent us from a solid diagnosis. Some relate to PTSD and some to aging. Research and clinical experience indicate that for many older victims at least PTSD symptoms are present, either right after the trauma or "de novo" decades later. The longitudinal effects of trauma are complex. These include PTSD symptoms, all the mediating variables discussed in previous chapters, as well as functionally autonomous symptoms or syndromes of depression and anxiety. The developmental issues of aging and trauma also interact. Noted above also, the concepts of trauma—loss, meaning-making, accepting reality, achieving ego integrity—are very close to those of aging. How these interface with trauma responses is complex indeed.

Additionally, the assessment of PTSD can be confusing for the clinician. On the one hand, those who experience chronic trauma also experience severe chronic stress and emotional deprivation, forcing the clinician to appreciate the multimodal influence on the continuance of PTSD. On the other, it is likely that many older people will not report symptoms because they do not see them as symptoms. Somatic problems and emotional numbing are especially problems. Often too symptoms are secondary to other problems or disorders and many are secondary symptoms to the DSM presentation.

We do not yet know what seems to potentiate problems for the most common variety of the aging victims, the appearance of PTSD symptoms after remitted periods: Do trauma symptoms occur as a result of age-related coping decline, recent stressful events, or is it just the nature of the disorder? As an older person with trauma problems often has "carried" PTSD baggage over time, we do not always know the lifespan developmental influences on the expression of the trauma. The admixture of transition process and the psychiatric symptoms make for interesting bedfellows.

There is much we do not know in a scientific or real clinical sense. What is PTSD at later life really? What does PTSD and depression mean if a patient is in a hospital and feels helpless and is not sleeping or eating? If this patient has a few Category B (intrusive) and D (arousal) symptoms but no evident Category C problems, what does that mean? Always the value or meaning of a symptom in the context of PTSD for an older person requires a clinical ear.

We know too that clients with the same problem are different, always. Clients differ in the amount and way that they meet the requirements of any diagnosis, not to mention comorbid diagnoses or personality issues. Diagnosis alone underspecifies pathology, especially with regard to treatment. Variations of a given disorder are intrinsically confusing. PTSD has many varieties, several of which are subclinical and often influenced by different forms of depression or other comorbidities. Any generalization of findings is achieved by theory-based thinking and the application by replication on a case-by-case basis. Theory-based, question-driven, single case practice in which disconfirmation remains a real possibility is a necessary skill within psychotherapy practice. Much of this "actuarial" process is in the clinician's head (both the science of the area and the messiness of the client). Millon (1999) stated:

> The purpose is not to put persons in the classification system, but instead to reorient the system with respect to the person by determining how his or her unique, ontological constellation of attributes overflows and exceeds it. The classification thus becomes a point of departure for comparison and contrast, a way station in achieving total understanding of the complexity of the whole, not a destination in itself. When in the course of an assessment the clinician begins to feel that the subject is understood at a level where ordinary diagnostic labels no longer adequately apply, the classification system is well on its way to be falsified relative to the individual, and a truly idiographic understanding of the person is close at hand, ready to be approached in a comprehensive and systematic way therapeutically. (p. 109)

In the use of our technologies of assessment and psychotherapy, we are somewhere between dust bowl, total open-ended, anything goes data input, and dogma. We are between naive interviewing and established surgery. As such, we need to be open at times and to be direct at others. A reasonable practice of assessment of PTSD defers to the former, but not at the expense of the latter. In the beginning, it is best to add to the search, opening eyes in all directions. The knowledge that the influence of the target population can sometimes be more qualitative and subtle and requires science and sensitivity in understanding (and as such extensive testing) can be disconcerting in the scientific sense but empowering in the human sense.

☐ The Players

We advocate for a multimethod approach. The most abused form of "understanding" of a trauma victim is the mono-method approach of one clinician. The patient talks to the therapist and the therapist forms a theory. The result is error, method variance, and distortion. Clinicians are advised to avoid a clinical hermeneutics error and to avoid the necessities of business-as-usual with a complex person who has age and trauma to contend with. While an older victim can exist in a vacuum, they cannot be treated in one.

Criterion A

"The concept of 'trauma' may not be needed. What is needed, instead, is a detailed characterization of the exposure—in terms of both continuous dimensions and nominal scale characteristics—for each individual. A multivariate analysis of the additive and interactive influences of the various dimensions of exposures on a particular outcome—together with an analysis of vulnerability factors—will adequately describe the pathogenic components of the exposure."
Kasl (1990, p. 1656)

Criterion A involves the trauma, a necessary feature for PTSD. Now clinicians are not required to have a trauma that is outside the realm of usual human experience (to meet DSM criterion). For starters, we note that this is a worthwhile exercise, as trauma is almost always related to PTSD intensity and frequency. We can take strength from the fact too that the evaluation of trauma serves as a context of a life review and as a developmental pointer. Resnick, Falsetti, Kilpatrick, and Freedy (1996) emphasized a number of important considerations in the assessment of Criterion A that are especially important for older persons. These include providing a context for the assessment, explaining the nature of extreme events, including behavioral specific operational definitions (e.g., asking a series of detailed questions about specific trauma events), assessing a broad range of potential events to which the respondents may have been exposed, including details of what happened, the ways in which the event are threatening, and others.

Ultimately, Criterion A is a stressor because it produces fear and with potential PTSD people alter life course at least for awhile. This means that the psychological portion of the definition is empowered. It is even conceivable that the person need have no physical threat that involves threat or injury. Carlson (1997) advocated for three conditions: (a) perception of the event as highly negative valence; (b) the suddenness of the experience; and (c) the inability to control the event leading to fear of safety and security.

For assessment, Norris (1990) has argued that six dimensions are required for all traumatic stress reactions: tangible loss, scope (others involved), threat to life and physical integrity, blame (self or others), familiarity, and post-traumatic reactions (cognitions and emotions tied to the event). Breslau, Davis, Andreski, and Peterson (1991) advocated for open-ended questions starting with available questions about exposure to "terrible experiences." If the answer is "no," another question regarding "great shock because something like that happened to someone close to you?" is asked. Those answering "yes" to that question are asked to describe the worst such event in their lives, which is coded into specific categories and then probed for "anything else like this," and then for "any other terrible or shocking experience" (Resnick, Falsetti, Kilpatrick, & Freedy, 1996). Of course this assessment is subject to all the problems of retrospective assessments and with older people, especially memory.

There are of course critical issues not addressed. We are still unclear about the extent of the subjective part versus the objective part of Criterion A; whether there should be one or greater numbers of traumas for the assessment of PTSD; whether patients have to attach Criterion B and C to the trauma event or they can be general; and what other symptoms can be let into the symptom mix before a "real" diagnosis is given, among others. We will just have to live with these.

Excessive but Good Trauma Scales   Two scales stand out as comprehensive, if not excessive. Brown and colleagues (1989) developed perhaps the Rolls Royce rating for trauma evaluation, the LEDS (Life Events and Difficulties Schedule). This is an intensive interview procedure that elicits respondents' descriptions not only of recent events but also past events and the context in which the event took place. For Brown, a panel ultimately rates the objective threat from a later rendition. Of interest is the fact that the meaning of the event is specially transcoded and with it the necessary components of hope and self-esteem are taken. This represents a "match" for each person depending on what is important (e.g., control, intelligence, perfection, etc). This applies also to personality styles, autonomous and sociotropy, as these have been shown to be related to vulnerability in distinct ways depending on the stressor.

The other scale is the ELS (Evaluation of Lifetime Stressors; Krinsley & Wheathers, 1995). This was developed at the National Center for PTSD on veterans with war trauma. As with the Brown scale, it is lengthy. Its advantage is that it assesses stressors across the lifespan, incorporating both objective and subjective elements of an experience required by the new DSM. It can serve as a kind of PTSD lifeline.

If we can use war trauma as a model, we come to the conclusion that an evaluation of exposure to the stressor represents an important area. Many measures of combat-related PTSD focus on detailing the intensity, frequency, and duration of the traditional combat experiences involving danger, loss of life, and severe physical injury (Green, Epstein, Krupnick, & Rowland, 1997). Again, using the domain of military experiences, we learn that the clinician should be inclusive. They should include war zone experiences outside of the realm of traditional trauma. This involves the context of combat-related experiences and the like, including the normal unpleasant parameters of military experience, the bad environment, food, and military support.

(For war trauma, there are also many self-report scales with reasonable psychometric properties. The most inclusive is the War Zone Stress Inventory [WZS; Kulka et al., 1990]. A shorter form is the Combat Exposure Scale [Keane, Newman, & Onsillo, 1996]. They require modification for older veterans.)

Other Trauma Scales   Other scales include the Adult Trauma Inventory (Saigh, 1989) and the Traumatic Stress Scale (TSS; Norris & Riad, 1996). The latter assesses 10 areas. The advantage of this scale is that it allows each individual to be further probed according to the extent of the loss produced, its scope, threat to life and physical integrity, whether the individual was blamed, and familiarity with the trauma.

We mention the PSEI (Potential Stressful Events Interview; Resnick, Kilpatrick, Ransky, Saunders, & Bert, 1993) also, as it was used in the DSM-IV field trials. This measure has been used in treatment settings. It is an example of how a research instrument can be used for clinical purposes. It consists of modules that assess stressor type, subjective-behavioral characteristics of the stressor, and subjective reaction of the stressor. It was the instrument that allowed for the broadening of the criteria for a stressor for the current DSM.

Additionally, there are a wide variety of measures that assess childhood stressors—Traumatic Events Scale (Elliot & Briere, 1992) and the Trauma Symptom Checklist for Children (Briere, 1996). Surprisingly, this issue is important in 25% of older war trauma samples (Hyer & Summers, 1994). Note also needs to be given to Axis IV of the current DSM. This axis specifies the severity of the psychosocial stressor. This stressor, however, is to have occurred within the past year and to have contributed to the onset, recurrence, or exacerbation of a disorder (either Axis I or Axis II). However it can be used as a marker of the problem.

Clinical Recommendation   Brief pre-assessment measures assist in the sensitization of the trauma telling. Green, Epstein, Krupnick, and Roland (1997) specified that an event inventory or similar screening device may be more important than other detailed procedures in the initial phases of the diagnostic process. Once the trauma has been discovered, a clear follow-up assessment plan should be developed. One option is to schedule a follow-up visit within a short period of time to explore and evaluate the trauma exposure and the impact of the symptoms and course of treatment.

We recommend a generic measure of Criterion A, followed by a description of the event. One brief scale, sensitive to many situations, is the Traumatic Events Questionnaire (TEQ; Lauterbach & Vrana, 1996). This assesses 11 stressors relevant to Criterion A: combat, larger fires or explosions, serious industrial or farm accidents, sexual assaults or rapes, natural disasters, violent crimes, adult abusive relationships, physical or sexual child abuse, witnessing someone being mutilated, seriously injured or violently killed, other life-threatening experiences, and violent or unexpected death of a loved one. Added to this is any other event or one that can't be told.

One other scale that assesses the subjective side of problems is the Modifiers and Perceived Stress Scale (MAPS; Linn, 1986). This scale has been used with older samples. It measures 41 different stressors, emphasizing the stressor experience of the person by addressing issues related to the person: perceived stress, unexpectedness of events, perceived responsibility, and degree of social support. This has been used with older populations.

Interviewer-Rated PTSD Measures

In a review chapter on PTSD scales, Norris and Riad (1997) stated that the field of trauma at this point should forgo temptation for generating new and largely similar scales and assessed the psychometrics of the existent ones. Perhaps we can concentrate on scales that show reasonable consistency for measurement. Blake et al. (1995) identified six criteria that could be used to evaluate PTSD measures in this regard:

1. Corresponds to established diagnostic criteria.
2. Provides dichotomous and continuous data about symptoms and disorder.
3. Can be administered by trained paraprofessionals.
4. Possesses adequate reliability and validity.
5. Provides clear and concise questions that include behavioral anchored rating descriptions.
6. Assumes a multidimensional view of severity and carefully delineates current and lifetime diagnostic life time frames.

Current "better" measures or scales are anchored in various ways to the DSM. A number of structured interviews are now available for diagnosing PTSD. These include stand-alone interviews, such as the Structured Interview for PTSD (SI-PTSD; Davidson, Kudler, Saunders, & Smith, 1990; Davidson, Smith, & Kudler, 1989), the PTSD interviews (PTSD-I; Watson, Juba, Manifold, Kucala, & Anderson, 1991), the PTSD Symptom Scale—Interview (PSS-1; Foa, Riggs, Dancu, & Rothbaum, 1993), and the Clinician-Administered PTSD Scale—Version 1 (CAPS-1; Blake et al., 1990; Blake et al., 1992), as well as PTSD modules of comprehensive diagnostic interviews, such as the Diagnostic Interview Schedule (DIS; Helzer, Robins, & McEvoy, 1987), the Structured Clinical Interview for DSM-IV (SCID; Spitzer & Williams, 1985; Spitzer, Williams, Gibbon, & First, 1990), and the Anxiety Disorders Interview Schedule—Revised (ADIS–R; DiNardo & Barlow, 1988).

The module of the DSM-IV SCID for PTSD is probably the standard-bearer. This is more popular and used more than the DIS or the ADIS–R, each with limitations. The SCID PTSD module corresponds to current diagnostic criteria. It has adequate reliability and validity. However, it lacks explicit rating descriptors; it yields primarily dichotomous information; it does not assess separate dimensions of severity; and the SCID developers strongly suggest that it be used only by experienced professionals or highly trained and clinically sophisticated paraprofessionals (cf. Spitzer, Williams, Gibbon, & First, 1990).

Recommendation The scale that has received the most interest empirically is the CAPS-1 (Clinician Administered PTSD Scale). This is an interviewer-rated scale on the frequency and intensity of the 17 diagnostic symptoms of PTSD drawn from the DSM, along with 8 other correlative PTSD symptoms. The time period addressed is the past month. There is also a lifetime frame. Recent studies on the CAPS (Blake, Weathers, Nagy, et al., 1995), carefully assessed the psychometric properties (on Vietnam veterans) and found adequate reliability (Weathers & Litz, 1994). Weathers, Ruscio, and Keane (1999) assessed nine scoring rules for the CAPS. All demonstrated good to excellent reliability and correspondence with PTSD diagnosis and SCID ratings. However, some rules were better suited for screening and others, for diagnosis. The standard "1-2" rule of frequency and intensity appear adequate for older victims (Hovens, et al., 1994; Summers, Hyer, & Boyd, 1993).

There are several advantages of this instrument. A victim can meet criteria for the current PTSD or have symptoms below the threshold (partial PTSD). Subclinical or past designations are interesting and probably distinct clinical states. No one knows fully what they mean, only that they can be prevalent in Vietnam trauma victims (Kulka et al., 1990). Perhaps, as we change criteria or levels of criteria in the DSM, the partial categories will provide increasing clinical information. Additionally, the CAPS-1 is one procedure that provides a measure of stress-related symptom clusters that can be evaluated against the "broader domain" of the person, personality, and other symptom disorders.

In a sample at a VA Medical Center, of 200+ treatment-seeking combat veterans, 39% had a full PTSD and 61% had a no PTSD based on the CAPS-1. These were veterans who had no psychosis or organic mental disorders and were largely from medical clinics. Out of the 200+ cases, only 9 are misclassified using the SCID as the base measure (92.8% efficiency). Strikingly, half of these veterans have two or more avoidant or hyperarousal symptoms some 50 years later, and $\frac{2}{3}$ have at least one arousal symptom. Most of these men had never used a psychiatric clinic.

A forward logistic regression equation was performed using the 17 CAPS items as predictors and the SCID–PTSD diagnosis as the criterion. This analysis shows the best set of variables with this population. Five variables with a overall hit rate of 91% resulted (Box 12-2). These are given in Box 12-2. These 5 CAPS-1 items had an overall hit rate of 91%.

This analysis (subject to cross validation) suggested that a full PTSD diagnosis would result among older combat veterans if these five items were rated as symptoms. Additionally, according to the criteria of Blake et al. above, the CAPS-1 rated an "A", fully satisfying the standard in each area. Increasingly it is being administered by trained paraprofessional. Weathers, Ruscio, and Keane (1997) have now identified nine

---

Box 12-2
Most Efficient CAPS-1 Variables

B-3 (Feeling/acting as if the trauma were occurring)
C-2 (Avoidance of activities)
C-6 (Restricted affect)
D-1 (Sleep problems)
D-4 (Hypervigilance)

scoring rules for use with the CAPS. It should be noted that the CAPS-1 does have other shortcomings. It does not carefully inventory Criterion A (i. e., the stressor). It takes at least 45 minutes and the frequency and intensity scheme for each item introduces a self-report scale.

Self-Report PTSD Measures

Self-report scales of PTSD have been many and varied. For the most part, these measures have bypassed Criterion A and assessed symptoms. Typically they involve alternative strategies to assess symptoms of PTSD. As with the interviewer scales, there are several that are attached to the current DSM, although few have been used with an older population. Not surprisingly, investigators often cite criticisms of the self-report method, such as selection of events (Brown, 1990; Costa & McCrae, 1990), or social desirability of responses (see Carlson, 1997). Others argue that self-report confounds the stressor with the outcome of stress (Costa & McCrae, 1990; Krohne, 1990; Wagner, 1990; Watson & Clark, 1984). This is a biased look at important measures and only suggests that these measures should never be the sole method used.

Hyer et al. (1994) evaluated 114 elderly combat veterans of World War II and Korea on PTSD measures developed for use with Vietnam veterans. Criterion measures of PTSD were interviewer-rated scales that were independently corroborated. The self-report scales included the Mississippi Scale for Combat-Related PTSD, the MMPI-PK subscale (MMPI-2), the Impact of Event Scale (IES), and the PTSD Scale from the Symptom Checklist 90–Revised. As hypothesized, these PTSD measures discriminated between veterans with and without PTSD (full and no PTSD) with lower cutoff scores than applicable on other age groups. Correct classification ratios were also presented for each scale and were all above .90. These proved to be very good tests with this population.

An alternative strategy is to derive PTSD subscales from larger symptom inventories, such as the MMPI, MCMI, and the SCL-90. The first two of these have the distinct advantage of providing data on response styles, the importance of which cannot be overemphasized. The MCMI-III–R (PTSD) scale, consisting of 16 items and assessing symptoms of anxious arousal and avoidance associated with the trauma, has been used with older victims with success (Hyer & Boyd, 1996). In a sample of older outpatient combat veterans who were treatment-seeking in medical and psychiatric clinics, Hyer and Boyd confirmed that two personality styles (identified in other research as potentially reflective of PTSD) contributed to the problems of PTSD beyond those variables normally associated with the stressor combat and aging. These were the avoidant and passive-aggressive styles.

Finally, an important step in PTSD assessment involves identifying the purpose of the PTSD instrument being used along with the population for which it is most appropriate. Several scales, like the SCL-90–R (Saunders et al., 1990) are able to differentiate crime victims with or without PTSD, but not chronic PTSD. Also there are strategies to develop measures that are tailored to the other experiences and culturally relative outcomes of specific trauma populations, such as refugees (Norris & Raid, 1997). Careful assessment of a target population is necessary, as nuances with a given population are qualitative and subtle and require testing.

Clinical Recommendation   Most PTSD self-report scales are similar. Two scales often used are the PTSD Symptom Scale (PSS; Foa et al., 1993) and the Modified PTSD

Symptom Scale (MPSS-SR; Falsetti, Resick, Resnick, & Kilpatrick, 1991). Both are carbon copies of the DSM criteria and reliable. We recommend either of these.

Our preferred self-report battery, however, includes the IES, the Civilian Mississippi Scale for PTSD or the National Center for PTSD Checklist-M (PCL-M; Figure 12-2). The first measure is different from the other two and provides good convergent validation. The IES is now universally used in batteries and assesses intrusions and avoidance. Norms are available.

The other two assess the severity and frequency of the 17 PTSD symptoms. Each is designed to evaluate symptoms over the recent past and can be used for any stressor. It can be scored as dichotomous (positive or negative for PTSD) or continuous. The Mississippi scales have been evaluated extensively, including older victims. The Civilian Mississippi Scale (CMS) was developed by Keane and colleagues (Norris & Perilla, 1996). The participant is asked to think about the past event and to react in re-experiencing and situational avoidance, withdrawal and numbing, arousal, and guilt and suicide areas. There are no subscales and the items have five response choices that vary. It was used successfully in the National Vietnam Veterans Readjustment Study. The Revised Mississippi Scale was improved on by Norris and Perilla (1996). It consists of items from the original CMS and the TSS. It is anchored to an undefined trauma event.

Finally, we recommend the MCMI-III as it provides a validated measure of PTSD (intensity of) and yields other information on comorbidity, response style, and of course personality.

As a whole, we recommend the use of a semi-structured interview (the CAPS-1), the assessment of relevant history and comorbid disorders, and the MCMI-III. In general, a high score on many of these scales (high positive predictive power) is often most helpful clinically, as it in effect rules in PTSD problems, if not a diagnosis of PTSD.

Neuropsychological Assessment of Trauma

The clinical presentation of an older person with PTSD can be straightforward, conceptualized from a trauma perspective, or have several clinical symptoms that can be explained from a neuropsychological perspective. "Organic" factors, therefore, might produce mood and panic problems as well as other symptoms. It is not unusual that an older trauma victim might have a DSM-IV profile that includes multiple Axis I diagnoses, such as major depression, PTSD, and perhaps a few other anxiety disorders. An Axis II personality disorder may also be present. They also produce their own problems related to cognitive problems.

There are several reviews on the assessment of older people on the neuropsychology of the dementias (Albert & Moss, 1988; La Rue, 1992, 1995; Lezak, 1995; Puente & McCaffrey, 1992; Spreen & Strauss, 1991; Storandt & VandenBos, 1994), as well as the importance of assessment with older folks in general (Cummings & Benson, 1992; Katzman & Rowe, 1992; Segal, Coolidge, & Hensen, 1999). This now applies to the oldest-old (those older than 85; Ivnik et al., 1992a, 1992b, 1992c; Maclec, Invik, & Smith, 1993; Van Gorp, Satz, Kiersch, & Henry, 1986). The import of these is that this area needs consideration at later life especially with something like a trauma.

Regarding trauma, let us say that PTSD may be exacerbated by several neurological conditions (Knight, 1997). These included traumatic head injury, neurotoxic exposure, hypoxic/anoxic episodes, pre-existing PTSD exacerbated by the onset of a neurological condition, neurological factors increasing the risk for experiencing trauma and developing PTSD, neuropsychological effects of substance abuse (especially alcoholism

The National Center for PTSD's self-report questionnaire (sample below) can assist providers in thoroughly assessing PTSD.

PCL-M Instructions: Below is a list of problems that veterans sometimes have in response to stressful military experiences. Please read each one carefully, then circle one of the numbers to the right to indicate how much you have been bothered by that problem *in the past month*.

	Not at all	A little bit	Moder- ately	Quite a bit	Extremely
1. Repeated, disturbing *memories, thoughts,* or *images* of a stressful military experience?	1	2	3	4	5
2. Repeated disturbing *dreams* of a stressful military experience?	1	2	3	4	5
3. Suddenly *acting* or *feeling* as if a stressful military experience *were happening* again (as if you were reliving it)?	1	2	3	4	5
4. Feeling *very upset* when *something reminded you* of a stressful military experience?	1	2	3	4	5
5. Having *physical reactions* (e.g., heart pounding, trouble breathing, sweating) when *something reminded you* of a stressful military experience?	1	2	3	4	5
6. Avoiding *thinking about* or *talking about* a stressful military experience or avoiding *having feelings* related to it?	1	2	3	4	5
7. Avoiding *activities* or *situations* because *they reminded you* of a stressful military experience?	1	2	3	4	5
8. Trouble *remembering important parts* of a stressful military experience?	1	2	3	4	5
9. *Loss of interest* in activities that you used to enjoy?	1	2	3	4	5
10. Feelings *distant* or *cut off* from other people?	1	2	3	4	5
11. Feeling *emotionally numb* or being unable to have loving feelings for those close to you?	1	2	3	4	5
12. Feeling as if your *future* will somehow be *cut short*?	1	2	3	4	5
13. Trouble *falling* or *staying asleep*?	1	2	3	4	5
14. Feeling *irritable* or having *angry outbursts*?	1	2	3	4	5
15. Having *difficulty concentrating*?	1	2	3	4	5
16. Being "*super-alert*" or watchful or on guard?	1	2	3	4	5
17. Feeling *jumpy* or easily startled?	1	2	3	4	5

Weathers, Litz, Huska, & Keane, National Center for PTSD.

FIGURE 12-2. PTSD Checklist

and stimulant abuse), and multiple comorbidity. Additionally, problems due to recent sleep quality and sleep patterns; residual effects of peripheral physical damage, as a result of the traumatic experience (motor vehicle accidents, damage from explosions etc.); medication and psychoactive substance abuse; the role of compensation, litigation and secondary gain; and evaluating attentional problems are present.

With older persons especially, a pre-existing PTSD that is exacerbated by the onset of a neurological condition may be a special problem. Exacerbation may result from the added effects of neurological conditions to the existing trauma symptoms, direct triggering of trauma content, or indirectly as a threat to health. Also, any health problem may diminish the patient's capabilities for suppressing negatively balanced memories and affect.

Recommendation   In general, clinicians should always be concerned about classic neuropsychological symptoms: rapid forgetting, verbal intrusions, low verbal fluency, anomia, attention or concentration problems, and executive functions. These may be especially at risk with trauma victims especially ones with a chronic history. Interestingly for the older victim, Knight (1997) also noted: "Although various studies detected these problems, as a group the studies reviewed did not consistently find impairments in these domains" (p. 455).

Unfortunately, there is little that is specific to the problems of trauma. Although van der Kolk (see Knight, 1997) and others argued for specific parts of the brain sensitive to the effects of trauma (increased anterior cingulate and decreased hippocampus and Broca's area, for example), these are not evident on many victims. There is no PTSD profile. Pointedly, the tasks of the clinician for issues of trauma of an older person are ones specific to the trauma itself, possible cognitive or neuropsychological sequelae, and other issues that are more troublesome at later life, social support, coping, and physical health.

The assessment of older folks with possible neurological problems is still an art/science. Even with MRI, fMRI, SPECT, PET, or CAT scans, the importance of a neuropsychological is highlighted. These scans are not isomorphic to behavior and there is less than perfect validation. The rule of common sense applies: Be suspect, measure, monitor (over time), resist premature (and seductive) closure, and treat the person. The context of the trauma deserves this respect.

Significant Others

There are two issues here. First, a collateral informant regarding the older person's PTSD symptoms almost always is helpful. In fact, if the person has one, the clinician is strongly advised to interview this person, alone or with the patient, or both. This provides information that cannot be obtained via self-reports, tests, or diagnostic interview procedures. The clinician can do this formally as in the use of a collateral measure (e.g., Significant Other NEO-PI-NP) or more informally with this person, often a spouse.

The second involves our old friend, social support. This is a multidimensional construct that has been defined as the comfort, assistance, and information received through formal or informal contacts with others. Interest in this construct has permeated both the aging and the PTSD literature. Results of several studies of victims have shown that social support plays a major role in the etiology, development, and maintenance of PTSD. Largely positive influences have been found in three areas of trauma: combat, sexual assault, and battering. There appears to be a consistent negative correlation between post-military adjustment, for example, and PTSD symptomatology (see Hyer et al., 1994).

In general, the more vulnerable the person, the greater the positive impact of helpful social input. Recently, the effect of social support on trauma victims is now better understood as regards the nature of the social interactions, along with the mediating or buffering effects on stress, the associated influence of support on human physiology, and the importance of social support in trauma and recovery.

Recommendation   In regard to the significant other, the clinician is advised to interview this person. We do recommend one scale that has been helpful. This is the PACL (Personality Adjective Checklist; Strack, 1990). This can be performed in five minutes and the person receives a printout on the coping styles of the person. This is often a most helpful insight and understanding into extant patterns of behavior.

Measures of social support are plentiful. The Social Adjustment Scale (SAS; Weissman & Prusoff, 1978) assesses functioning in the major role areas in the 2 weeks prior to evaluation. Subscale scores can be obtained on work, social and leisure, extended family, marital, parental, family unit, and economic. Additionally Proscidano and Heller's (1983) Social Support from Friends (PSS-fr) and Family (PSS-fa) (58) has been used with older victims to good ends.

☐ Psychophysiology

We also recommend one other measure, psychophysiological responses, when possible. It is virtually universal that a trauma victim is reactive to their trauma script. Using an older combat sample we (Hyer & Summers, 1997) noted that, if a veteran had greater than one PTSD problem and said that he had a hard time talking about this, the chances of high physiological arousal and high scores on self-report scales were quite good. Davidson noted that many stress victims often deny that stress is a problem for them but have left frontal lobe activation (motivation-enhancing section of the brain). This is hardly a stress free person, as it takes work to tame or inhibit negative feelings and maintain positive ones. This "upbeat denial" may occur in many older veterans.

Recommendation   A trauma reaction is discernable on physiological measures. This especially applies to heart rate. The simple use of a portable heart monitor may be of use.

☐ Measures of Comorbid Issues

Because other chapters addressed the aging-related issues, we briefly consider only their measurement here.

Depression

As we indicated, depression appears omnipresent with trauma at later life. Its nature, severity, and duration should be assessed. Several depression scales are used routinely with this population. The Beck Depression Inventory (BDI; 21 items) has been found to adequately assess depression and have acceptable reliability and validity with older adults (Rapp et al., 1988). Even shorter versions are used (see Dozers, Dobron, & Ahnberg, 1998). The Geriatric Depression Scale (GDS) is a 30-item scale assessing the psychological features of depression, de-emphasizing the somatic symptoms of depression. Caution is warranted in assessing victims with cognitive problems (Kosniak, 1996).

The Hamilton Rating Scale for Depression (HRSD) has 17- and 21-item versions, with symptoms rated as to severity. These are clinician-rated scales. This has been used successfully with older populations. Adequate guidelines for using the HRSD have been developed (Williams, 1988).

We note one other scale that shows promise. Jaminson and Scogin (1992) developed the Geriatric Depression Rating Scale (GDRS) to combine the format of the HRSD for severity rating purposes with the content of the GDS, thus de-emphasizing somatic items that can be problematic. The GDRS has 35 items, with 6 added to conform to the RDC for major depression. This scale appears to have acceptable psychometric properties (Jamison & Scogin, 1992).

There are three obvious problems here. First, inventories are not particularly well-suited to identifying dysthymic disorder or for capturing a lifetime history of depressive disorder. This is best done via the interview. However, the more symptoms, the greater the assurance of the depression/anxiety. Second, it may be best to be aware of the differential diagnostic items that are on the border of depression and neuropsychological problems. These two issues cause more problems in the treatment of older people than any other disorders.

Thirdly, the somatic influence of an illness is tightly pressed against both depression and PTSD. It may well be that having PTSD or depression mediates health behaviors on the way to an illness (Green, Epstein, Krupnick, & Rowland, 1997). Older people with PTSD or depression do not practice healthy behaviors and thereby are at risk. Box 12-3 provides questions relating to physical illness in the consideration of depression.

Recommendation   We recommend using a self-report instrument, such as the BDI or the GDS, with a cutoff score set low to maximize sensitivity. Few false negatives will occur, and false positives can be identified. The administration of a depression "screener" should be followed by a diagnostic or clinical interview. A semi-structured DSM-IV set of questions for establishing major depression, dysthymic disorder, depressive disorder not otherwise specified, and adjustment disorder with depressed features is recommended.

Coping

Theories of coping have emphasized its multidimensional aspects, focusing on two aspects particularly, the focus (problem- or emotion-focused) and the method (cognitive or behavioral) of coping. We can understand much of the process of PTSD and its problems through this traditional way of viewing coping. Adaptation is facilitated by the use of more active coping resources (Moos, 1993). In general, the type, severity, and appraisal of stressors influence coping responses. PTSD participants who experience more negative life events in the past year, for example, react with a coping response pattern of both approach and avoidant styles, or simply use avoidant coping. In fact, the reliance on more avoidant coping (especially emotional discharge) and less on problem solving is almost a universal finding with depression and PTSD groups (Fondacaro & Moos, 1990).

Box 12-3
Questions Pertaining to Physical Illness and Depression

1. How do you disentangle depression from symptoms of illness?
2. When does depression occur relative to an illness, when does it appear?
3. In what diseases is depression likely to reoccur (as in COPD) over the life of the disorder)?
4. When is depression ecologically based in a biological illness and when reactive? (Parkinson's Disease depression occurs in right hemisphere problem patients and more with the onset of motor symptoms than with ADL problems.)
5. When is a depressive symptom a depression symptom? In cancer this is a problem. Anorexia, for instance, is a symptom in mastectomy but not necessarily in liver cancer.
6. Is there a difference between older age complaints and life problems and subclinical depression? Should the clinician treat this subclinical state?
7. Is there a psychological depression, neurological depression, and remote depression at later life?

Less is known about the connection between the coping of the (potential) victim during the actual stressor and any eventual trauma response. After the stressor, however, it appears that this construct has something to offer and applies especially to older people, if not victims. Several studies (e.g., Fairbank, Hansen, & Fittenberg, 1991) have documented that PTSD victims use poorer coping techniques for managing trauma memories than for other stressors. Poor coping pervades trauma situations: excessive self or other blame, avoidance strategies of all kinds, substance abuse, cynicism and excessive pessimism, and prolonged social isolation among others (Hobfoll et al., 1991).

Effective coping methods are worth knowing about clinically: breaking down problems into manageable parts, setting small goals, rewarding self for small wins, actively helping others, being active and consistent in requesting help, balancing both intimate and social support, applying distinctive coping strategies where appropriate (e.g., emotion focused vs. problem-focused), among others.

Coping may indeed be a marker variable: It interacts with just about every variable that we have addressed. More educated, higher income, and more self-confident people, for example, use problem-solving coping when confronted with a stressor. In fact, like aging, it is a carrier variable: It carries other variables.

Susan Folkman (2000) has studied coping among AIDS caregiving. Her issue of greatest concern is: How do people under such conditions remain sane? By means of coping measures she was able to identify several coping mechanisms of positive reappraisal, problem-focused coping, and obtaining positive meaning in normal events.

Recommendation   Coping is situated in the psychological space of variables such that it provides much information on the patterns of interaction. It is less permanent than personality (and thereby less dispositional) but clearly reflective of the person(ality) as well as the situation. Coping then lies in the borderland between personality trait and the situation. When one measures personality, in part one is also measuring coping.

A coping profile can assist in the examination of the connection of appraisal and coping resources, the variation in coping associated with the type of stressful event, and the way in which new and ongoing stressors may alter an individual's coping responses. It can also identify the risk and resistance factors involved in the process of remission and relapse of psychiatric disorders (Moos, 1993). Box 12-4 presents the usual coping profile of a PTSD victim based on the Coping Strategy Indicator (Moos, 1993). Use of a measure like the Moos is recommended.

Health Status

Health status among the elderly is the number one contributor to the quality of life. In fact, it has been argued that no study should evaluate the many components of "living" with a later life sample without addressing health. Health status has also been found to be an important variable for younger veterans, following exposure to combat-related trauma (Green et al., 1997). At one VA Medical Center, participants in various studies averaged just under 4 chronic medical problems and 6.1 medications. Older veterans with current full PTSD have more chronic medical problems and require more medications than other groups.

One other aspect of health status involves a somatic focus. A major channel for the expression of emotional problems is through the body. In fact, this is modal. It is estimated that 20–84% of patients presenting to primary care physicians report symptoms for which no significant organic pathology can be attributed (American Association of Geropsychiatry, 1996). Perhaps one reason for this involves the lack of clarity of somatoform problems (disorders) and confusion around the interplay of medical and psychological problems. In fact, so much controversy exists that somatoform diagnoses are rarely used (Escobar et al., 1998).

Box 12-4
Typical (Poor) Coping Response Inventory Pattern

Approach-coping responses:
1. Low logical analysis: not understand and prepare for stressor.
2. Low positive reappraisal: not positively restructure problem.
3. Medium seeking guidance and support: does not seek information and support.
4. Low problem-solving: no action to deal with stressor.

Avoidance-coping responses:
5. High cognitive avoidance: avoid thinking realistically about problem.
6. Medium acceptance or resignation: does not react to problem by acceptance.
7. Low alternative reward seeking: not involved with other activities.
8. High emotional discharge: does not reduce tension by expressing negative feelings.

Nonetheless it is not uncommon for physical illnesses to increase the occurrence of emotional problems and vice versa. Ford (1995) reviewed medical use patterns and noted that a sizable percentage of patients who have psychiatric distress seek medical care under the guise of a physical symptom. It is estimated that the incidence of severe medical problems is over 50% and the contribution to these states is substantial, even more in the elderly.

The problem with health status is not that clinicians are not alert. Rather there are too many problems with its measurement. How do you ask a person these issues, what do you measure in a person, what organ system(s), how many times, at what cost, and so on. That said, a scale that measures a spectrum of health-related behaviors, quality-of-life indicators, and medical history (Health Risk Appraisal, 1988) may be appropriate. Yet these too naturally leave something to be desired, not the least of which is time.

Recommendation   Any older patient should receive an assessment from the primary care physician. This always provides a wealth of information. This is the objective side of things. We also recommend a health perception by a question that has been used in the literature with considerable success: For your age would you say that your health is (1 = *bad*, 2 = *poor*, 3 = *fair*, 4 = *good*, 5 = *excellent*?). When in doubt, an ADL scale may be considered (as these are significantly related to health) or a significant other can be interviewed. Other scales have been developed that tap into the issue of daily behaviors, likes, and dislikes (see Spreen & Strauss, 1998). Although this is not an ADL scale, they are most helpful and are highly correlated with depression and other aging disorders.

Various scales measure different features of the somatoform problems. We do not recommend any one, but we do recommend a sensitivity to this issue. In addition, we recommend the SCL-90-R, MMPI-2, MCMI-II or III , or the Personality Assessment Inventory (PAI; Morey, 1996), personality scales with somatic scales that also provide a context for the assessment of the person. These have merit also because of response styles scales.

Additionally, the Structured Diagnostic Interview for the DSM-IV (SCID) should be considered. This has been shown to be reliable and to have discriminant validity (see Spreen & Strauss, 1998). Of interest too, Escobar et al. (1998) used an abbreviated somatization index, based on specific symptom thresholds. This abridged somatization was most usable and predicted unexplained symptoms and subsequent disability and psychopathology.

Finally, the clinician should think factors. This is done in the context of PTSD. One grouping is especially relevant as it reflects a cognitive and behavioral approach: catastrophizing cognitions, intolerance of bodily complaints, bodily weakness, autonomic sensations, and health habits. In treatment, the clinician needs to perform a microanalysis on the cognitive and behavioral targets of somatic problems.

Dissociation

Dissociation, the non-disorder problem, deserves special mention also. Dissociative experiences are perhaps best conceptualized as reflecting a generalized hyperarousal of PTSD, involving both cognitive and affective states. Additionally, the phenomenon of dissociation probably leads to the symptoms of PTSD (i.e., flashbacks, nightmares, and the like may really be dissociative experiences, and denial, avoidance, and the like are attempts to avoid these; Marmar, Weiss, & Metzer, 1997). A flashback, therefore, may very well be a result of this poor processing of trauma as it potentiates avoidance and numbing responses for purposes of sanctuary. Also, dissociative experiences are part of the experience of Acute Stress Disorder.

Briere (1997) described *dissociation* as a continuum of coping mechanisms that ranges from simple to more complex patterns of behavior. These mechanisms include (a) disengagement, which involves "cognitive separation," "time out" from, or "spacing out" in response to an abusive environment; (b) detachment or numbing, or the removal of oneself from emotions to distance oneself from the full impact of pain; (c) observation, which entails avoiding the full impact of stress by watching personal events as if one is outside the self; (d) amnesia, or unconsciously avoiding awareness by banishing information from awareness; and (e) multiple personality disorder, which involves the creation of two or more distinct personalities as "a protective shield from complete awareness and thus from the posttraumatic pain that otherwise would follow" (Brier, 1992). The first three categories (a–c) represent features of depersonalization disorder, the fourth mechanism (d) is labeled *dissociative amnesia*, and the fifth category (e) is now labeled *dissociative identity disorder* (DSM-IV, 1994).

In general, victims who frequently have dissociative experiences score in a more pathological direction on a variety of measures, including level of PTSD intrusions, flashbacks, sleep problems, and nightmares, as well as many basic personality scores and depression scales (Hyer, Albrecht, Boudewyns, Woods, & Brandsma, 1993). When these symptoms occur, the victim requires special treatment—at the least an awareness of this condition, anchors or bridges between the "now" and "then," some ability to use a safe place, ability to read stress triggers, and a supportive environment that "permits" this symptom to run its course. The goal is to be able to access trauma memories so they are under the control of the victim.

Dissociative phenomena are then annoyingly and pervasively a part of the chronic PTSD experience. Who gets these, with what other symptoms, and what they portend for treatment, have unknown answers. This lack of definitive knowledge is a grim reminder that PTSD may be something else.

Probably older trauma victims have fewer intrusion symptoms than younger ones. But there are virtually no scientific data on dissociation, except that it is a feature of Acute Stress Disorder and sometimes seen with older victims. This symptom is, however, so insidious as to warrant special consideration.

Recommendation   No scales exist for this measure in older victims. Despite this, we recommend one interviewer-rated scale and two self-report scales. First, the SCID-D (Sternberg, 1997) (Box 12-5) was developed to assess dissociative disorders. It has more than 250 items, many of which are open-ended. It evaluates five core dissociative symptoms: amnesia, depersonalization, derealization, identity confusion, and identity alteration. Ratings are based on symptom frequency, duration, distress, and level of impairment or dysfunction. This scale provides diagnoses for the DSM-IV dissociative disorders.

Two (largely) self-report scales are used. The first is the Dissociative Experiences Scale (DES). This is an analogue measure of dissociative experiences that is used more than any other scale. It has been factored now on several occasions with depersonalization, absorption, and amnesia as factors. Second, the Peritraumatic Dissociative Experiences Questionnaire (Marmar, Weiss, Metzler, & Delucchi, 1996) is a report of this experience during the trauma. This is considered a risk factor for later PTSD. Actually there are various versions of this, in both self-report and interviewer format.

Box 12-5
Key Questions on SCID-D

1. Amnesia
   Have you found yourself in a strange place and had no explanation?
   Do you lose sense of time for long periods?
   Have you forgotten basic facts about yourself?
2. Depersonalization
   Have you ever felt you were able to observe yourself from a point outside your body?
   Have you ever felt like a stranger to yourself?
   Have you ever had the feeling that your body was disconnected from yourself?
   Have you ever felt as though you were two different people with one part observing the other?
3. Derealization
   Has there ever been a time when familiar people/places seemed unfamiliar or unreal?
   Has there been a time when you were unable to recognize close friends, relatives, or your own home?
   Have you ever felt puzzled as to what is real and what is unreal in your surroundings?
4. Identity confusion
   Have you ever felt as if there were a struggle going on inside you as to who you really are?
   How you ever felt confused about who you are?
5. Identity alteration
   Have you ever been told by others that you seem like a different person?
   Have you ever referred to yourself by different names?
   Have you ever found things that obviously belonged to you, that you do not remember buying or bringing home?
   Are there any inner dialogues with yourself?

Therapy

Therapy in the 21st century requires some form of measurement. There are many issues of measurement that apply here. Our effort, however, is based on simplicity and minimally adequate psychometrics, reliability, and concurrent validity.

There are several reliable and valid measures that evaluate therapy. These include the Basis-32, OQ-45, among others (see Dornelas et al., 1996). The point is that these measures can provide a way to discern the efficacy of efforts and whether one should switch tactics. At our outpatient clinics (University of Medicine and Dentistry in New Jersey), we use the Basis-32 and are able to isolate the patient that is at risk for non-compliance, for resistance to change, and for added treatment effort. This effort on the part of the therapist is important and opens the door for efficacy and a lot more, including satisfaction, transference reactions, and compliance.

Box 12-6
Rating Psychotherapy

7	6	5	4	3	2	1
Much Better		**Good**	**The Same**	**Poorer**	**Much Worse**	

PTSD Symptoms:

Re-experiencing: _____

Avoidance: _____

Arousal: _____

Overall Problems:

Anxiety: _____

Depression: _____

Anger: _____

Outlook:

Feel happy: _____

Sense of control: _____

Overall:

Health: _____

Pain: _____

Sleep: _____

Appetite: _____

Relationships in general:

Affection and caring: _____

Intimacy and closeness: _____

Support from others: _____

Personal effort for therapy:

Energy (for exercises) after the therapy: _____

Use therapy ideas in week: _____

Therapy itself:

Trust the therapist: _____

Felt understood: _____

Recommendation Pragmatic assessment of outcomes should assess the overall treatment as well as the session-by-session treatment based on patient variables (Is there change?), and therapist variables (Is the therapist liked and delivering the correct strategy?). As noted, we use the Basis-32 on the first and every fifth session, as well as at termination (Box 12-7). This provides us with a "care trajectory" that is relevant for the efficacy of treatment.

Session-by-session evaluation involves something different. The client becomes like an operator online and establishes a "continual process improvement." The monitoring can act as a model to reduce excess and define an optimal balance for the issue at hand. David Burns (1999) says that any such scales are required to be comfortable for the patient, convenient for the therapist, and show basic reliability. We provide measures of PTSD (DSM-IV categories) symptoms, including anger, outlook, health, relationship, self-effort, and the therapeutic alliance. This is a self-report scale (Box 12-6). All items are rated on a 7-point scale. We find that these areas subserve many others that are related to care, such as anxiety and the relationship. The entire effort takes 2 minutes and is done between sessions.

Importantly, the therapist has immediate feedback on the course of treatment. We find that this feedback can be beneficial for both as it is used at the beginning of each session for an understanding of the course of treatment. It is now clear also that

---

Box 12-7
Recommended Core Assessment Battery

Criteria A
  Verbal Reception
  MAPS
Screen
  IES
  PCL-M
Personality Measure
  MCMI-III
Structural Interview
  CAPS-I
Neuropsychological Evaluation
  MMSE
Necessary Other
  GDS
  DES
"Nice" Other
  Physiological Indicies
    Especially Heartbeat
  Significant Other (PACL)
Therapy
  Basis 32
Psychotherapy Rating
  Box 12-6

compliance with homework, outside the therapy work, makes an independent and significant contribution to change in therapy (Burns & Spangler, 1988).

Finally, we are not adverse to having the patient experiment with monitoring. The patient can be given a golf counter and count the number of intrusions or avoidance behaviors. Additionally, we liberally apply self-report measures (as well as a standard fare of readings). We want the patient to monitor and in so doing this becomes an intervention itself (an experiment). As noted in a previous chapter, we also apply a "survival guide" roughly half way through the session for the progress made and coping needed.

☐ Conclusion

Perhaps the key to assessment is that the clinician is not assessing symptoms, but a person that has symptoms. The pivotal role of the case history in geriatric mental health assessment has been professed: "Biography can be as important as biology." We are evaluating people.

Psychological assessment, as traditionally used, has received little support in the emerging managed health care environments. Psychologists report devoting 14% of their time or less to these activities (Watkins, 1991). Largely assessment has been criticized for its conceptual confusion and inappropriate psychometric criteria (Hayes, Nelson, & Jarrett, 1987), and is considered to be one of the more expendable aspects of health care (Moreland, Fowler, & Honaker, 1994). It is paradoxical that, when given the choice, clinicians would rather rely on their unsubstantiated clinical judgments than on a formal "test."

If nothing else, the measure of PTSD is straightforward. A person has a trauma, the DSM components of PTSD are applied, as well as its ancillary issues, intensity, and the existence of the several constructs noted here—but this is never enough. The person is complex, so the clinician mixes and matches the empirically validated measures of the disorder with the empirically validated treatment components of trauma. The matches are never fully met or even discovered. It will no doubt be this way for some time.

In this chapter we have provided a temporary sanctuary for understanding.

REFERENCES

Aaron, H. (1996). End of an era. *The Brooklings Review, 14*(1), 335–37.

Aarts, P. G., & Op den Velde, W. (1996). Prior traumatization and the process of aging: Theory and clinical implication. In B. A. van der Kolk, A. C. McFarlane, & L. Weisaeth (Eds.), *Traumatic Stress: The effects of overwhelming experience on mind, body, and society* (pp. 155–181). New York: The Guilford Press.

Abeles, N. A. (1997). *What practitioners should know about working with older adults.* Washington: American Psychological Association.

Abrams, R. C., & Horowitz, S. V. (1996). Personality disorders after age 50: A meta-analysis. *Journal of Personality Disorders, 10*(3), 271–281.

Abrams, R. C., & Horowitz, S. V. (1999). Personality disorders after age 50: A meta-analytic review of the literature. In E. Rosowsky, R. C. Abrams, & R. A. Zweig, *Personality disorders in older adults: Emerging issues in diagnosis and treatment* (pp. 55–68). Mahwah, NJ: Lawrence Erlbaum Associates.

Abrams, R. C., Alexopoulos, G. S., & Young, R. C. (1987). Geriatric depression and DSM-III-R personality disorder criteria. *Journal of the American Geriatric Society, 35,* 383–386.

Abrams, R. C., Horowitz, S. V., & Alexopoulos, G. S. (1995). *Personality and quality of life in old depressives.* New Research Abstracts presented at the annual meeting of the American Psychiatric Association, Miami, FL.

Abrams, R. C., Rosendahl, E., Card, C., & Alexopoulos, G. S. (1994). Personality disorder correlates of late and early onset depression. *Journal of American Geriatric Society, 42,* 1–5.

Abrams, R. C., Spielman, L. A., Alexopoulos, G. S., & Klausner, E. (1998). Personality disorder symptoms and functioning in elderly depressed patients. *American Journal of Geriatric Psychiatry, 6*(1), 24–30.

Abramson, L. Y., Metalsky, G. I., & Alloy, L. B. (1989). Hopelessness depression: A theory-based subtype of depression. *Psychological Bulletin, 96,* 358–372.

Abramson, L., Seligman, M., & Teasdale, J. (1978). Learned helplessness in humans: critique and reformulation. *Journal of Abnormal Psychology, 87,* 49–74.

Acierno, R., Hersen, M., Van Hasselt, V. B., Tremont, G., & Meuser, K. T. (1994). Review of the validation and dissemination of Eye-movement Desensitization and Reprocessing: A scientific and ethical dilemma. *Clinical Psychology Review, 14*(4), 287–299.

Adams, J. (1984). Reminiscence in the geriatric ward: An undervalued resource. *Oral history, 12*(2), 54–9.

Adams-Westcott, J., Dafforn, T., & Sterne, P. (1993). Escaping victim life stories and co-constructing personal agency. In S. Gilligan & R. Price (Eds.), *Therapeutic conversations* (pp. 258–271). New York: Norton.

Adler, A. (1927). *Understanding human nature.* Garden City, NY: Doubleday Anchor.

Affleck, G., Tennen, H., & Gershman, K. (1985). Cognitive adaptations to high-risk infants: The search for mastery, meaning, and protection from future harm. *American Journal of Mental Deficiency, 89,* 653–656.

Agronin, M. E. *Personality disorders in the elderly: An overview.*

Albert, M. S., & Moss, M. B. (Eds.) (1988). *Geriatric neuropsychology.* New York: Guilford Press.

Aldwin, C. M. (1993). Coping with traumatic stress. *PTSD Research Quarterly, 4*(3).

Aldwin, C. (1990). Change and stability in mental health over the life-span (abstract). *The Gerontologist, 30,* 333A–334A.

Aldwin, C. M. (19??). The role of stress in aging and adult development. *The Cutting Edge,* pg. 3.

Aldwin, C. M. (1992). Aging, coping and efficacy: Theoretical framework for coping in lifespan development context. In Wykle, M. L., Kahana, E., & Kowal, J. (Eds.), *Stress and Health Among the Elderly* (pp. 96–113). New York: Springer.

Aldwin, C. M., Levenson, M. R., & Spiro, A. III (1994). Vulnerability and resilience to combat exposure: Can stress have lifelong effects? *Psychology and Aging, 9,* 34–44.

Aldwin, C. M., Levenson, M. R., Spiro, A., & Bosse, R. (1989). Does emotionality predict stress? Findings from the Normative Aging Study. *Journal of Personality of Social Psychology, 56,* 618–624.

Aldwin, C. A., & Stokols, D. (1988). The effects of environmental change on individuals and groups: Some neglected issues in stress research. *Journal of Environmental Psychology, 8:*67–75.

Alexander, F., & French, T. M. (1947). *Psychoanalytic therapy: Principles and applications.* Ronald Press. NOTE: BOOK CHAPTER LISTS 1946 WHILE REFERENCE AT END LISTS 1947.

American Psychiatric Association (1994). *Diagnostic and statistical manual of mental disorders (4th ed. revised).* Washington, DC.

Amen, D. A. (1998). *Change your brain, change your life.* New York: Times Books.

Diagnosis and treatment of late-life depression: Making a difference. Monograph by ???. American Association for Geriatric Psychiatry (1996).

Ames, A., & Molinari, V. (1994). Prevalence of personality disorders in community living elderly. *Journal of Geriatric Psychiatry and Neurology, 7,* 189–194.

Anderson, H. (1990). Then and now: A journey from "knowing" to "not knowing." *Contemporary Family Therapy, 12*(3), 193–197.

Anderson, H., & Goolishian, H. (1988). Human systems as linguistic systems: Preliminary and evolving ideas about the implications for clinical theory. *Family Process, 27,* 371–393.

Anderson, H., & Goolishian, H. (1990a). Beyond cybernetics: Comments on Atkinson and Heath's "Further thoughts on second-order family therapy." *Family Process, 29,* 157–163.

Anderson, H., & Goolishian, H. (1992). The client is the expert: A not-knowing approach to therapy. In S. McNames & K. J. Gergen (Eds.), *Therapy as social construction.* Newbury Park, CA: Sage.

Anderson, R., & Newman, J. F. (1973). Societal and individual determinants of medical care utilization in the United States. *Millbank Memorial Fund Quarterly/Health in Society, 51,* 95–124.

Anderson, T. (1991b, May 10–12). Relationship, language, and pre-understanding in the reflecting process. Read at the Houston-Galveston Institute's Conference, "Narrative and Psychotherapy: New Directions in Theory and Practice for the 21st Century," Houston.

Ansbacher, H. L., & Ansbacher, R. R. (Eds.). (1973). *Superiority and social interest: A collection of later writings.* New York: Viking.

Anthony, E. J. (1974). The syndrome of the psychologically invulnerable child. In E. J. Anthony & C. Koupernik (Eds.), *The child in his family: Vol. 3. Children at psychiatric risk* (pp. 529–544). New York: John Wiley & Sons.

Antonovsky, A. (1987). *Unraveling the mystery of health: How people manage stress and stay well.* San Francisco: Jossey Bass.

Atchley, R. C. (1991). The influence of aging or frailty on perceptions and expressions of the self: Theoretical and methodological issues. In J. E. Birren & J. E. Lubben (Eds.), *The concept and measurement of quality of life in the frail elderly* (pp. 207–225). San Diego: Academic Press.

Auerhahn, N. C., Laub, D., & Peskin, H. (1993). Psychotherapy with Holocaust survivors. *Psychotherapy, 30,* 434–442.

Bagge', R., & Brandsma, J. (1994). PTSD and grief: Traumatic Grief. In L. Hyer (Ed.), *Trauma victim: Theoretical Issues and practical suggestions.* Muncie IN: Accelerated Press.

Baltes, P. B. (1987). Theoretical propositions of life-span psychology: On the dynamics between growth and decline. *Developmental Psychology, 23,* 611–626.

Baltes, P. B., Reese, H. W., & Lipsitt, C. P. (1980). Lifespan developmental psychology. *Annual Review of Psychology, 31,* 65–110.

Baltes, P. B., & Staudinger, U. M. (1993). The search for a psychology of wisdom. *Current directions in psychological science, 2*, 75–80.

Bamberg, M. (Ed.), (2000). *Narrative development: Six approaches.* Mahwah, NJ: Lawrence Erlbaum Associates.

Bandura, A. (1977). Self-efficacy: Toward a unifying theory of behavioral change. *Psychological Review, 84*, 191–215.

Barclay, C. R. (1986). Schematization of autobiographical memory. In D. C. Rubin (Ed.), *Autobiographical memory* (pp. 82–99). New York: Cambridge University Press.

Barlow, D. H. (1988). *Anxiety and its disorders: The nature and treatment of anxiety and panic.* New York: The Guilford Press.

Barlow, D. H., (discussant) Symposium: Comparison of medication, psychotherapy, and combination treatment for chronic depression. Presented at 108th annual convention of the American Psychological Association at Washington, DC, August 5, 2000.

Barrera, M., Sandler, I. N., & Ramsay, T. B. (1981). Preliminary development of a scale of social support: Studies on college students. *American Journal of Community Psychology, 9*, 435–447.

Basseches, M. (1984). *Dialectical thinking and adult development.* Norwood, NJ: Ablex.

BAUM ET AL. NOT IN REFERENCES

Baumeister, R. F. (1991). *Meanings of life.* New York: Guilford Press.

Beardslee, W. R. (1986). The role of self understanding in resilient individuals. The development of a perspective. *American Journal of Orthopsychiatry, 59*, 266–278.

Beardslee, W. R., & Podorefsky, D. (1986). Resilient adolescents whose parents have serious affective and other psychiatric disorders: Importance of self-under-standing and relationships. *American Journal of Psychiatry, 145*, 63–69.

Beck, A., & Freeman, A. (1990). *Cognitive therapy of personality disorders.* New York: Guilford.

Beck, J. S. (1995). *Cognitive Therapy: Basics and beyond.* New York: Guilford.

Blake, D., Nagy, L., Kaloupek, D., Klauminzer, G., Charney, D., & Keane, T. (September, 1990). A Clinical Rating Scale for Assessing current and lifetime PTSD: CAPS-1. *The Behavior Therapist.* September, 1987–188.

Beckham, E. E. (1989). Improvement after evaluation in psychotherapy of depression: Evidence of a placebo effect? *Journal of Clinical Psychology, 45*, 945–950.

Behland, H. (1988). Alteration of the ego due to defensive processes and the limitations of psychoanalytic treatment. *International Journal of Psychoanalysis, 69*(2), 189–205.

Bengtson, V. L., Reedy, M. N., & Gordon, C. (1985). Aging and self-conceptions: In J. E. Birren & K. W. Schaie (Eds.). *Handbook of the Psychology of Aging,* New York: Van Nostrand Reinhold.

Benjamin, L. S. (1993). Every psychopathology is a gift of love. *Psycotherapy Research, 3*, 1–24.

Benson, H. (1975). *The relaxation response.* New York: William Morrow.

Berezin, M. A. (1972). Psychodynamic considerations of aging and the aged: An overview. *American Jouornal of Psychiatry, 128*, 33–41.

Berg, I. (1990). Solution-focused approach to family based services. Milwaukee: Brief Family Therapy Center.

Berman, S., Price, S., & Gusman, F. (1982). An inpatient program for Vietnam combat veterans in a Veterans Administration Hospital. *Hospital and Community Psychiatry, 33*, 919–927.

Bernstein, E. M., & Putnam, F. W. (1986). Development, reliability and validity of a dissociation scale. *Journal of Nervous and Mental Disease, 174*, 570–578.

Berwick, D. M. (1989). Continuous improvement as an ideal in health care. *New England Journal of Medicine, 320*, 53–36.

Beutler, L., & Clarkin, J. F. (1990). *Systematic treatment selection: Toward targeted therapeutic interventions.* New York: Brunner/Mazel.

Beutler, L. E. (1991). Have all won and must all have prizes? Revisiting Luborsky, et. al.'s verdict. *Journal of Consulting and Clinical Psychology, 59*, 226–232.

Beutler, L. E. (1991). Selective treatment matching: Systematic eclectic psychotherapy. *Psychotherapy, 28*, 457–462.

Beutler, L. E., & Hill, C. E. (1992). Process and outcome research in the treatment of adult victims of childhood sexual abuse: Methodological issues. *Journal of Consulting and Clinical Psychology, 60*(2), 204–212.

Beutler, L. E., Kim, E. J., Davison, E., & Karno, M. (Summer, 1996). Research contributions to improving managed health care outcomes. *Psychotherapy, 33*, 197–206.

Beutler, L. E., Machado, P. P. P., Engle, D., & Mohr, D. (1993). Differential patient X treatment maintenance of treatment effects among cognitive, experiential, and self-directed psychotherapies. *Journal of Psychotherapy Integration, 3*, 15–31.

Beutler, L. E., Scogin, F., Kirkish, P., Schretlen, D., Corbishley, A., Hamblin, D., Meredith, K., Potter, R., Bamford, C. R., & Levenson, A. I. (1987). Group cognitive therapy and alprazolam in the treatment of depression in older adults. *Journal of Consulting and Clinical Psychology, 55*, 550–557.

Beutler, L. E., Williams, R. E., Wakefield, P. J., & Entwistle, S. R. (1995). Bridging scientist and practitioner perspectives in clinical psychology. *American Psychologist, 50*, 984–994.

Billings, A. G., & Moos, R. H. (1984). Coping, stress, and social resources among adults with unipolar depression. *Journal of Personality and Social Psychology, 46*, 877–891.

Binder, J. Key elements of psychotherapy. Workshop presented at 107th annual meeting of the American Psychological Association at Boston, MA, August 1999.

Birren, J. E., & Deutchman, D. E. (1991). *Guiding Autobiography Groups for Older Adults*. London: Johns Hopkins University Press.

Blackman, D. K., Howe, M., & Pinkston, E. M. (1976). Increasing participation in social interactions of the institutionalized elderly. *The Gerontologist, 16*, 69–76.

Blake, D. D., Cook, J. D., & Keane, T. M. (1992). Psychological coping patterns and PTSD in veterans seeking medical treatment. *J. Clinical Psychology, 48*, 695–704.

Blake, D. D., Weathers, F. W., Nagy, L. M., Kaloupek, D. G., Gusman, F. D., Charney, D. S., & Keane, T. M. (1995). The Development of a Clinician-Administered PTSD Scale. *Journal of Traumatic Stress, 8*, No. 1, 1995.

Blake, D. D., Weathers, F. W., Nagy, L. M., Kaloupek, D. G., Klauminzer, G., Charney, D. S., & Keane, T. M. (1990). A clinician rating scale for assessing current and lifetime PTSD: The CAPS-1. *Behavior Therapy, 13*, 187–188.

Blanchard, E. B., & Hickling, E. J. (1998). Motor vehicle accident survivors and PTSD. *PTSD Research Quarterly, 9*(3), 1–3.

Blanchard, E. B., Hickling, E. J., Taylor, A. E., Loos, W. R., Forneris, C. A., & Jaccard, J. (1996). Who develops PTSD from motor vehicle accidents? *Behavior Research and Therapy, 34*, 1–10.

Blanchard, E. B., Hickling, E. J., Taylor, A. E., Loos, W. R. (1995). Psychiatric morbidity associated with motor vehicle accidents. *Journal of Nervous and Mental Disease, 183*, 495–504.

Blank, A. (1994). Clinical detection, diagnosis and differential diagnosis of PTSD. *Psychiatric Clinics of North America* 359–383.

Blazer, D. (1998). *Emotional problems in later life*. New York: Springer.

Blazer, D. G., George, L. K., Londerman, R., Pennybacker, M., Melville, M. L., Woodbury, M., Manton, K. G., Jordan, K., & Locke, B. (1985). Psychiatric disorders, a rural/urban comparison. *Archives General Psychiatry, 42*, 651–656.

Bleuler, M. (1978). *The schizophrenic disorders: The long term patient and family studies*. Translated by S. M. Clemens. New Haven, Yale University Press.

Block, J. (1971). *Lives through time*. Berkeley, CA: Bancroft Books.

Block, J. (1981). Some enduring and consequential structures of personality, pp. 27–43. *In Further Explorations in Personality*. New York: John Wiley & Sons.

Borderline personality disorder in later years (letter). *American Journal of Psychiatry, 140*, 271–272.

Bornat, J. (1994). *Reminiscence reviewed: perspectives, evaluations, achievements*. Great Britain: Biddles Limited, Guildford and Kings Lynn.

Bornat, J. (Ed.). (1994). Reminiscence reviewed: Perspectives, evaluations, achievements. Buckingham: Open University Press.

Bortz, G., & O'Brien, K. (1997). Psychotherapy with older adults: Theoretical issues, empirical findings, and clinical applications. In P. D. Nussbaum (Ed.). *Handbook of neuropsychology and aging*. New York: Plenum.

Borysenko, J. (1988). *Minding the body: Mending the mind*. New York: Bantam.

Botwinick, J. (1977). Intellectual abilities. In J. E. Birren & K. W. Schaie (Eds.), *Handbook of the Psychology of Aging* (pp. 580–605). New York: Van Nostrand Reinhold.

Botwinick, J. (1984). *Aging and Behavior.* New York: Springer.

Botwinick, J., & Thompson, L. W. (1967) Depressive affect, speed of response, and age. *Journal Consulting Psychology, 31,* 106.

Boudewyns, P., & Hyer, L. (1990). Changes in psychophysiological response to war memories among Vietnam veteran PTSD patients treated with direct therapeutic exposure. *Behavior Therapy, 21,* 63–87.

Boudewyns, P., & Hyer, L. (1997). Eye movement desensitization and reprocessing (EMDR) as treatment for post-traumatic stress disorder (PTSD). *Clinical Psychology and Psychotherapy.*

Boudewyns, P. A., Hyer, L., Peralme, L., Touze, J., & Kiel, A. (1995, May). Eye Movement Desensitization and Reprocessing for Combat-Related PTSD: An early look. In S. Lazrove (Chair), *Eye movement desensitization and reprocessing: Evidence pro and con.* Symposium conducted at the convention of the American Psychiatric Association, Miami, FL.

Boudewyns, P., Woods, M., Hyer, L., & Albrecht, W. (1990). Chronic combat-related PTSD and concurrent substance abuse: Implications for treatment of this frequent "dual diagnosis." *Journal of Traumatic Stress, 4,* 549–560.

Boudewyns, P. A., Albrecht, J. W., Talbert, F. S., Hyer, L. (1994). Co-morbidity and treatment outcome in inpatients with chronic combat-related PTSD. *Hospital and Community Psychiatry, 42,* 63–87.

Boudewyns, P. A., Hyer, L. A. (in press). Eye Movement Desensitization and Reprocessing (EMDR) as treatment for post-traumatic stress disorder (PTSD). *British Journal of Psychiatry.*

Boudreaux, E., Kilpatrick, D. G., Resnick, H. S., Best, C. L., & Saunders, B. E. (1998). Criminal victimization, posttraumatic stress disorder, and comorbid pschopathology among a community sample of women. *Journal of Traumatic Stress, 11*(4), 665–678.

Bower, G. (1981). Mood and Memory. *American Psychologist, 36,* 129–148.

Bowlby, J. (1980). *Attachment and loss volume III, Loss.* New York: Basic Books.

Brandsma J., & Hyer, L. (in press). *Resolution of traumatic grief.* NCS Newsletter.

Brandsma, J., & Hyer, L. (1995). The treatment of grief in PTSD. NCP: *Clinical Newsletter, 5.*

Brandsma, J. M. (1998). Forgiveness. In Benner, D. G., & Hill, P. C. (Eds.), *Baker's Encyclopedia of Psychology* (2nd ed.). Grand Rapids, MI: Baker Book House.

Braun, B. (1988). The BASK model of dissociation. *Dissociation, 1,* 4–15.

Bremner, J. D., Southwick, S. M., & Charney, D. S. (1991). Animal models for the neurobiology of trauma. *PTSD Research Quarterly, 2*(4), 1–3.

Breslau, L. (1980). The faltering therapeutic perspective toward narcissistically wounded institutionalized aged. *Journal of Geriatric Psychiatry, 13,* 193–206.

Breslau, N., & Davis, G. C. (1992). Posttraumatic stress disorder in an urban population of young adults: Risk factors for chronicity. *American Journal of Psychiatry, 149,* 671–675.

Breslau, N., Davis, G., Andreski, P., & Peterson, E. (1991). Traumatic events and PTSD in an urban population of young adults. *Arch. Gen. Psychiat., 48,* 216–222.

Breunlin, D., Schwartz, R., & Kune-Karrer Mac, B. (1992). *Metaframeworks: Transcending the models of family therapy.* San Francisco: Jossey-Bass.

Brewer, W. F. (1986). What is autobiographical memory? In D. Rubin (Ed.), *Autobiographical memory* (pp. 25–49). New York: Cambridge University Press.

Brewin, C. R., Andrews, B., & Gotlib, I. H. (1993). Psychopathology and early experience: A reappraisal of retrospective reports. *Psychological Bulletin, 113,* 82–98.

Brewin, C. R., Andrews, B., & Valentine, J. D. (2000). Meta-analysis of risk factors for posttraumatic stress disorder in trauma-exposed adults. *Journal of Consulting and Clinical Psychology, 68*(5), 748–766.

Brewin, C. R., Dalgleish, T., & Joseph, S. (1996). A dual representation theory of posttraumatic stress disorder. *Psychological Review, 103,* 670–686.

Brewin, C. R., Joseph, S., & Kuyken, W. (1993). PTSD and depression: what is their relationship. Paper presented at the meeting of the British Psychological Society, Belfast.

Brewin, C. R., & Lennard, H. (1999). Effects of mode of writing on emotional narratives. *Journal of Traumatic Stress, 12*(2), 355–361.

Briere, J. (1989). *Therapy for adults molested as children.* New York: Springer.

Briere, J. (1994 May). Working with abuse survivors in the age of denial: Dissociation, "repressed memories," and "false memory syndrome." Paper presented at the continuing education conference sponsored by the Iowa Coalition Against Sexual Assault, Des Moines, IA.

Briere, J. N. (1992). *Child abuse trauma: Theory and treatment of the lasting effects.* Newbury Park, CA: Sage.

Brigham, D. D., Davis, A., & Cameron-Sampey, D. (1994). *Imagery for getting well: Clinical applications of behavioral medicine.* New York: W. W. Norton & Company.

Brink, T. L. (1978). Geriatric rigidity and its psychotherapeutic implications. *Journal of the American Geriatrics Society, 26*(6), 274–277.

Britton, P. G., & Savage, R. D. (1966). The MMPI and the aged: Some normative data from a community sample. *British Journal of Psychology, 112,* 941–943.

Brody, E. M., Kleban, M. H., Lawton, M. P., & Silverman, H. A. (1971). Excess disabilities of mentally impaired aged: Impact of individual treatment. *The Gerontologist 11,* 124–133.

Brody, C. M., & Semel, V. G. (1993). *Strategies for therapy with the elderly.* New York: Springer.

Brody, H. (1987). *Stories of sickness.* New Haven, CT: Yale University Press.

Brokaw, T. (1998). *The greatest generation.* New York: Random House.

Bromley, D. B. (1988). *Human ageing: An introduction to gerontology.* Harmondsworth: Penguin.

Brown, A. Gatchel, R. J., & Schaeffer, M. A. (1989). *Life events and illness.* New York: Guilford Press.

Brown, G. W. (1990). What about the real world? Hassles and Richard Lazarus. *Psychological Inquiry, 1,* 19–22.

Bryant, R. A. (2000). Acute stress disorder. *PTSD Research Quarterly, 11*(2), 1–3.

Bruner, J. (1987). *Actual minds, possible worlds.* Cambridge, MA: Harvard University Press.

Bruner, J. S. (1990). *Acts of meaning.* Cambridge: Harvard University Press.

Bugental, J. F. T. (1987). *The Art of the Psychotherapist.* New York: W. W. Norton & Company.

Burgess, C., Morris, T., & Pettingale, K. W. (1988). Psychological response to cancer: Evidence for coping styles. *Journal of Psychosomatic Research, 32,* 263–272.

Burish, T. G., & Carey, M. P. (1986). Conditioned average responses in cancer chemotherapy patients: Theoretical and developmental analysis. *Journal of Consulting and Clinical Psychology, 54*(5), 593–600.

Burish, T. G., Snyder, S., & Jenkins, R. A. (1991). Preparing patients for cancer chemotherapy: Effect of coping preparation and relaxation intervention. *Journal of Counseling and Clinical Psychology, 59*(4), 518–525.

Burish, T. G., & Carey, M. P., Krozely, M. G., & Greco, F. A. (1987). Conditioned side effects induced by cancer chemotherapy: Prevention through behavioral treatment. *Journal of Consulting and Clinical Psychology 55*(1), 42–48.

Burish, T. G., Carey, M. P., Wallston, K. A., Stein, M. J., Jamison, R. N., & Lyles, J. N. (1984). Health locus of control and chronic disease: An external orientation may be advantageous. *Journal of Social and Clinical Psychology, 2*(4), 326–332.

Burish, T. G., Vasterline, J. J., Carey, M. P., Matt, D. A., & Krozely, M. G. (1988). Posttreatment use of relaxation training by cancer patients. *The Hospice Journal, 4*(2), 1–9.

Burns, D. (1999). *The feeling good handbook.* New York: Plume.

Burns, D. D., & Nolen-Hoeksema, S. (1992). Therapeutic empathy and recovery from depression in cognitive behavioral therapy: A structural equation model. *Journal of Consulting and Clinical Psychology, 60,* 441–449.

Burns, D. D., & Spangler, D. (1988). Does homework lead to recovery in cognitive behavioral therapy? Or does recovery lead to homework compliance? (manuscript under review).

Burville, P. W., Hall, W. D., Stampfer, H. G., & Emmerson, J. P. (1989). A comparison of early-onset and late-onset depressive illness in the elderly. *British Journal of Psychiatry, 155,* 673–679.

Busse, E. (1975). Aging and psychiatric diseases in late life. M. Reiser (Ed.), *American handbook of psychiatry, 4.* New York: Basic Books.

Busse, E. W., & Blazer, D. G. (Eds.). (1989). *Geriatric psychiatry.* Washington, DC: American Psychiatric Press.

Butler, R. N. (1963). The life review: An interpretation of reminiscence in the aged. *Psychiatry, 26,* 65–76.

Byrne, D. G., & White, H. M. (1980). Life events and myocardial infarction revisited: The role of measures of individual impact. *Psychosomatic Medicine, 42,* 1–9.

Calhoun, L. G., & Tedeschi, R. G. (1989–1990). Positive aspects of critical life problems: Recollections of grief. *Omega, 20,* 265–272.

Calhoun, L. H., & Tedeschi, R. G. (1998). Posttraumatic growth: Future directions. In R. G. Tedeschi, C. L. Park, & L. G. Calhoun, *Posttraumatic Growth.* Mahwah, NJ: Lawrence Erlbaum.

Campbell, L. F. (Summer, 1996). *Psychotherapy, 33,* 190–196.

Campbell, R., Sefl, T., Barnes, H. E., Courtney, E. Ahrens, Wasco, S. M., & Zaragoza-Diesfield, Y. (1999). Community services for rape survivors: Enhancing psychological well-being or increasing trauma? *Journal of Consulting and Clinical Psychology, 67*(6), 847–858.

Cantor, N., & Kihlstrom, J. F. (1987). *Personality and social intelligence.* Englewood Cliffs, NJ: Prentice-Hall.

Card, J. J. (1983). *Lives After Vietnam: The Personal Impact of Military Service.* Lexington, MA: Lexington Books.

Carey, M. P., & Burish, T. G. (1987). Providing relation training to cancer chemotherapy patients: A comparison of three delivery techniques. *Journal of Consulting and Clinical Psychology, 55*(5), 732–777.

Carey, M. P., & Burish, T. G. (1988). Etiology and treatment of the psychological side effects associated with cancer chemotherapy: A critical review and discussion. *Psychological Bulletin, 104*(3), 307–325.

Carlsen, M. B. (1988). *Meaning-making: Therapeutic processes in adult development.* New York: W. W. Norton.

Carlson, E. B. (1997). *Trauma assessments: A clinician's guide.* New York: Guilford.

Carstensen, L. L. (1988). The emerging field of behavioral gerontology. *Behavior Therapy, 19,* 259–281.

Carver, C. S., & Gaines, J. G. (1987). Optimism, pessimism, and post-partum depression. *Cognitive Therapy and Research, 11,* 449–462.

Carver, C. S., Scheier, M. F., & Weintraub, J. K. (1989). Assessing coping strategies: A theoretically based approach. *Journal of Personality and Social Psychology, 56,* 267–283.

Casarjian, R. (1992). *Forgiveness.* New York: Bantam.

Casey, D. A., & Schrodt, C. J. (1989). Axis II diagnoses in geriatric inpatients. *Journal Geriatric Psychiatry & Neurology, 2,* 87–88.

Casey, E. (1987). *Remembering: A Phenomenological Study.* Bloomington, Ind: Indiana University Press.

Casey, J. (1999). *The half life of happiness.* New York: Vintage Books.

Casey, M. P., & Burish, T. G. (1985). Anxiety as a predictor of behavioral therapy outcome of cancer chemotherapy patients. *Journal of Consulting and Clinical Psychology 53*(6), 860–865.

Casey, P. (1988). The epidemiology of personality disorder. In P. Tyrer (Ed.), *Personality disorders: Diagnosis, management and course* (pp. 74–81). London: John Wright.

Caspi, A., Bem, D. J., & Elder, G. H. (1989). Character type and character organization. *Journal of the American Psychoanalytic Association, 37*(3), 655–688.

Cassiday, K. L., McNally, R. J., & Zeitlin, S. B. (1992). Cognitive processing of trauma cues in rape victims with posttraumatic stress disorder. *Cognitive Therapy and Research, 16,* 283–295.

Castonguay, L. G. (2000). A common factors approach to psychotherapy training. *Journal of Psychotherapy Integration, 10*(3), 263–282.

Cath, S. H. (1965). Some dynamics of middle and later years. A study of depletion and restitution. In M. Berezin & S. H. Cath (Eds.), *Geriatric Psychiatry: Grief, Loss, and Emotional Disorders in the Aging Process* (pp. 21–72). New York: International Universities Press.

Cautela, J. R., & Mansfield, L. (1977). A behavioral approach to geriatrics. In W. D. Gentry (Ed.), *Geropsychology: A model of training and clinical service.* Cambridge, MA: Ballinger Publishing Company.

Charme, S. L. (1984). *Meaning and myth in the study of lives: A Sartrean perspective.* Philadelphia: University of Pennsylvania Press.

Charney, D. S., & Heninger, G. R. (1986). Abnormal regulation of noradrenergic function in panic disorder. *Arch. Gen. Psychiat., 43,* 1042–1058.

Chaudhury, H. (1999). Self and reminiscence of place: A conceptual study. *Journal of Aging and Identity, 4*(4), 231–253.

Chemtob, C. M., Hamada, R. S., Roitblat, H. L., & Muraoka, M. Y. (1994). Anger, impulsivity, and anger control in combat-related posttraumatic stress disorder. *Journal of Consulting and Clinical Psychology, 62,* 827–832.

Chinen, A. B. (1984). Modal logic: A new paradigm of development and late life potential. *Human Development, 27,* 52–56.

Chinen, A. (1986). Elder tales revised: Forms of transendence in later life. *The Journal of Transpersonal Psychology, 26,* 171–192.

Chiriboga, D. A., & Cutler, L. (1980). Stress and adaptations: Life span perspectives. In R. W. Poon (Ed.), *Aging in the 1980's* (pp. 347–362). Washington, DC: Gerontological Society.

Choca, J. P., Shanley, L. A., & Van Denberg, E. (1992). *Interpretive Guide to the Millon Clinical Multiaxial Inventory,* Washington, DC: American Psychological Association.

Chowanec, G. D. (1994). Continuous quality improvement: Conceptual foundations and application to mental health care. *Hospital and Community Psychiatry, 45,* 789–793.

Ciarlo, J. A., Brown, T. R., Edwards, D. W., Kiresuk, T. K., & Newman, F. L. (1986). *Assessing mental health treatment outcome measurement techniques. Series FN No. 9. DHHS Pub. No. (ADM)8-1301.* Washington, DC: U.S. Government Printing office.

Clay, R. A. (2000). Psychotherapy is cost-effective. *Monitor on Psychology, 31*(1), 40–41.

Cohen, J. (1988). *Statistical power analysis for the behavioral sciences.* NY: Erlbaum Associates.

Cohen, R. (1992). *Psychodynamic theories of recovery from adult trauma: An empirical study.* Paper presented at the 100th Annual Convention of the American Psychological Association. Washington, DC.

Cohler, B. J. (1982). Personal narrative and the life course. In P. Baltes & O. G. Brim, Jr. (Eds.), *Life-span development and behavior: 4,* New York: Academic Press.

Colarusso, C. A., & Nemiroff, R. A. (1981). *Adult development: A new dimension in psychodynamic theory and practice.* New York: Plenum.

Coleman, P. G. (1986). *Ageing and Reminiscence Processes: Social and Clinical Implications.* Chichester: John Wiley.

Coleman, P. G. (1986). *Ageing and Reminiscence Processes: Social and Clinical Implications.* Chichester: John Wiley.

Commons, M. L., & Richards, F. A. (1982). A general model of stage theory. In J. L. Commons, F. A. Richards & S. Armon (Eds.), *Beyond formal operations: Late adolescent and adult cognitive development.* New York: Praeger.

Compas, B. E., Banez, G. A., & Malcarne, V. (1991). Perceived control and coping with stress: A developmental perspective. *Journal of Social Issues, 47,* 357–364.

Cook, A., & Dworkin, D. (1992). *Helping the bereaved: Therapeutic interventions for children, adolescence and adults.* USA: Basic Books.

Cooper, N. A., & Clum, G. A. (1989). Imaginal flooding as a supplementary treatment for PTSD in combat veterans: A controlled study. *Behavior Therapy, 20,* 381–391.

Cornelius, S. W., & Caspi, A. (1987). Everyday problem solving in adulthood and old age. *Psychology and Aging, 2,* 144–153.

Cornell, W. F., & Olio, K. A. (1991). Integrating affect in treatment with adult survivors of physical and sexual abuse. *American Journal of Orthopsychiatry, 61,* 50–69.

Cornell, W. F., & Olio, K. A. (1992). Consequences of childhood bodily abuse: A clinical model for affective interventions. *Transactional Analysis Journal, 22,* 131–143.

Costa, P. T., Gatz, M., Neugarten, B. L., Salthouse, T. A., & Siegler, I. C. (1994). *The adult years: Continuity and change.* Washington, DC: American Psychological Association.

Costa, P., & McCrae, R. (1990). Personality disorders and the five-factor model of personality. *Journal of Personality Disorders, 4,* 362–371.

Costa, P. T., Jr., & McCrae, R. R. (1984). Personality as a life long determinant of well-being. In C. Malatesta & C. Izard (Eds.), *Affective processes in adult development and aging* (pp. 190–204). Beverly Hills, CA: Sage.

Costa, P. T., & McCrae, R. R. (1978). Objective personality assessment. In M. Storandt, I. C. Siegler, & M. F. Elias (Eds.), *The Clinical Psychology of Aging* (pp. 119–143). New York: Plenum.

Costa, P. T., & McCrae, R. R. (1984). Personality as a life-long determinant of well-being. In C. Z. Malatesta & C. E. Izard (Eds.), *Emotions in Adult Development* (pp. 141–157). Beverly Hills, CA: Sage.

Costa, P. T., & McCrae, R. R. (1988). From catalog to classification: Murray's needs and the five-factor model. *Journal of Personal and Social Psychology, 55*, 258–265.

Costa, P. T., & McCrae, R. R. (1992). The five-factor model of personality and its relevance to personality disorders. *Journal of Personality Disorders, 6*, 343–359.

Costa, P. T., Jr., & McCrae, R. E. (1993). Psychological stress and coping in old age. In L. Goldberger & S. Breznitz (Eds.), *Handbook of stress: Theoretical and clinical aspects* (2nd ed.) (pp. 403–413). New York: Free Press.

Costa, P. T., Jr., & McCrae, R. R. (1985). *The NEO Personality Inventory manual.* Odessa, FL: Psychological Assessment Resources.

Costa, P. T., McCrae, R. R., Zonderman, A. B., Barbano, H. E., Lebowitz, B., & Larson, D. M. (1986). Cross-sectional studies of personality in a national sample: 2. Stability in neuroticism, extroversion, and openness. *Psychology and Aging, 1*, 144–149.

Costa, P. T., & Widiger, T. A. (1994). *Personality disorders and the five-factor model of personality.* Washington, DC: American Psychological Association.

Costa, P. T., Zonderman, A. B., McCrae, R. R., Cornoni-Huntley, J., Locke, B. Z., & Barbano, H. E. (1987). Longitudinal analysis of psychological well-being in a national sample: Stability of mean levels. *Journal of Gerontology, 42*, 50–55.

Courtois, C. (1988). *Healing the incest wound.* New York: Norton.

Courtois, C. (1992). The memory retrieval process in incest survivor therapy. *Journal of Child Sexual Abuse, 1*(1), 15–31.

Cox, D. S., Taylor, A. G., & Nowacek, S. (1984). The relationship between psychological stress and insulin-dependent diabetic blood glucose control: Preliminary investigations. *Health Psychology, 3*, 63–75.

Creamer, M., Burgess, P., & Pattison, P. (1992). Reaction to trauma: A cognitive-processing model. *J. Abn. Psych., 01*, 452–459.

Cronbach, L. J. (1989). Construct validation after thirty years. In R. L. Linn (Ed.), *Intelligence: Measurement, theory, and public policy* (pp. 147–171). Urbana, IL: University of Illinois Press.

Cumming, E., & Henry, W. (1961). *Growing Old.* New York: Basic Books.

Cummings, J. L., & Benson, D. F. (1992). *Dementia: A clinical approach* (2nd ed.). Boston: Butterworths-Heinemann.

Cummings, N., & Sayama, M. (1995). *Focused psychotherapy.* New York: Brunner/Mazel.

Daldrup, R. J., Beutler, L. E., Engle, D., & Greenberg, L. S. (1988). *Focused expressive psychotherapy: Freeing the overcontrolled patient.* New York: Guilford.

Davidson, J., Kudler, H., Saunders, E., & Smith, R. (1990). Symptom and comoribidity patterns in World War II and Vietnam veterans with posttraumatic stress disorder. *Comparative Psychiatry, 31*, 162–170.

Davidson, J., Smith, R., & Kudler, H. (1989). Validity and reliability of the DSM-III criteria for Post-traumatic Stress disorder: Experience with a structured interview. *Journal of Nervous and Mental Disease, 177*, 336–341.

Davidson, J. R. T., & van der Kolk, B. A. (1996). The psychopharmacological treatment of posttraumatic stress disorder. In B. A. van der Kolk, A. C. McFarlane, & L. Weisaeth (Eds.), *Traumatic Stress: The effects of overwhelming experience on mind, body, and society* (pp. 511–524). New York: The Guilford Press.

Davies, J. M., & Frawley, M. G. (1994). *Treating the adult survivor of childhood sexual abuse: A psychoanalytic perspective.* New York: Basic Books.

de Rivera, J. (1984). Development and the full range of emotional expression. In C. Z. Malatesta & C. E. Izard (Eds.), *Emotion in adult development* (pp. 45–63). Beverly Hills, CA: Sage.

Delongis, A., Folkman S., & Lazarus, R. S. (1988). The impact of daily stress on mood, psychological, and social resources as mediators. *Journal of Personality and Social Psychology, 54*, 486–495.

Deming, W. E. (1986). *Out of the crisis.* Cambridge, MA: MIT Center for Advanced Engineering Study.

Demorest, A. P., & Alexander, I. E. (1992). Affective scripts as organizers of personal experience. *Journal of Personality, 60,* 645–663.

Depue, R. A., & Monroe, S. M. (1986). Conceptualization and measurement of human disorder in life stress research: The problem of chronic disturbance. *Psychological Bulletin, 99,* 36–51.

Derogatis, L. R., Morrow, G. R., Felting, J., Penman, D., Piasetsky, S., Schmale, A. M., Henrichs, M., & Carnicke, C. L. M. (1983). The prevalence of psychiatric disorder among cancer patients. *Journal of the American Medical Association, 249,* 752–757.

DeRubeis, R. J., & Hollon, S. D. (1995). Explanatory style in the treatment of depression. In G. M. Buchanan & M. E. P. Seligman (Eds.), *Explanatory style* (pp. 99–111). Hillsdale, NJ: Erlbaum.

De Shazer, S. (1988). *Clues: Investigating solutions in brief therapy.* New York: Norton.

deVries, B., Blando, J. A., & Walker, L. J. (1995). An exploratory analysis of the content and structure of the life review. In B. Haight & J. D. Webster (Eds.). *The art and science of reminiscing: Theory, research, methods and applications* (pp. 123–137). Washington, DC: Taylor & Francis.

Dibner, S. C. (1978). The psychology of normal aging. In M. Spencer & C. Dorr (Eds.). *Understanding aging: A multidisciplinary approach.* New York: Appleton-Century-Croft.

Dick, L. P., & Gallagher-Thompson, D. (1995). Cognitive therapy with the core beliefs of a distressed, lonely caregiver. *Journal of Cognitive Psychotherapy: An International Quarterly,* 215–227.

DiNardo, P. A., & Barlow, D. H. (1988). *Anxiety disorders interview scale-revised.* Albany, NY: Center for Phobia and Anxiety Disorders.

Dobson, CASE (1989). A meta-analysis of the efficacy of cognitive therapy for depression. *Journal Consulting Clinical Psychology, 57,* 414–419.

Dohrenwend, B. S., & Dohrenwend, B. P. (Eds.). (1981). *Stressful life events and their context.* New York: Neale Watson.

Dorfman, R. A., & Walsh, K. E. (1996). Theoretical dimensions of successful aging. *Journal of Aging and Identity, 1*(3), 165–176.

Dornelas, E. A., Correll, R. E., Lothstein, L, Wilber, C., & Goethe, J. W. (1996). Designing and implementing outcome evaluations: Some guidelines for practitioners. *Psychotherapy, 33*(2), 237–245.

Douglas, K., & Arenberg, D. (1978). Age changes, cohort differences, and cultural change on the Guilford-Aimmerman Temperament Survey. *Journal Gerontology, 33,* 737–747.

Drozd, J. F., & Goldfried, M. R. (Summer, 1996). A critical evaluation of the state-of-the-art in psychotherapy outcome research. *Psychotherapy, 33.*

Duffin, P. (1992). *Then and now: A training pack for Reminiscence work.* Manchester: Gatehouse Books.

Dye, E., & Roth, S. (1991). Psychotherapy with Vietnam veterans and rape and incest survivors. *Psychotherapy, 28,* 103–120.

Edinberg, M. A. (1985). *Mental Health Practice with the Elderly.* Englewood Cliffs, NJ: Prentice-Hall.

Egendorf, A. (1995). Hearing people through their pain. *Journal of Traumatic Stress, 8*(1), 5–28.

Eisen, S. V., & Dickey, B. (Summer 1996). Mental health outcome assessment: The new agenda. *Psychotherapy, 33,* pp. 181–189.

Elder, G. H., & Clipp, E. C. (1989). Combat experience and emotional health: Impairment and resilience in later life. *Journal of Personality, 57,* 311–341.

Elder, G. H., Shanahan, M. J., & Clipp, E. C. (1994). When war comes to men's lives: Life course patterns in family, work, and health. *Psychology and Aging, 9,* 5–16.

Elder, L., & Caspi, A. (1990). Studying lives in a changing society: Sociological and personological explanations. In A. Rabin, R. Zucker, R. Emmons, & S. Frank (Eds.), *Studying persons and lives* (pp. 201–247). New York: Springer.

Elder, G. H., Jr. (1987). War mobilization and the life course: A cohort of World War II veterans. *Sociological Forum, 2:*449–71.

Elder, G. H., & Clipp, E. C. (1988). Wartime losses and social bonding: Influences across forty years in men's lives. *Psychiatry, 51,* 177–188.

Elliott, D. M., & Briere, J. (1992). Sexual abuse trauma among professional women: Validating the Trauma symptom Checklist-40 (TSC-40). *Child Abuse and Neglect, 16*, 391–398.

Emery, G. (1981). Cognitive therapy with the elderly. In G. Emery, S. D. Holton, & R. C. Bedrosian (Eds.), *New directions in cognitive therapy* (pp. 84–98). New York: Guilford Press.

Emery, P., & Emery, V. (1989). Psychoanalytic considerations on post-traumatic stress disorders. *Journal Contemporary Psychotherapy, 19*, 19–53.

Emery, V., Emery, P., Shama, D., Quiana, N., & Jassani, A. (1991).

Emmons, R. A. (1986). Personal strivings: An approach to personality and subjective well-being. *Journal of Personality and Social Psychology, 51*, 1058–1068.

Engels, G. I., & Vermey, M. (1997). Efficacy of nonmedical treatments of depression in elders: A quantitative analysis. *Journal of Clinical Geropsychology, 3*(1), 17–35.

Engels, G. I., Garnefski, N., & Diekstra, R. E. W. (1993). Self-statement modification with adults: A meta-analysis. *Journal of Consulting and Clinical Psychology, 61*, 1083–1090.

Enright, R. E., Eastin, D. L., Golden, S., Sarinopoulos, S., & Freedman, S. (1992). Interpersonal forgiveness within the helping professions: An attempt to resolve differences of opinion. *Counseling and Values, 36*, 84–103.

Ensel, W. M. (1991). "Important" life events and depression among older adults: The role of psychological and social resources. *Journal of Aging and Health, 3*, 546–566.

Epstein, S. (1978). The self-concept revised or a theory of a theory. *American Psychologist*, 404–409.

Epstein, S. (1990). Beliefs and symptoms in maladaptive resolutions of the traumatic neurosis. In D. Ozer, J. M. Healy, & A. J. Stewart (Eds.), *Perspectives on personality, Vol. 3*. London: Jessica Kingsley, Publishers.

Epstein, S. (1991). The self-concept, the traumatic neurosis, and the structure of personality. In D. Ozer, J. M. Healy, Jr., & A. J. Stewart (Eds.), *Perspectives on personality, 3*. London: Jessica Kingsley.

Epston, D. (1993a). Internalizing discourses versus externalizing discourses. In S. Gilligan & R. Price (Eds.), *Therapeutic conversations* (pp. 161–177). New York: Norton.

Erikson, E. H. (1950). *The Dynamics of Anxiety and Hysteria*. London: Routledge & Kegan Paul.

Erikson, E. H. (1963). *Childhood and society*. New York: MacMillan.

Erikson, E. (1975). *Life history and the historical movement*. New York: Norton Press.

Everly, G. (1989). *A clinical guide to the treatment of the human stress response*. New York: Plenum.

Eysenck, H. J. (1957). *The dynamics of anxiety and hysteria*. London: Routledge & Kegan Paul.

Eysenck, H. J. (1981). *A model for personality*. New York: Springer.

Eysenck, S. B. G., Pearson, P. R., Easting, G., & Allsopp, J. F. (1985). Age norms for impulsiveness, venturesomeness, and empathy in adults. *Personal & Individual Differences, 6*, 613–619.

Fairbank, J. A., & Keane, T. M. (1982). Traumatic memories. *Associates for the Advancement of Behaviour Therapy, 13*, 449–510.

Fairbank, J. A., Hansen, D. J., & Fitterling, J. M. (1991). Patterns of appraisal and coping across different stressor conditions among former prisoners of war with and without posttraumatic stress disorder. *Journal of Consulting and Clinical Psychology, 59*, 274–281.

Falk, B., Hersen, M. H., Van Hasselt, V. (1994). Assessment of Post-traumatic stress disorder in older adults: A critical review. *Clinical Psychology Review, 14*(5), 383–415.

Fava, G., Grandi, S, Zielezn, M, Rafanelli, C., & Canestrari, R. (1996). Four-year outcome for cognitive behavioral treatment of residual symptoms in major depression. *American Journal of Psychiatry, 153*, 945–947.

Fenichel, O. (1945). *The psychoanalytic theory of neurosis*. New York: W. W. Norton & Company.

Fenton, W. S., & McGlashan, T. H. (1991). Natural history of schizophrenia subtypes: II. Positive and negative symptoms and long-term course. *Archives of General Psychiatry, 48*, 978–986.

Field, D., & Millsap, R. E. (1991). Personality in advanced old age: Continuity or change? *Journals of Geronology: Psychological Sciences, 48*, P299–P308.

Fielden, M. A. (1990). Reminiscence as a therapeutic intervention with sheltered housing residents: A comparative study. *British Journal of Social Work, 20*(1), 21–44.

Figley, C. R. (Ed.) (1989). *Treating stress in families*. New York: Brunner/Mazel.

Figley, C. R., Bride, B. R., Mazza, N., (Eds.) (1997). *Death and trauma: The traumatology of grieving*. Washington, DC: Taylor and Francis.

Finch, E. E., & Hayflick, L. (Eds.) (1977). *Handbook of the biology of aging*. New York: van Nostrand Reinhold.

Finn, S. E. (1996). *Manual for using the MMPI-2 as a therapeutic intervention*. Minneapolis, MN: University of Minnesota Press.

Finney, J. C. (1985). Anxiety: Its measurement by objective personality tests and self-report. In A. H. Truma & J. Maser (Eds.), *Anxiety and the anxiety disorders* (pp. 645–673). Hillsdale, NJ: Lawrence Erlbaum Associates, Publishers.

Fisher, S., & Greenberg, R. P. (1989). *The limits of biological treatments for psychological distress: Comparisons with psychotherapy and placebo*. Hillsdale, NJ: Lawrence Erlbaum Associates.

Flannery, R. B. (1990). Social support and psychological trauma: A methodological review. *Journal of Traumatic Stress, 3*, 593–612.

Fleming, S., & Robinson, P. (1990). The application of cognitive therapy to the bereaved. In T. Vallis (Ed.), *The challenge of cognitive therapy: Application to nontraditional populations* (pp. 135–157). New York: Plenum.

Floyd, M., & Scogin, F. (1998). Cognitive-behavior therapy for older adults: How does it work? *Psychotherapy: Theory, Research, Practice, Training, 35*(4), 459–463.

Foa, E., & Kozak, M. (1986). Emotional processing of fear: Exposure to corrective information. *Psychological Bulletin, 99*, 20–35.

Foa, E., & Kozak, M. (1991). Emotional processing: Theory, research, and clinical implications for anxiety disorders. In J. Safran & L. Greenberg (Eds.), *Emotions, psychology and change* (pp. 31–49). New York: Guilford Press.

Foa, E. B., Molnar, C., & Cashman, L. (1995). Change in rape narratives during exposure therapy for posttraumatic stress disorder. *Journal of Traumatic Stress, 8*(4), 675–690.

Foa, E., Steketee, G., & Rothbaum, B. (1989). Behavioral/cognitive conceptualizations of post-traumatic stress disorder. *Behavior Therapy, 20*, 155–176.

Foa, E., Zimbarg, R., & Rothbaum, B. (1992). Uncontrollability and unpredictability of PTSD: An anima model. *Psychological Bulletin, 12*(2), 218–238.

Foa, E. B., & Kozak, M. J. (1986). Emotional processing of fear: Exposure to corrective information. *Psychological Bulletin, 99*, 20–31.

Foa, E. B., & Kozak, M. J. (1991). Emotional processing: Theory, research and clinical implications for anxiety disorders. In J. D. Safran & L. S. Greenberg (Eds.), *Emotion, psychotherapy, and change*, pp, 21–49. New York: Guilford Press.

Foa, E. B. (1996). Failure of emotional processing: Post-trauma psychopathology and its treatment. Presented at the 104th Annual Convention of the American Psychological Association, Toronto.

Foa, E. B., & Kozak, M. J. (1986). Emotional processing of fear: Exposure to corrective information. *Psychological Bulletin, 99*, 20–35.

Foa, E. B., & Kozak, M. J. (1986). Treatment of anxiety disorders: Implications for psychopathology. In A. H. Tuma & J. Maser (Eds.), *Anxiety and the Anxiety Disorders* (pp. 421–452). Hillsdale, NJ: Lawrence Erlbaum Associates.

Foa, E. B., Feski, U., Murdock, T. B., Kozak, M. M., & McCarthy, P. R. (1991). Processing of threat-related information in rape victims. *Journal of Abnormal Psychology, 100*, 156–162.

Foa, E. B., Freund, B. F., Hembree, E., Dancu, C. V., Franklin, M. E., Perry, K. J., Riggs, D. S., & Molnar, C. (1994). Efficacy of short term behavioral treatments of PTSD in sexual and nonsexual assault victims. Paper presented at the annual meeting of the Association for Advancement of Behavior Therapy, San Diego, CA.

Foa, E. B., Keane, T. M., & Friedman, M. J. (2000). *Effective treatments for PTSD: Practice guidelines from the International Society for Traumatic Stress Studies*. New York: Guilford.

Foa, E. B., & Meadows, E. A. (1997). Psychosocial treatments for posttraumatic stress disorder: A critical review. *Annual Review of Psychology, 48*, 449–480.

Foa, E. B., Molnar, C., & Cashman, L. (1995). Change in rape narratives during exposure therapy for posttraumatic stress disorder. *Journal of Traumatic Stress, 8*(4), 675–690.

Foa, E. B., Riggs, D. S., Dancu, C. V., & Rothbaum, B. O. (1993). Reliability and validity of a brief instrument for assessing post-traumatic stress disorder. *Journal of Traumatic Stress, 6*, 4459–473.

Foa, E. B., Rothbaum, B. O., Riggs, D. S., & Murdock, T. B. (1991). Treatment of posttraumatic stress disorder in rape victims: A comparison between cognitive-behavioral procedures and counseling. *Journal of Consulting & Clinical Psychology, 59,* 712–715.

Fogel, B. S., & Westlake, R. (1990). Personality disorder diagnoses and age in inpatients with major depression. *Journal of Clinical Psychiatry, 51,* 232–235.

Fontana, A., & Rosenheck, R. (1993). A causal model of the etiology of war-related PTSD. *Journal of Traumatic Stress, 6,* 475–500.

Fontana, A., & Rosenheck, R. (1994). Traumatic war stressors and psychiatric symptoms among World War II, Korean, and Vietnam War veterans. *Psychology and Aging, 9(1),* 27–33.

Ford, J. (1995). Object relations and PTSD treatment outcomes. Paper presented at the ISTSS Conference. Boston, MA.

Fox, R. E. (March 1994). Training professional psychologists for the twenty-first century. *American Psychologist, 49(3),* 200–206.

Fox, R. E., Barclay, A. G., & Rogers, D. A. (1982). Proposals for a revolution in the preparation and regulation of professional psychologists. *American Psychologist, 40,* 1042–1050.

Foy, D. W. (1992). *Treating Ptsd: Cognitive-behavioral strategies. Treatment manuals for practitioners.* New York: Guilford.

Foy, D. W., Osato, S. S., Houskamp, B. M., & Neumann, D. A. (1992). Etiology of posttraumatic stress disorder. In A. P. Goldstein, L. Krasner, & S. L. Garfield (Eds.), *Posttraumatic stress disorder,* pp. 28–49. New York: MacMillan Publishing Company.

Frances, A., Clarkin, J., & Perry, S. (1984). *Differential therapeutics in psychiatry: The art and science of treatment selection.* New York: Brunner/Mazel.

Frank, E., Anderson, B., Stewart, B. D., Dancu, C., Hughes, C., & West, D. (1988). Efficacy of cognitive behavior therapy and systematic desensitization in the treatment of rape trauma. *Behavior Therapy, 19,* 403–420.

Fransella, F. (1984). Dellu's constructs and Durkheim's representations. In R. Farr & S. Doscovici (Eds.)., *Social representation.* Towerbridge: Redwood Burn.

Freedman, J., & Combs, G. (1996). *Narrative therapy.* New York: W. W. Norton & Company.

Freedy, J. R., Shaw, D. L., Jarrell, M. P., & Masters, C. R. (1992). Towards an understanding of the psychological impact of natural disasters: An application of the conservation resources stress model. *Journal of Traumatic Stress, 5,* 441–444.

Freeman, A. (1999). Cognitive behavior therapy in brief treatment. Presentation at University of Medicine and Dentistry of New Jersey, University Behavioral Health Care, Brief Treatment Services, New Brunswick, NJ, May 15, 1999.

Freud, M. J. (1984). Masson J. Freud and the seduction theory. *Atlantic Monthly,* Feb: 30–60.

Friedman, M. J. (2000). A guide to the literature on pharmacotherapy for PTSD. *PTSD Research Quarterly, 11(1)* 1–3.

Friedman, S. (1993). *The new constructive collaboration language in psychotherapy of change.* New York: The Guilford Press.

Frueh, B. C., Turner, S. M., Beidel, D. C., Mirabella, R. F., & Jones, W. J. (1996). Trauma management therapy: A preliminary evaluation of a multicomponent behavioral treatment for chronic combat-related PTSD. *Behav. Res. Ther., 34(7),* 533–543.

Fry, P. S. (1983). Structured and unstructured reminiscence training and depression among the elderly. *Clin. Gerontol., 1,* 15–37.

Gallagher, D., Rose, J., Rivera, P., Lovett, S., & Thompson, L. W. (1989). Prevalence of depression in family caregivers. *The Gerontologist, 29,* 449–456.

Gallagher, D., & Thompson, L. W. (1981). *Depression in the elderly: A behavioral treatment manual.* Los Angeles: USC Press.

Gallagher, D., & Thompson, L. W. (1982). Treatment of Major Depressive Disorder in older adult outpatients with brief psychotherapies. *Psychotherapy: Theory, Research, and Practice, 19,* 482–490.

Gallagher, D., & Thompson, L. W. (1983). Effectiveness of psychotherapy for both endogenous and nonendogenous depression in older adult outpatients. *Journal of Gerontology, 38,* 707–712.

Gallagher-Thompson, D., & Thompson, L. W. (1995). Psychotherapy with older adults in theory and practice. In B. Boner & L. Beutler (Eds.), *Comprehensive textbook of psychotherapy* (pp. 357–379). New York: Oxford University Press.

Gallagher-Thompson, D., & Thompson, L. W. (1996). Applying cognitive-behavioral therapy to the psychological problems of later life. In S. H. Zarit & B. G. Knight (Eds.), *A guide to psychotherapy and aging* (pp. 61–82). Washington, DC: American Psychological Association.

Gallagher-Thompson, D., Hanley-Peterson, P., & Thompson, L. W. (1990). Maintenance of gains versus relapse following brief psychotherapy for depression. *Journal of Counseling and Clinical Psychology, 58,* 371–374.

Gallagher-Thompson, D., & Thompson, L. W. (1996). Applying cognitive-behavioral therapy to the psychological problems of later life. In S. H. Zarit & B. G. Knight (Eds.), *A guide to psychotherapy and aging.* Washington, DC: American Psychological Association.

Ganz, F., Gallagher-Thompson, D., & Rodman, J. (1992). Inhibited grief. In A. Freeman & F. Datillio (Eds.), *Comprehensive textbook of cognitive therapy* (pp. 201–209). New York: Penum.

Garb, R., Bleich, A., & Lerer, B. (1987). Bereavement in combat. *The Psychiatric Clinics of North America, 10*(3).

Garfein, A. J., Ronis, D. L., & Bates, E. W. (1993). *Toward a case-mix planning model for the VA mental health outpatient system: Factors affecting diagnostic case-mix.* Ann Arbor, MI: Great Lakes HSR&D Field Program.

Garland, J. (1994). What splendor, it al coheres: Life review therapy with older people. In J. Bornat (Ed.), *Reminiscence reviewed: Perspectives, evaluations, achievements* (pp. 21–31). Bristol, PA: Open University Press.

Garmezy, N. (1987). Stress, competence and development: Continuities in the study of schizophrenic adults, children vulnerable to psychopathology and the search for stress-resistant children. *American Journal of Orthopsychiatry, 57*(2), 159–174.

Garmezy, N. (1987). Stress, competence and development: Continuities in the study of schizophrenic adults, children vulnerable to psychopathology and the search for stress-resistant children. *American Journal of Orthopsychiatry, 57*(2), 159–174.

Gaston, L., Marmar, C. R., Gallagher, D., & Thompson, L. W. (1989). Impact of confirming patient expectations of change processes in behavioral, cognitive, and brief dynamic psychotherapy. *Psychotherapy, 26,* 296–302.

Gaston, L., Marmar, C. R., Thompson, L. W., & Gallagher, D. (1988). Relation of patient pretreatment characteristics to the therapeutic alliance in diverse psychotherapies. *Journal of Consulting and Clinical Psychology, 56,* 483–489.

Gatz, M. (1994). Application of assessment to therapy and intervention with older adults. In M. Storandt & G. R. VandenBos, (Eds.), *Neuropsychological assessment of dementia and depression in older adults: A clinician's guide.* Washington, DC: American Psychological Association.

Gatz, M., Hopkin, S., Pino, C., & van den Bos, G. (1995). Psychological interventions with older adults. In J. E. Birren & K. W. Schaie (Eds.), *Handbook of the Psychology of Aging.* (pp. 755–785). New York: Van Nostrand Reinhold.

Gatz, M. (1999). Acute stress disorder. Paper presented at the 52nd annual convention of Gerontological Society of America at San Francisco, November 1999.

Gatz, M., Popkin, S., Pino, C., & VandenBos, G. (1985). Psychological interventions with older adults. In J. E. Birren & K. W. Schaie (Eds.), *Handbook of the psychology of aging* (2nd ed.) (pp. 755–788). New York: Van Nostrand Reinhold.

Gatz, M., Siegler, I. C., & Dibner, S. S. (1979). Individual and community: Normative conflicts in the development of a new therapeutic community for older persons. *International Journal of Aging and Human Development, 10,* 249–263.

Gendlin, E. T. (1962). *Experiencing and the creation of meaning: A philosophical and psychological approach to the subjective.* New York: Free Press of Glencoe.

Gendlin, E. T. (1981), *Focusing.* New York: Bantam.

Gendlin, E. (1991). On Emotion in Therapy. In J. D. Safran & L. S. Greenberg (Eds.), *Emotion, Psychotherapy, & Change* (pp. 255–279). New York: Guilford Press.

Gendlin, E. T. (1996). *Focusing-oriented psychotherapy.* New York: Guilford.

George, L. (1981). Predicting service utilization among the elderly. Paper presented at the annual meeting of the Gerontological Society of America, Toronto, Ontario.

Gibbs, M. (1989). Factors in the victim that mediate between disaster and psychopathology: A review. *Journal of Traumatic Stress, 2*, 4, 489–514.

Giddens, A. (1991). *Modernity and self-identity: Self and society in the late modern age.* Stanford, CA: Stanford University Press.

Gill, M. (1991). A re-experiencing therapy. In M. Kahn (Ed.), *Between therapist and client: The new relationship.* New York: W. H. Freeman & Company.

Gilligan, C. (1982). *In a different voice: Psychological theory and women's development.* Cambridge, MA: Harvard University Press.

Gitlin, M. J. (1990). *The psychotherapist's guide to psychopharmacology* (2nd ed.). New York: The Free Press.

Glanz, M. D. (1989). Cognitive therapy with the elderly. In: *Comprehensive Handbook of Cognitive Therapy* (pp. 467–489). New York: Plenum.

Golden, W. L. (1989). Resistance and change in cognitive-behavior therapy. In W. Dryden & P. Trower (Eds.), *Cognitive psychotherapy: Stasis and change* (pp. 3–13.) New York: Springer.

Goldfarb, A. I. (1955). Psychotherapy of aged persons. *Psychoanalytic Review, 42*, 180–187.

Goldfried, M. (2000). *Integrating affective & relational interventions in cognitive behavior therapy.* Presentation for New Jersey Association of Cognitive Therapists at Kennilworth, NJ, March 5, 2000.

Goldfried, M. R., & Davison, G. (1976). *Clinical behavior theory.* New York: Holt.

Goldfried, M. R. (1980). Toward the delineation of therapeutic change principles. *American Psychologist, 35*, 991–999.

Goldfried, M. R. (1993). Commentary on how the field of psychotherapy can facilitate psychotherapy integration. *Journal of Psychotherapy Integration, 3*, 353–360.

Goldfried, M. R., Greenberg, L., & Marmar, C. (1990). Individual psychotherapy: Process and outcome. *Annual Review of Psychology, 41*, 659–688.

Goldstein, E. G. (1992b). Narcissistic personality disorder. In F. J. Turner (Ed.), *Mental Health and the Elderly.* New York: Free Press.

Goldstein, S. E., & Birnbom, F. (1976). *Hypocondriasis and the elderly.*

Goldstein, G., van Kammen, W., Shelly, C., Miller, D. J., & van Kammen, D. P. (1987). Survivors of imprisonment in the Pacific Theater during World War II. *American Journal of Psychiatry, 144*, 1210–1213.

Goleman, D. (1995). *Emotional intelligence.* New York: Bantam.

Goodman, G. S., Hirschman, J. E., Hepps, D., & Rudy, L. (1991). Children's memory for stressful events. *Merrill-Palmer Quarterly, 37*(1), 109–158.

Goolishian, H., & Anderson, H. (1990). Understanding the therapeutic process: From individuals and families to systems in language. In F. Kaslow (Ed.), *Voices in family psychology.* Newbury Park, CA: Sage.

Goolishian, H. (1990). Therapy as a linguistic system: Hermeneutics, narrative and meaning. *The Family Psychologist, 6*, 44–45.

Gortmaker, S., Eckenrode, J., & Gore, S. (1982). Stress and utilization of health services: A time-series analysis and cross-sectional analysis. *Journal of Health and Social Behavior, 43*, 25–38.

Gould, R. L. (1978). *Transformations: Growth and change in adult life.* New York: Simon and Schuster.

Gray, J. A. (1991). Neural systems, emotion and personality. In J. Madden (Ed.). *Neurobiology of learning, emotion and affect.* New York: Raven.

Gray, J. (1992). *Men are from Mars; women are from Venus.* New York: Harper Collins.

Greeberg, L. S., & Safran, J. D. (1987b). *Emotion in psychotherapy: Affect and cognition in the process of change.* New York: Guilford Press.

Green, B. (1991). Evaluating the effects of disasters. *Psychological Assessment: A Journal of Consulting and Clinical Psychiatry, 3*, 538–546.

Green, B. L. (1994). Psychological research in traumatic stress: an update. *Journal of Traumatic Stress, 7*, 341–362.

Green, B. Epstein, S., Kruptnick, J., & Rowland, J. (1997). Trauma and medical illness: Assessing trauma-related disorders in medical settings. In J. Wilson & T. Keane (Eds.), *Assessing psychological trauma and PTSD* (pp. 160–191). New York: Guilford.

Green, B. L., Lindy, J. D., & Grace, M. C. (1994). Psychological effects of toxic contamination. In R. J. Ursano, B. G. McCaughey, & C. S. Fullerton (Eds.), *Individual and community responses to trauma and disaster* (pp. 154–176). Cambridge: Cambridge University Press.

Green, B. L., Lindy, J. D., & Grace, M. C. (1985). Posttraumatic stress disorder: Toward DSM-IV. *Journal of Nervous and Mental Disease, 173*(7), 406–411.

Green, B. L., Wilson, J. P., & Lindy, J. D. (1985). Conceptualizing PTSD: A psychosocial framework. In C. R. Figley (Ed.), *Trauma and its wake.* NY: Brunner/Mazel.

Greenberg, L. S., & Johnson, S. M. (1988). *Emotionally focused therapy for couples.* New York: Guilford Press.

Greenberg, L. S., & Rhodes, R. H. (1991). Emotion in the change process. In R. C. Curtis & G. Stricker (Eds.), *How people change: Inside and outside therapy* (pp. 39–59). New York: Plenum.

Greenberg, L. S., & Safran, J. D. (1987). *Emotion in psychotherapy.* New York: Guilford Press.

Greenberg, L. S. (1979). Resolving splits: The two-chair techniques. *Psychotherapy: Theory, Research and Practice, 16,* 310–318.

Greenberg, L. S., Rice, L. N., & Elliott, R. (1993). *Facilitating Emotional Change.* New York: Guilford.

Gregg, C. H. (1980). Rehabilitation implications of sexual and reproductive problems in diabetes. *Journal of Applied Rehabilitation Counseling, 11*(2), 76–79.

Griffin, B. P., & Grunes, J. M. (1990). A developmental approach to psychoanalytic psychotherapy with the aged. In R. A. Nemiroff & C. A. Colarusso (Eds.), *New Dimensions in Adult Development* (pp. 267–287). New York: Basic Books.

Grilo, C. M. (1993). An alternative perspective regarding "Non-compliance: What to do?" *the Behavior Therapist, 16*(8), 219–220.

Grossman, F. K., & Moore, R. P. (1994). Against the odds: Resiliency in a adult survivor of childhood sexual abuse. In C. E. Franz & A. J. Stewart (Eds.), *Women creating lives: Identities, resilience, and resistance.* New York: Guilford Press.

Grotjahn, M. D. (1978). Group communication and group therapy with the aged. A promising project. In L. F. Jarvik (Ed.), *Aging to the Twenty-First Century* (pp. 113–121). New York: Gardner Press.

Grove, D. J., & Panzer, B. I. (1991). *Resolving traumatic memories.* New York: Irvington Publishers.

Guidano, V. F. (1991). Affective change events in a cognitive system approach. In J. Safran & L. Greenberg (Eds.), *Emotion, Psychotherapy, & Change* (pp. 50–79). New York: Guilford Press.

Gurian, B., & Miner, J. (1991). Clinical presentation of consulting in the elderly. In C. Salzman & B. Lebowitz (Eds.), *Anxiety in the elderly; Treatment and research* (pp. 31–40). New York: Springer.

Gurin, G., Veroff, J., & Feld, S. (1960). *Americans view their mental health.* New York: Basic Books.

Gurland, B. J. (1984). Personality disorders of old age. In D. W. K. Kay & G. D. Burrows (Eds.), *Handbook of studies on psychiatry and old age.* New York: Elsevier.

Gurvits, T., Lakso, N., Schachter, S., Kuhne, A., Orr, S., & Pitman, R. (1993). Neurological status of Vietnam veterans with chronic posttraumatic stress disorder. *Journal of Neuropsychiatry and Clinical Neurosciences, 5,* 183–188.

Gutman, G. M. (1966). A note on the MMPI: Age and sex differences in extroversion and neuroticism in a Canadian sample. *British Journal Social & Clinical Psychology, 5,* 128–129.

Gutmann, D. (1987). *Reclaimed powers: Toward a new psychology of men and women in later life.* New York: Basic Books.

Gutmann, D. (1990). Psychological development and pathology in later adulthood. In R. A. Nemiroff & C. A. Colarusso (Eds.), *New Dimensions in Adult Development* (pp. 170–185).

Gutmann, D. L. (1980). Psychoanalysis and aging: A developmental view. In S. I. Greenspan & G. H. Pollock (Eds.), *The course of life: Psychoanalytic contributions towards understanding personality development. vo. iii: Adulthood and the aging process* (pp. 489–517). Washington, DC: US Department of Health and Human Services.

Gutmann, D. L. (1987). *Reclaimed Powers: Toward a new psychology of men and women in later life.* New York: Basic Books.

Gynther, M. D. (1979). Aging and personality. In J. N. Butcher (Ed.), *New developments in the use of the MMPI* (pp. 36–68). Minneapolis: University of Minnesota Press.

Hagman, G. (1995). Bereavement and neurosis. *Journal of the Academy of Psychoanalysis, 23,* 635–653.

Haley, W. E. (1996). The medical context of psychotherapy with the elderly. In S. H. Zarit & B. G. Knight (Eds.), *A guide to psychotherapy and aging: Effective clinical interventions in a life-stage context.* Washington, DC: American Psychological Association.

Hall, J. M., Kondora, L. L., 1997. Beyond "True" and "False" Memories: Remembering and Recovery in the Survival of Childhood Sexual Abuse. *Adv Nurs Sci, 19*(4), 37–54.

Halligan, S. L., & Yehuda, R. (2000). Risk factors for PTSD. *PTSD Research Quarterly, 11*(3), 1–3.

Hamera, E. K., & Shontz, F. C. (1987). Perceived positive and negative effects of life-threatening illness. *Journal of Psychosomatic Medicine, 22,* 419–424.

Hammaraberg, M., & Silver, S. (1994). Outcome of treatment for posttraumatic stress disorder in a primary care unit serving Vietnam veterans. *Journal of Traumatic Stress, 7*(2), 195–216.

Hammen, C., Marks, T., Mayol, A., & Demayo, R. (1985). Depressive self-schemas, life stress and vulnerability to depression. *Journal of Abnormal Psychology, 94,* 308–319.

Hankin, C. S., Abueg, F. R., Gallagher-Thompson, D., & Laws, A. (1996). Dimensions of PTSD among older veterans seeking outpatient care: A pilot study. *Journal of Clinical Geropsychology, 2*(4), 239–246.

Hanley-Peterson, P., Futterman, A., Thompson, L., Zeiss, A. M., Gallagher, D., & Ironson, G. (1990). Endogenous depression and psychotherapy outcome in an elderly population [abstract]. *Gerontologist, 30,* 51A.

Hann, N., Millsap, R., & Hartka, E. (1987). As time goes by: Change and stability in personality over fifty years. *Psychology and aging,* 220–232.

Harding, C. M. (1988). Course types in schizophrenia: An analysis of European and American studies. *Schizophrenia Bulletin, 14,* 633–643.

Harding, C. M., Brooks, G. W., Ashikaga, T., Strauss, J. S., & Breier, A. (1987). The Vermont longitudinal study: II. Long-term outcome for subjects who retrospectively met DSM-III criteria for schizophrenia. *American Journal of Psychiatry, 144,* 727–735.

Hare-Mustin, R. (1994). Discourses in the mirrored room: A postmodern analysis of therapy. *Family Process, 33,* 19–35.

Harter, S. (1983). Developmental perspectives on the self-system. In P. H. Mussen (Ed.), *Handbook of child psychology: Vol 4, socialization, personality, and social development* (4th ed.) (pp. 275–386). New York: Wiley.

Harvey, M. (1996). An ecological view of psychological trauma and trauma recovery. *Journal of Traumatic Stress, 9,* 2–24.

Harvey, J., Orbuch, T., Chivalisz, K., & Garwood, G. (1991). Coping with sexual assault: The roles of account making and confiding. *Journal of Traumatic Stress, 4,* 515–532.

Havens, K. (1999). Acute stress disorder. Paper presented at the 52nd annual convention of Gerontological Society of America at San Francisco, November 1999.

Havens, L. (1999). Personality and aging: A psychotherapist reflects late in his own life. In E. Rosowsky, R. C. Abrams, & R. A. Zweig, *Personality disorders in older adults: Emerging issues in diagnosis and treatment* (pp. 17–30). Mahwah, NJ: Lawrence Erlbaum Associates.

Havinghurst, R. J. (1977). Life-style and leisure patterns. In R. A. Kalish (Ed.), *The later years,* Monterey, CA: Brooks/Cole.

Hayes, S. C., Nelson, R. P., & Jarrett, R. B. (1987). The treatment utility of assessment: A functional approach to evaluate assessment quality. *American Psychologist, 42,* 963–974.

Hazan, H. (1988). Course versus cycle: On the understanding of aging. *Journal of Aging Studies, 2*(1), 1–11.

Hazan, C., & Shaver, P. (1990). Love and work: An attachment-theoretical perspective. *Journal of Personality and Social Psychology, 59,* 270–280.

Hebl, J. H., & Enright, R. D. (1993). Forgiveness as a psychotherapeutic goal with elderly females. *Psychotherapy, 30,* 658–667.

Helzer, J. E., Robins, L. N., & McEvoy, L. (1987). Post-traumatic stress disorder in the general population: findings of the epidemiologic catchment area survey. *The New England Journal of Medicine, 317,* 1630–1634.

Hendin, H. (1983). Psychotherapy for Vietnam veterans with PTSD. *American Journal of Psychotherapy, 37,* 86–99.

Hendin, H., Pollinger, A., Singer, P., & Ulman, R. B. (1981). Meaning of combat and the development of posttraumatic stress disorder. *American Journal of Psychiatry, 138,* 1490–1493.

Henry, W. P., Strupp, H. H., Butler, S. F., Schacht, T. E., & Ginder, J. L. (1993). Effects of training in time-limited dynamic psychotherapy: Changes in therapist behavior. *Journal of Consulting and Clinical Psychology, 61,* 434–440.

Herbert, J. D., & Meuser, K. T. (1992). Eye movement desensitization: A critique of the evidence. *Journal of Behavior Therapy and Experimental Psychiatry, 23,* 169–174.

Herman, J. L. (1992a). Complex PTSD: A syndrome in survivors of prolonged and repeated trauma. *Journal of Traumatic Stress, 5,* 377–391.

Herman, J. L. (1993). Sequelae of prolonged and repeated trauma: Evidence for a complex posttraumatic syndrome (DESNOS). In J. R. T. Davidson & E. B. Foa (Eds.), *Posttraumatic stress disorder: DSM-IV and beyond* (pp. 213–228). Washington, DC: American Psychiatric Press.

Hermans, H. (1995). *Self-narratives: The construction of meaning in psychotherapy.* New York: Guilford.

Hermans, H. J. M., & Hermans-Jansen, E. (1995). *Self-narratives: The construction of meaning in psychotherapy.* New York: The Guilford Press.

Hermans, H. J. M., & Kempen, H. J. G. (1993). *The dialogical self: Meaning as movement.* San Diego: Academic Press.

Heron, A., & Chown, S. M. (1967). *Age and function.* London: Churchill.

Hiley-Young, B. (1992). Trauma reactivation assessment and treatment. *Journal of Traumatic Stress, 5*(4), 545–555.

Herzog, C. Overview of skills among the aged. Presentation at The Georgia Consortioum on Aging at Athens, GA, April 1997.

Hilliard, R. B. (1993). Single case methodology in psycho-therapy process and outcome research. *Journal of Consulting and Clinical Psychology, 61*(3), 371–372.

Hobfoll, S., Spielberger, C., Breznitz, S., Figley, C., Folkman, S., Lepper-Green, B., Meichenbaum, D., Milgram, A., Sandler, I., Sarason, I., & van der Kolk, B. (1991). War related stress: Addressing the stress of war and other traumatic events. *American Psychologist, 46,* 848–855.

Hochschild, A. R. (1975). Disengagement theory: A critique and proposal. *American Sociological Review, 40,* 553–569.

Hoffman, L. (1991). Foreword. In T. Andersen (Ed.), *The reflecting team: Dialogues and dialogues about the dialogues* (pp. ix–xiv). New York: Norton.

Holahan, C. K., & Holahan, C. K. (1987). Life stress, hassles and self-efficacy in aging: A replication and extension. *Journal of Applied Social Psychology, 17,* 574–592.

Hollon, S. D. (1996). The efficacy and effectiveness of psychotherapy relative to medications. *American Psychologist, 51*(10), 1025–1030.

Holmbeck, G. N., & Updegrove, A. L. (Spring, 1995). Clinical developmental interface: Implications of developmental research for adolescent psychotherapy. *Psychotherapy, 32.f.*

Holmes, R. H., & Rahe, R. R. (1967). The social Readjustment Rating Scale. *Journal of Psychosomatic Research, 11,* 213–218.

Horowitz, M. J. (1975). Intrusive and repetitive thoughts after experimental stress. *Archives of General Psychiatry, 32,* 1457–1463.

Horowitz, M. J. (1986). *Stress response syndromes.* New York: Jason Aronson.

Horowitz, M., Marmar, C., Krupnick, J., Wilner, N., Kaltreider, N., & Wallerstein, R. (1984). *Personality styles and brief psychotherapy.* New York: Basic Books.

Horowitz, M., Stinson, C., & Fridhandler, B. (1993). Pathological grief: An intensive case study. *Psychiatry Interpersonal and Biological Processes, 56*(4), 56–374.

Horowitz, M. J., & Wilner, N. (1980). *Life events, stress and coping. Aging in the 1980's.* American Psychological Association, Washington, DC.

Horowitz, R., Bonanno, G., & Holen, A. (1993). Pathological grief: Diagnosis and explanation. *Psychosomatic Medicine, 55*(3), 260–273.

Hossack, A., & Bentall, R. P. (1996). Elimination of posttraumatic symptomatology by relaxation and visual-kinesthetic dissociation. *Journal of Traumatic Stress, 8*(1).

Houck, P., George, C., & Kupfer, D. (1995). Complicated grief and bereavement-related depression as distinct disorders: Preliminary empirical validation in elderly bereaved spouses. *American Journal of Psychiatry, 152*(1), 22–30.

Hovens, J. E., van Der Ploeg, H. M., Klaarenbeek, M. T., Bramsen, I., Schreuder, J. H., & Rivero, V. V. (1994). The assessment of posttraumatic stress disorder with the Clinician Administered PTSD Scale: Dutch results. *Journal of Clinical Psychology, 50*(3), 325–336.

Howard, G. (1991). Culture tales: A narrative approach to thinking, cross-cultural psychology, and psychotherapy. *American Psychologist, 46,* 187–197.

Howard, K. I., Brill, P. L., & Lueger, R. J. (1992). (NOTE 1993 IS IN TEXT WHILE 1992 IS ONLY REFERENCE) *Integra outpatient tracking assessment: Psychometric properties.* Radnor, PA: Integra.

Howard, K. I., Orlinsky, D. E., & Lueger, R. J. (1994). *British Journal of Psychiatry, 165,* 4–8.

HUMAN CHANGE PROCESSES: The Scientific Foundations of Psychotherapy. Michael J. Mahoney.

Hussian, R. A. (1981). *Geriatric psychology: A behavioral perspective.* New York: Van Nostrand Reinhold.

Hyer, L., & Associates (1994). *Trauma victim: Theoretical considerations and practical suggestions.* Muncie, IN: Accelerated Development Inc.

Hyer, L., & Brandsma, J. (1997). EMDR minus eye movements equals good psychotherapy. *Journal of Traumatic Stress, 10*(3), 515–523.

Hyer, L., & Stanger, E. (1997). The interaction of posttraumatic stress disorder and depression among older combat veterans. Psychological Reports.

Hyer, L. (1994). *Trauma victim: Theoretical considerations and practical suggestions.* Munice, IN: Accelerated Press, Inc.

Hyer, L. (1994). Treatment outcome study of PTSD among rape trauma victims. National Institute of Mental Health (RO1).

Hyer, L. (1995). Use of EMDR in a "dementing" PTSD survivor. *Clinical Gerontologist, 16,* 70–74.

Hyer, L., & Summers, M. (1995). *An understanding of combat trauma at later life.* VA Merit Review. Augusta, GA.

Hyer, L., Swanson, G., & Lefkowitz, R. (1990). Cognitive schema model with stress groups at later life. *Clinical Gerontologist. Special Issue: Group Therapy in Nursing Homes, 9*(3/4), 145–190.

Hyer, L., Swanson, G., Lefkowitz, R., Hillesland, D., Davis, H., & Woods, M. (1990). The application of the cognitive behavioral model to two older stressor groups. *Clinical Gerontologist, 9*(3/4), 145–190.

Hyer, L. A. The status of psychological treatment with older adults. Presentation at Consortium on Aging, at Athens, GA, April, 1998.

Hyer, L., & Boudewyns, P. (1985). The 8-2 code among Vietnam veterans. *PTSD Newsletter, 4,* 2.

Hyer, L. A., Sohnle, S. J. Nielsen, N. Psychotherapy with older people: CTB versus the alliance. Paper presented at the 53rd Annual Scientific Meeting of the Gerontological Society of America at Washington, DC, November 18, 2000.

Iezzoni, L. I., Restuccia, J. D., Schwartz, M., Schaumburg, D., Coffman, G. A., Kreger, B. E., Buterly, J. R., & Selker, H. (1992). The utility of severity of illness information in assessing the quality of hospital care. The role of the clinical trajectory. *Medical Care, 30,* 428–444.

Jacobowitz, J., & Newton, N. (1990). Time, context, and character: A life-span view of psychopathology during the second half of life. In R. A. Nemiroff & C. A. Colarusso (Eds.), *New Dimensions in Adult Development.* New York: Basic Books:

Jacobowitz, J., & Newton, N. A. (1999). Dynamics and treatment of narcissism in later life. In M. Duffy (Ed.). *Handbook of counseling and psychotherapy with older adults.* New York: John Wiley and Sons.

Jacobson, E. (1964). *Anxiety and tension control*. Philadelphia, PA: J. B. Lippincott.

Jacobson, N. S. (1994). Behavior therapy and psychotherapy integration. *Journal of Psychotherapy Integration, 4*, 105–119.

James, W. (1963). *Psychology*. Greenwich, CT: Fawcett. (Original work published 1892).

Janet, P. (1909). *Les nervoses*. Paris: Flammarion.

Janet, P. (1911). *L'etat mental des hysteriques* (2nd ed.). Paris: Alcan.

Janoff-Bulman, R. (1985). The aftermath of victimization: Rebuilding shattered assumptions. In C. R. Figley (Ed.), *Trauma and its wake, Vol I. The study and treatment of post-traumatic stress disorder* (pp. 15–35). New York: Brunner Mazel.

Janoff-Bulman, R. (1989). Assumptive worlds and the stress of traumatic events: Application of the schema construct. *Social Cognition, 7*, 113–136.

Jenkins, R. (1990). Toward a system of outcome indicators for mental health care. *British Journal of Psychiatry, 157*, 500–514.

Jensen, J. A. (1994). An investigation of Eye Movement Desensitization and Reprocessing (EMD/R) as a treatment for posttraumatic stress disorder (PTSD) symptoms of Vietnam combat veterans. *Behavior Therapy, 25*, 311–325.

Jensen, M. P., Turner, J. A., Romano, J. M., & Karoly, P. (1991). Coping with chronic pain: A critical review of the literature. *Pain, 47*(3), 249–253.

Jeste, D., Alexopoulos, G., Bartels, S., Jeffrey, L., Cummings, J., Gallo, J., Gotlieb, G., Halpain, M., Palmer, B., Patterson, T., Reynolds, C., & Lebowitz, B. (1999). Consensus statement on the upcoming crisis in geriatric mental health. *Archives of General Psychiatry, 56*, 848–854.

Johnson, F. (1991). Psychotherapy of the elderly anxious patient. In C. Saltzman & B. Lebowitz (Eds.), *Anxiety in the elderly: Treatment and research* (pp. 215–248). New York: Springer.

Johnson, D., Feldman, S., Southwick, S., & Charney, D. (1994). The concept of the second generation program in the treatment of post-traumatic stress disorder among Vietnam veterans. *Journal of Traumatic Stress, 7*(2), 217–236.

Joint Commission on Accreditation of Healthcare Organizations (1991). *An introduction to quality improvement in health care*. Oakbrook Terrace, IL.

Jongedijk, R. A., Carlier, I. V. E., Schreuder, Bas, J. N., & Gersons, Berthold P. R. (1996). Complex Posttraumatic Stress Disorder: An Exploratory Investigation of PTSD and DES NOS Among Dutch War Veterans. *Journal of Traumatic Stress, 9*(3).

Joseph, S., Williams, R., & Yule, W. (1995). Psychosocial perspectives on post-traumatic stress disorder. *Clinical Psychology Review, 15*, 515–544.

Jung, C. G. (1959). Mandalas. *In Collected works, Vol. 9, Part 1*. Princeton: Princeton University Press.

Jung, C. G. (1971). "The Stages of Life." In the Portable Jung. New York: Viking Press.

Juran, J. M. (1988). *Juran on planning for quality*. New York: Free Press.

Kagan, J. (1980). Perspectives on continuity. In O. G. Brim, Jr., & J. Kagan (Eds.), *Constancy and change in human development* (pp. 26–74). Cambridge, MA: Harvard University Press.

Kahana, R. J., & Bibring, F. L. (1964). Personality types in medical management. In N. E. Zimberg (Ed.), *Psychiatry and medical practice in a general hospital*. New York: International Universities Press.

Kahn, M. (1991). Between therapist and client: The new relationship. New York: W. H. Freeman and Company.

Kleinknecht, R. A., & Morgan, M. P. (1992). Treatment of posttraumatic stress disorder with eye movement desensitization and reprocessing. *Journal of Behavior Therapy and Experimental Psychiatry, 23*, 43–49.

Kaiser, R. T., & Ozer, D. J. (1996). *The structure of personal goals and their relation to personality traits*. Manuscript submitted for publication.

Kalson, L. (19??). Chapter 5 Group therapy with the aged.

Kanter, F. H., & Schefft, K. K. (1988). *Guiding the process of therapeutic change*. Champaign, IL: Research Press.

Karasu, T. B. (1986). The specificity versus nonspecificity dilemma: Toward identifying therapeutic change agents. *American Journal of Psychiatry 143*, 687–695.

Kastenbaum, R. (1985). Dying and death: A life-span approach. The psychological construction of the life span. In J. E. Birren & K. W. Shaie, *Handbook of psychology and aging* (pp. 594–618). New York: Van Nostrand Reinhold.

Kastenbaum, R. (1987). Prevention of age-related problems. In L. L. Carstensen & B. A. Edelstein (Eds.), *Handbook of Clinical Gerontology* (pp. 322–334). New York: Pergamon Press.

Kastenbaum, R. J. (1978). Personality theory, therapeutic approaches, and the elderly client. In M. Storandt, I. C. Siegler, & M. F. Elias (Eds.), *The clinical psychology of aging*. New York: Plenum Press.

Kaszniak, A. W. (1996). Techniques and instruments for assessment of the elderly. In S. H. Zarit & B. G. Knight (Eds.), *A guide to psychotherapy and aging* (pp. 163–219). Washington, DC: American Psychological Association.

Katzman, R., & Rowe, J. W. (Eds.) (1992). *Principles of geriatric neurology*. Philadelphia: F. A. Davis.

Kaufman, S. R. (1986). *The Ageless Self: Sources of Meaning in Later Life*. Madison, WI: University of Wisconsin Press.

Keane, T. A., & Kaloupek, D. G. (1982). Brief Reports. Imaginal flooding in the treatment of Posttraumatic Stress Disorder. *Journal of Consulting and Clinical Psychology, 50*, 138–140.

Keane, T. M., Fairbank, J. A., Caddell, J. M., & Zimering, R. T. (1989). Implosive (flooding) therapy reduces symptoms of PTSD in Vietnam combat veterans. *Behavior Therapy, 20*, 245–260.

Keane, T. M., & Kolb, L. C. (1988). A psychological study of chronic PTSD in Vietnam veterans. VA Cooperative Study.

Keane, T., & Wolfe, J. (1990). Comorbidity in posttraumatic stress disorder: an analysis of community and clinical studies. *Journal of Applied Social Psychology, 20*, 1776–1788.

Kegan, R. (1983). *The evolving self*. Cambridge: Harvard University Press.

Keller, M. B., Lavori, P. W., Mueller, T. I., Endicott, J., Coryell, W., Hirschfeld, R. M. A., & Shea, T. (1992). Time to recovery, chronicity, and levels of psychopathology in major depression: A 5-year prospective follow-up of 431 subjects. *Archives of General Psychiatry, 49*, 809–816.

Kelly, G. (1963). *A theory of personality*. New York: Norton.

Kelly, G. A. (1955). *The psychology of personal constructs*. New York: Norton.

Kelly, G. A. (1969). The psychotherapeutic relationship. In B. Maher (Ed.), *Clinical psychology and personality: The selected papers of George Kelly* (pp. 216–223). New York: Wiley.

Kendall, P. C., & Southam-Gerow, M. A. pg 706. Beutler, L. E. (1991). Selective treatment matching: Systematic eclectic psychotherapy. *Psychotherapy, 28*, 457–462.

Kenrick, D. T., & Funder, D. C. (1988). Profiting from controversy: Lessons from the person-situation debate. *American Psychologist, 43*, 23–34.

Kessler, R. C., Sonnega, A. Bromet, E., Hughes, M., & Nelson, C. B. (1995). Posttraumatic stress disorder in the National Comorbidity Survey. *Archives of General Psychiatry, 52*, 1048–1060.

Kiecolt-Glasser, J., Dura, J. R., Speicher, C. E., Trask, O. J., & Glaser, R. (1991). Spousal caregivers of dementia victims: Longitudinal changes in immunity and health. *Psychosomatic Medicine, 53*, 345–362.

Kiecolt-Glaser, J. K., & Glaser, R. (1991). Stress and immune functions in humans. In R. Adler, D. L. Felton, & N. Cohen (Eds.), *KPsychoneuroimmunology, 2nd ed.* (pp. 175–189). San Diego, CA: Academic Press.

Kiesler, D. J. (1966). Some myths of psychotherapy research and the search for a paradigm. *Psychological Bulletin, 65*, 110–136.

Kilpatrick, D., & Resnick, H. (1992). PTSD associated with exposure to criminal victimization in clinical and community populations. In J. Davidson & E. Foa (Eds.), *Post-traumatic stress disorder in review: Recent research and future directions*. Washington, DC: American Psychiatric Press.

Kilpatrick, D. G., Resnick, H. S., Freedy, J. R., Pelcovitz, D., Resick, P., Roth, S., & van der Kolk, B. (1994). The posttraumatic stress disorder field trial: emphasis on criterion A and overall PTSD diagnosis. In T. A. Widiger (Ed.), *DSM-IV sourcebook*, (Vol. 5). Washington, DC: American Psychiatric Press.

Kilpatrick, D., Saunders, B., Veronen, L., Best, C., & Von, J. (1987). Criminal victimization: Lifetime prevalence, reporting to police, and psychological impact. Paper presented at the meeting of the Association for the Advancement of Behavior Therapy, Boston, MA.

Kilpatrick, D. G., & Veronen, L. J. (1983). Treatment for rape-related problems: Crisis intervention is not enough. In L. H. Cohen, W. L. Claiborn, & G. A. Specter (Eds.), *Crisis intervention.* New York: Human Sciences Press.

Kitchell, M. A., Barnes, R. F., Veith, R. C., Okimoto, J. T., Raskind, M. A. (1982). Screening for depression in hospitalized geriatric medical patients. *Journal of the American Geriatrics Society, 30,* 174–177.

Kleinman, A. (1988). *The illness narratives.* New York: Basic Books.

Klerman, G. L., Weissman, M. M., Rounsaville, B. J., & Chevron, E. S. (1984). *Interpersonal psychotherapy for depression.* New York: Basic Books.

Klerman, G. L., & Weissman, M. M. (1993). *New applications of interpersonal therapy.* Washington, DC: American Psychiatric Press.

Kluckhohn, C., & Murray, H. A. (1953). Personality formation: The determinants. In C. Kluckhohn, H. A. Murray, & D. M. Schneider (Eds.), *Personality in nature, society, and culture* (pp. 53–67). New York: Knopf.

Knight, B. G. (1996). *Psychotherapy with older adults* (2nd ed.). Newbury Park, CA: Sage.

Knight, B. G., Teri, L., Wohlford, P., & Santos, J. (1995). *Mental Health Services for Older Adults.* American Psychiatric Association.

Knight, B. (1986) *Psychotherapy with older adults.* London: Sage Publications.

Knight, J. (1997). Neuropsychological assessment in postratumatic stress disorder. In J. Wilson and T. Keane (Eds.), *Assessing psychological trauma and PTSD* (448–492). New York: Guilford Press.

Kobasa, S. C. (1979). Stressful life events, personality, and health: An inquiry into hardiness. *Journal of Personality and Social Psychology, 37,* 1–11.

Kogan, N. (1990). Personality and aging. In: *Handbook of the Psychology of Aging* (pp. 330–346). J. E. Birren & K. W. Schaie (Eds.). San Diego, CA: Academic Press.

Kohut, H. (1984). *How does analysis cure?* Chicago, IL: University of Chicago Press.

Kolhberg, I. (1973). The claim to moral adequacy of a highest stage of moral development. *Journal of Philosophy, 70,* 630–646.

Kopta, S. M., Howard, K. I., Lowry, J. L., & Beutler, L. E. (1994). Patterns of symptomatic recovery in psychotherapy. *Journal of Consulting and Clinical Psychology, 62,* 1009–1016.

Kordy, H. (1995). Does psychotherapy research answer the questions of practitioners, and should it? *Psychotherapy Research, 5*(2), 128–130.

Kotre, J. (1995). *White gloves: How we create ourselves through memory.* New York: The Free Press.

Kovach, C. (1990). Promise and problems in reminiscence research. *Journal of Gerontological Nursing, 16*(4), 10–14.

KRANTZ ET AL. (1987) NOT IN REFERENCES

Krinsley, K. E., & Weathers, F. W. (Summer, 1995). The assessment of trauma in adults. *PTSD Research Quarterly, 6*(3), 1–3.

Krivenko, C. A., & Chodroff, C. (1994). The analysis of clinical outcomes: Getting started in benchmarking. *Journal of Quality Improvement, 20,* 260–266.

Kroessler, D. (1990). Personality disorder in the elderly. *Hospital Community Psychiatry, 41,* 1325–1329.

Krohne, H. W. (1990). Personality as a mediator between objective events and their subjective representation. *Psychological Inquiry, 1,* 26–19.

Kruse, A. (1987). Coping with chronic disease, dying and death. A contribution to competence in old age. *Comparative Gerontology, 1,* 1–11.

Krystal, H. (1968). *Massive psychit trauma.* New York: International Universities Press.

Kubany, E. (1994). A cognitive model of guilt typology in combat-relalated PTSD. *Journal of Traumatic Stress, 7*(1), 3–19.

Kulka, R. A., Schlenger, W. E., Fairbank, J. A., Hough, R. L., Jordan, B. K., Hough, R. L., Marmar, C. R., & Weiss, D. S. (1990). *Trauma and the Vietnam War generation.* Brunner/Mazel: New York.

Kundera, M. (1984). *The unbearable lightness of being.* New York: Harper & Row.

Kunik, M. E., Mulsant, B. H., Rifai, A. H., Sweet, R. A., Pasternak, R., Rosen, J., & Zubenko, G. S. (1993). Personality disorders in elderly inpatients with major depression. *American Journal of Geriatric Psychiatry, 1,* 38–45.

Kunik, M. E., Mulsant, B. H., Rifal, A. H., Sweet, R. A., Pasternak, R., & Zubenko, G. S. (1994). Diagnostic rate of comorbid personality disorder in elderly psychiatric inpatients. *American Journal of Psychiatry, 151,* 603–605.

Kuypers, J. A. (1974). Ego functioning in old age: Early adult life antecedents. *International Journal of Againg and Human Development, 5,* 157–178.

Kwentus, J. A., Harkins, S. W., Lignon, N., & Silverman, J. J. (1985). Current concepts of geriatric pain and its treatment. *Geriatrics, 40*(4), 48–57.

Labouvie-Vief, G. (1982a). Dynamic development and mature autonomy. *Human Development, 25,* 161–191.

Labouvie-Vief, G. (1982b). Growth and aging in life-span perspective. *Human Development, 25,* 65–78.

Labouvie-Vief, G., DeVoe, M., & Bulka, D. (1989). Speaking about feeelings: Conceptions of emotion across the life span. *Psychology and Aging, 4,* 425–437.

Lam, J. N., & Grossman, F. K. (1997). Resiliency and adult adaptation in women with and without self-reported histories of childhood sexual abuse. *Journal of Traumatic Stress, 10*(2).

Landau, R., & Litwin, H. (2000). The effects of extreme early stress in very old age. *Journal of Traumatic Stress, 13*(3), 473–488.

Larson, R. (1978). Thirty years of research on the subjective well-being of older Americans. *Journal of Gerontology, 33,* 109–125.

LaRue, A. (1992). *Aging and neuropsychological assessment.* New York: Plenum Press.

Lauterbach, D., & Vrana, S. (1996). Three studies on the reliability and validity of a self-report measure of posttraumatic stress disorder. *Assessment, 3,* 17–25.

Lawrence, J., & Mace, J. (1992). *Remembering in Groups: Ideas from Reminiscence and Literacy Work.* London: Oral History Society.

Lawton, M. P., Kleban, M. H., & Dean, J. (1993). Affect and age: Cross-sectional comparisons of structure and prevalence. *Psychology and Aging, 8,* 165–175.

Lawton, M. P., Kleban, M. H., Rajagopal, D., & Dean, J. (1992). Dimensions of affective experience in three age groups. *Psychology of Aging, 7,* 171–184.

Layden, M. A., Newman, C. F., Freeman, A., & Morse, S. B. (1993). *Cognitive therapy of borderline personality disorder.* Boston: Allyn and Bacon.

Lazarus, A. The use of imagery in psychotherapy. Presentation to New Jersey Association of Cognitive Therapists at Garwood, NJ, September 24, 2000.

Lazarus, R. S., & Delongis, A. (1983). Psychological stress and coping in aging. *American Psychologist, 38,* 245–254.

Lazarus, R. S., & Folkman, S. (1984). *Stress, appraisal, and coping.* New York: Springer.

Lazarus, R. S., & Folkman S. (1989). *Manual for the study of daily hassles.* Palo Alto, CA: Consulting Psychologists Press.

Lazarus, R. S. (1984). Puzzles in the study of daily hassles. *Journal of Behavioral Medicine, 7,* 375–389.

Lazarus, R. S. (1990). Theory-based stress measurement. *Psychological Inquiry, 1,* 3–13.

Leads, A. Resource installation in EMDR. Workshop presented in Westfield, NJ, October 15, 1999.

LeDoux, J. E. (1992). Emotion as memory: Anatomical systems underlying indelible neural traces. In S. A. Christianson (Ed.), *Handbook of emotion and memory.* Hillsdale, NJ: Erlbaum.

Lee, K. A., Vaillant, G. E., Torrey, W. C., & Elder, G. H. (1995). A 50-year prospective study of the psychological sequelae of World War II combat. *American Journal of Psychiatry, 152,* 516–522.

Leebov, W., & Ersoz, C. J. (1991). *The health care manager's guide to continuous quality improvement.* Chicago: American Hospital Publishing.

Lehman, D. R., Davis, C. G., Delongis, A., Wortman, C., Bluck, S., Mandel, D. R., & Ellard, J. H. (1993). Positive and negative life changes following bereavement and their relations to adjustment. *Journal of Social and Clinical Psychology, 12,* 90–112.

Leitenberg, H., Greenwalk, E., & Cado, S. (1992). A retrospective study of long-term methods of coping with having been sexually abused during childhood. *Child Abuse and Neglect: The International Journal, 16,* 399–407.

Leon, G. R., Gillum B., Gillum, R., & Gouze, M. (1979). Personality Stability and Change over a 3 year period middle age to old age. *Journal of Consulting and Clinical Psychology, 47,* 517–524.

Lepore, S., Silver, R., & Wortman, C. (1996). Social constraints, intrusive thoughts, and depressive symptoms among bereaved mothers. *Journal of Personality and Social Psychology, 70*(2), 271–282.

Levanthal, H. (1982). The integration of emotion and cognitions: A view from the perceptual-motor theory of emotion. In M. S. Clark & S. T. Fiske (Eds.), *Affect and Cognition.* Hillsdale, NJ: Lawrence Erlbaum.

Levenson, H. (1995). *Time-limited dynamic psychotherapy,* New York: Basic.

Levenson, R. W., Carstensen, L. L., Friesen, W. V., & Ekman, P. (1991). Emotion, physiology, and expression in old age. *Psychology and Aging, 6,* 28–35.

Leventhal, H., Leventhal, E. A., & Schaefer, P. M. (1992). Vigilant coping and health behavior. In M. G. Ory, R. P. Abeles, & P. D. Lipman (Eds.), *Aging, health, and behavior.* Newbury Park, CA: Sage.

Leventhan, H. (1999). *Role of health factors in psychological assessment.* Invited address, University of Medicine and Dentistry of New Jersey, Robert Wood Johnson Medical School.

Levin, C., Grainger, R., Allen-Byrd, L., & Fulcher, G. (1994, August). Efficacy of eye movement desensitization and reprocessing for survivors of Hurricane Andrew: A comparative study. Paper presented at the 102nd annual meeting of the American Psychological Association, Los Angeles, CA.

Levin, S. (1977). Normal psychology of the aging process, revisited–II: Introduction. *Journal of Geriatric Psychiatry, 10,* 3–17.

Levinson, D. J. (1978). *The seasons of a man's life.* New York: Knopf.

Levy, S. M., Derogatis, L. R., Gallagher, D., & Gatz, M. (1985). *Intervention with older adults and the evaluation of outcome.*

Lewinsohn, P. M. (1974). A behavioral approach to depression. In R. Friedman & M. Katz (Eds.), *The psychology of depression.* New York: John Wiley.

Lewinsohn, P. M., Biglan, A., & Zeiss, A. (1979). Behavioral treatment of depression. In P. Davidson (Ed.), *Behavioral management of anxiety, depression, and pain* (pp. 91–146). New York: Brunner/Mazel.

Lewinsohn, P. M., Munoz, R. F., Youngren, M. A., & Zeiss, A. M. (1978). *Control your depression.* Englewood Cliffs, NJ: Prentice Hall.

Lewis, C. N. (1973). The adaptive value of reminiscence in old age. *Journal of Geriatric Psychiatry, 6*(1): 117–21.

Lewis, M. I., & Butler, R. N. (1974). Life-review therapy: Putting memories to work in individual and group psychotherapy. *Geriatrics, 29,* 165–173.

Lezak, M. D. (1995). *Neuropsychological assessment* (3rd ed.). Baltimore: Johns Hopkins University Press.

Lichstein, K. L., & Johnson, R. S. (1993). Relaxation for insomnia and hypnotic medication use in older women. *Psychology and Aging, 8,* 103–111.

Lieberman, M. A., & Gourash, N. (1979). Evaluating the effects of change groups on the elderly. *International Journal of Group Psychotherapy, 29,* 283–304.

Lieberman, M. A., & Tobin, S. S. (1983). *The experience of old age: Stress, coping and survival.* New York: Basic Books.

Lifton, J. (1993). From Hiroshima to the Nazi doctors: The evolution of Psychoformative approaches to understanding traumatic stress syndromes. In J. P. Wilson & B. Raphael (Eds.), *International handbook of traumatic stress syndromes* (pp. 11–23). New York: Plenum Press.

Lifton, R. (1992). *Home from the Vietnam war: Learning from Vietnam veterans.* Boston: Beacon Press.

Lindenberger, U., & Baltes, P. B. (1994). Sensory functioning and intelligence in old age: A strong connection. *Psychology and Aging, 6,* 416–425.

Lindsay, D. S., & Read, J. D. (1994). Psychotherapy and memories of childhood sexual abuse: A cognitive perspective. *Applied Cognitive Psychology, 8,* 281–338.

Linehan, M. M. (1993). *Cognitive-behavioral treatment of borderline personality disorders*. New York: Guilford.

Lingiardi, V., Madeddu, F., Fossati, A, & Maffei, C. (1994). Reliability and validity of the Personality Functioning Scale (PFS). *Journal of Personality Disorders, 8*, 111–120.

Lipchik, E. (1988). *Interviewing with a constructive ear*. Dulwich Centre Newsletter, Winter, 3–7.

Lipchick, E., & de Shzer, S. (1986). The purposeful interview. *Journal of Strategic and Systemic Therapies, 5*(1), 88–99.

Lipke, H. (1995). EMDR Clinician Survey. In F. Shapiro (Ed.), *Eye Movement Desensitization and Reprocessing* (pp. 376–386). The Guilford Press, NY.

Lipkin, J. O., Scurfield, R. M., & Blank, A. S. (1983). Post-traumatic stress disorder in Vietnam veterans: Assessment in forensic setting. *Behavioral Sciences and the Law, 1*, 51–67.

Litz, B. T., & Keane, T. M. (1989). Information processing in anxiety disorders: Application to the understanding of post-traumatic stress disorder. *Clinical Psychology Review, 9*, 243–257.

Litz, B. T., Weathers, F. W., Monaco, V., Herman, D. S., Wulfsohn, M., Marx, B., & Keane, T. M. (1996). Attention, Arousal, and Memory in Postrraumatic Stress Disorder. *Journal of Traumatic Stress, 9*(3).

Lockwood, K. A., Alexopoulos, G. S., Kakuma, T., & Van Gorp, W. G. (2000). Subtypes of cognitive impairment in depressed older adults. *American Journal of Geriatric Psychiatry, 8*(3), 201–208.

Loebel, J. P. (1990). Completed suicide in the elderly. In Abstracts of the Third Annual Meeting and Symposium, American Association for Geriatric Psychiatry, San Diego, CA.

Loevinger, J. (1976). *Ego development*. San Francisco: Jossey-Bass.

Loftus, E. F., & Davies, G. M. (1984). Distortions in the memory of children. *Journal of Social Issues, 40*, 51–67.

Logsdon, R. G. (1995). Psychopathology and treatment: Curriculum and research needs. In B. G. Knight, L. Terri, P. Wohlford, & J. Santos (Eds.), *Mental health services for older adults: Implications for training and practice in geropsychology* (pp. 41–51).

Lohr, J, Klienknecht, R., Tolin, D., & Barrett, R. (1995). The empirical status of the clinical application of eye movement desensitization and reprocessing. *Journal of Behavior Therapy and Experimental Psychiatry, 25*, 285–302.

Lohr, J. M., Kleinknecht, R. A., Conley, A. T., Cerro, S. D., Schmidt, J., & Sonntag, M. (1992). A methodological critique of the current status of eye movement desensitization. *Journal of Behavior Therapy and Experimental Psychiatry, 23*, 159–167.

Lopata, H. Z. (1973). Self-identity in marriage and widowhood. *Sociological Quarterly, 14*, 407–418.

Loranger, A. W., Susman, V. L., Oldham, J. M., & Russakoff, L. M. (1987). The personality disorder examination: A preliminary report. *Journal of Personality Disorders, 1*, 1–13.

Lowenthal, M. F., Thurnher, M., & Chiriboga, D. (1975). *Four stages of life*. San Francisco: Jossey-Bass.

Luborsky, L., & Crits-Christoph, P. (1991). *Understanding transference: The core conflictual relationship theme method*. New York: Basic.

Luborsky, L., Mark, D., Hole, A., Popp, C., Goldsmith, B., & Cacciola, J. (1995). Supportive-expressive dynamic psychotherapy of depression: A time-limited version. In J. P. Barber, & P. Crits-Christoph, *Dynamic therapies for psychiatric disorders: Axis I*. New York: Basic Books.

Lyddon, W. J., & Alford, D. J. (1993). Constructivist assessment: A developmental-epistemic perspective. In G. J. Neimeyer (Ed.), *Constructivist assessment: A casebook* (pp. 31–57). Newbury Park, CA: Sage.

Lyness, J. M., Caine, E. D., Conwell, Y., King, D. A., & Cox, C. (1993). Depressive symptoms, medical illness, and functional status in depressed psychiatric patients. *American Journal of Psychiatry, 150*, 910–915.

Lyons, J. A. (1991). Strategies for assessing the potential for positive adjustment following trauma. *Journal of Traumatic Stress, 4*, 93–112.

Maas, H. S., & Kuypers, J. A. (1974). *From thirty to seventy*. San Francisco: Jossey-Bass.

MacIntyre, A. (1984). *After virtue*. Notre Dame, IN: University of Notre Dame Press.

Maddox, G. L. (1976). Scope, concepts and methods in the study of aging. In R. Binstock & E. Shanas (Eds.), *Handbook of aging and the social sciences* (pp. 3–34). New York: Van Nostrand Reinhold.

Magai, C., & Cohen, C. I. (1998). Attachment style and emotion regulation in dementia patients and their relation to caregiver burden. *Journal of Gerontology: Psychological Sciences, 53b*(3), 147–154.

Magni, G. (1987). On the relationship between chronic pain and depression when there is no organic lesion. *Pain, 31*(1), 1–21.

Mahoney, M. J. (1991). *Human change processes.* Basic Books, New York, NY.

Mahoney, M. J. (1991). *Human change processes: The scientific foundations of psychotherapy.* New York: Basic Books, Inc.

Malatesta, C. Z., & Kalnok, M. (1984). Emotional experience in younger and older adults. *Journal of Gerontology, 39,* 301–308.

Malinak, D. P., Hoyt, M. F., & Patterson, V. (1979). Adults' reactions to the death of a parent. *American Journal of Psychiatry, 136,* 1152–1156.

Malt, U. F. (1988). The long term consequences of accidental injury. *British Journal of Psychiatry, 153,* 810–818.

Marengo, J., Harrow, M., Sands, J., & Galloway, C. (1991). European versus U.S. data on the course of schizophrenia. *American Journal of Psychiatry, 148,* 606–611.

Marin, R. S. (1997). Apathy-who cares?: An introduction to apathy and related disorders of diminished motivation. *Psychiatric Annals, 27,* 18–23.

Markus, H., & Nurius, P. (1986). Possible selves. *American Psychologist, 41,* 954–969.

Markus, H. R., & Herzog, A. R. (1991). The role of the self concept in aging. *Annual Review of Gerontology and Geriatrics, 11,* 110–143.

Marmar, C. R., Gaston, L., Gallagher, D., & Thompson, L. W. (1989). Alliance and outcome in late-life depression. *Journal of Nervous and Mental Disease, 177,* 464–472.

Marmar, C. R., Weiss, D. S., Metzler, T. J., & Delucchi, K. (1996). Characteristics of emergency services personnel related to peritraumatic dissociation during critical incident exposure. *American Journal of Psychiatry, 153,* 94–102.

Marmar, C. R., Weiss, D. S., & Metzler, T. J. (1997). The peritraumatic dissociative experiences questionnaire. In J. P. Wilson & T. M. Keane (Eds.), *Assessing psychological trauma and PTSD.* New York: Guilford.

Marmor, J. (1986). The corrective emotional experience revisited. *International Journal of Short-Term Psychotherapy, 1,* 43–47.

Marshall, R. D., Stein, D. J., Liebowitz, M. R., & Yehuda, R. (1996). A pharmacotherapy algorithm in the treatment of posttraumatic stress disorder. *Psychiatric Annals, 26*(4), 217–225.

Marwit, S. (1991). DSM-III grief reactions and a call for revisions. *Professional Psychology and Research, 22*(1), 75–79.

Mason, J., Giller, E., Kosten, T., & Wahby, V. (1990). Serum testosterone levels in posttraumatic stress disorder inpatients. *Journal of Traumatic Stress., 3,* 449–457.

Matsakis, A. (1994). *Post-traumatic stress disorder: A complete treatment guide.* Oakland, CA: New Harbinger.

Matt, D. A., Sementilli, M. E., & Burish, T. G. (1988). Denial as a strategy for coping with cancer. *Journal of Mental Health Counseling, 10*(2), 136–144.

Matt, G. E., Dean, A., & Wood, P. (1991). Identifying clinical syndromes in a community sample of elderly persons. *Psychological Assessment, 4,* 174–184.

Maughan, B., & Rutter, M. (1997). Retrospective reporting of childhood and adult psychopathology. *Journal of Personality Disorders, 11,* 19–33.

Mayou, R. Bryant, B., & Duthie, R. (1993). Psychiatric consequences of road traffic accidents. *British Medical Journal, 307,* 647–651.

Mazor, A., Gampel, Y., Enright, R. D., & Orenstein, R. (1990). Holocaust survivors: Coping with post-traumatic memories in childhood and 40 years later. *Journal of Traumatic Stress, 3,* 1–14.

McAdams, D. P. (1985). *Power, intimacy and the life story: Personological inquiries into identity.* New York: Guilford Press.

McAdams, D. P. (1987). A life-story model of identity. In R. Hogan & W. Jones (Eds.), *Perspectives in personality: 2.* Greenwich, CT: JAI Press.

McAdams, D. P. (1990). Unity and purpose in human lives: The emergency of identity as a life story. In I. Rabin, R. Zucker, R. Emmons, & S. Frank (Eds.), *Studying person and lives* (pp. 148–200). New York: Springer.

McAdams, D. P. (1993). *The stories we live by: Personal myths and the making of the self.* New York: Guilford.

McAdams, D. P. (1996). Personality, modernity, and the storied self: A contemporary framework for studying persons. *Psychological Inquiry, 7*(4), 295–321.

McCann, I., & Pearlman (1990). *Psychological Trauma and the Adult Survivor: Theory, Therapy and Transformation.* New York: Brunner/Mazel.

McCarthy, P., Katz, I., & Foa, E. (1991). Cognitive-behavioral treatment of anxiety in the elderly: A proposal model. In C. Saltzman & B. Lebowitz (Eds.), *Anxiety in the elderly: Treatment and research* (pp. 197–214). New York: Springer.

McClanahan, L. E., & Risley, T. R. (1974). Design of living environments for nursing home residents: Recruiting attendance at activities. *The Gerontologist, 14,* 236–240.

McClelland, D. C. (1981). *Is Personality Consistent? In Further Explorations in Personality.* New York: Little, Brown.

McCormick, R. A., Taber, J., & Kruedelbach, N. (1989). The relationship between attributional style and post traumatic stress disorder in addicted patients. *Journal of Traumatic Stress, 2,* 477–487.

McCrae, R. R., & Costa, P. T., Jr. (1986). Personality, coping and coping effectiveness in an adult sample. *Journal of Personality, 54,* 385–405.

McCrae, R. R. (1987). Neuroticism. In G. I. Maddox (Ed.), *Encyclopedia of Aging* (pp. 482–483). New York: Springer.

McCrae, R. R., & Costa, P. T., Jr. (1990). *Personality in adulthood.* NY: Guilford Press.

McCranie, E., Hyer, L., Boudewyns, P., & Woods, M. (1991). Negative parenting, combat exposure, and PTSD symptom severity: Test of a person/event interaction model. *Journal of Nervous and Mental Disease, 180,* 431–438.

McCranie, E., Hyer, L., Boudewyns, P., & Woods, M. (1991). Negative parenting, combat exposure, and PTSD symptom severity: Test of a person/event interaction model. *Journal of Nervous and Mental Disease.*

McCranie, E., Hyer, L., Woods, M., & Boudewyns, P. (1992). Negative parenting behavior, combat exposure and PTSD symptom severity: Test of person/event interaction model. *Journal of Nervous Disorder and Mental Disease.*

McCranie, E. W., & Hyer, L. A. (in press). *Self-critical depressive experience in Posttraumatic Stress Disorder.* Psychological Reports.

McCullough, M. E., & Worthington, E. L. (1994). Encouraging clients to forgive people who have hurt them: Review, critique, and research perspective. *Journal of Psychology and Theology, 22,* 3–20.

McFarlane, A. (1990). Vulnerability to posttraumatic stress disorder. In M. Wolf & A. Mosnaim (Eds.), *Posttraumatic stress disorder: Etiology, phenomenology, and treatment* (pp. 2–21). Washington, DC: American Psychiatric Press.

McFarlane, A. C. (1992). Avoidance and intrusion in posttraumatic stress disorder. *Journal of Nervous and Mental Disease, 180*(7), 439–445.

McFarlane, A. C., & Yehuda, R. (1996). Resilience, vulnerability, and the course of posttraumatic reactions. In B. A. van der Kolk, A. C. McFarlane, & L. Weisaeth (Eds.), *Traumatic Stress: The effects of overwhelming experience on mind, body, and society* (pp. 155–181). New York: The Guilford Press.

McNally, R. J. (1993). Self-representation in post-traumatic stress disorder: A cognitive perspective. In Segal, Z. V., & Blatt, S. J. (Eds.), *The self in emotional distress: Cognitive and psychodynamic perspectives* (pp. 71–91). New York: Guilford Press.

McNally, R. J., Kaspi, S. P., Reimann, B. C, & Zeitlin, S. B. (1990). Selective processing of threat cues in post-traumatic stress disorder. *Journal of Abnormal Psychology, 99,* 398–402.

McNally, R. J., Lasko, N. B., Macklin, M. L., Pitman, R. K. (1995). Autobiographical memory disturbance in combat-related posttraumatic stress disorder. *Behav. Res. Ther., 33*(6), 619–630.

Mehlman, R. D. (1977). Normal psychology of the aging process, revisited–II: Discussion. *Journal of Geriatric Psychiatry, 10,* 53–60.

Meichenbaum, D. (1985). *Stress Inoculation Training.* New York: Pergamon Press.

Meichenbaum, D., & Frizpatrick, D. (1991). A constructivist narrative perspective of stress and coping: Stress inoculation applications. In L. Goldberger & S. Breznitz (Eds.), *Handbook of stress.* New York: Free Press.

Meiselman, K. C. (1990). *Resolving the trauma of incest: Reintegration therapy with survivors.* San Francisco: Josse-Bass.

Melges, F. T. (1982). *Time and the inner future: A temporal approach to psychiatric disorders.* John Wiley and Sons.

Mellman, T. A., Randolph, C. A., Brawman-Mintzer, O., Flores, L. P., & Milanes, F. J. (1992). Phenomenology and course of psychiatric disorders associated with combat-related post-traumatic stress disorder. *American Journal of Psychiatry, 149,* 1568–1574.

Merleau-Ponty, M. (1964a). *The Primacy of Perception.* Evanston, IL: Northwestern University Press.

Messick, S. (1995). Validity of Psychological Assessment: Validation of inferences from persons' responses and performances as scientific inquiry into score meaning. *American Psychologist, 50*(9), 741–749.

Mezzich, T. E., Fabrega, H., Coffman, G. A., & Claven, Y. (1987). Comprehensively diagnosing geriatric patients. *Comprehensive Psychiatry, 28,* 68–76.

Mikulincer, M., & Solomon, Z. (1988). Attributional style and combat-related posttraumatic stress disorder. *Journal of Abnormal Psychology, 97,* 308–313.

Miller, M. D., Wolfson, L., Frank, E., Cornes, C., Silberman, R., Ehrenpreis, L., Zaltman, J., Malloy, J., and Reynolds, C. F. (3rd). Using interpersonal psychotherapy (IPT) in a combined psychotherapy/medication research protocol with depressed elders. A descriptive report with case vignettes. *Journal of Psychotherapy Practice & Research, 7*(1):47–55, 1997 Winter.

Millon, T. (1986). Personality prototypes and their diagnostic criteria. In: *Contemporary Directions in Psychopathology: Toward DSM-IV* (pp. 672–696). New York: The Guilford Press.

Millon, T. (1999). *Personality-guided therapy.* New York: John Wiley & Sons.

Millon, T. (2000). Toward a new model of integrative psychotherapy: Psychosynergy. *Journal of Psychotherapy Integration, 10*(1), 37–53.

Millon, T., & Davis, R. (1995). *Disorders of personality: DSM-IV and beyond.* New York: Wiley and Sons.

Mischel, W., & Shoda, Y. (1999). Integrating dispositions and processing dynamics within a unified theory of personality: The cognitive-affective personality system. In L. A. Pervin & O. P. John (Eds.), *Handbook of personality: Theory and research* (pp. 197–218). New York: Guilford.

Minsky, M. (1985, 1986). *The Society of Mind.* New York: Simon & Schuster.

Mitchell, S. A. (1994). Recent development in psychoanalytic theorizing. *Journal of Psychotherapy Integration, 4,* 93–103.

Molinari, V. Group therapy in the nursing home setting. Presented at 108th annual convention of the American Psychological Association at Washington, DC, August 6, 2000.

Molinari, V., & Reichlin, R. E. (1985). Life review reminiscence in the elderly: A review of the literature. *International Journal of Aging and Human Development, 20,* 81–92.

Monroe, S. M., Bromet, E. J., Connell, M. M., & Steiner, S. C. (1986). Social support, life events, and depressive symptoms: A 1-year prospective study. *Journal Consulting Clinical Psychology, 54,* 424–431.

Moody, H. R., & Carroll, D. (1997). *The five stages of the soul.* New York: Anchor.

Moore, J. T. (1985). Dysthymia in the elderly. *Journal of Affective Disorders, (Suppl.), 9,* S15–S21.

Moore, T. (1994a). *Care of the soul.* New York: Free Press.

Moore, T. (1994b). *Soul mates: Honoring the mysteries of love and relationship.* New York: Harper Perennial.

Moos, R. H. (1992). *Coping resources inventory: Professional manual.* Odessa, FL: Psychological Assessment Resources.

Moos, R., Brennan, P, Fondacaro, M, & Moos, B. (1990). Approach and avoidance coping responses among older problem and nonproblem drinkers. *Psychology and Aging, 5,* 31–40.

Moos, R. H., & Lemke, S. (1984). *Multiphasic environmental assessment procedure: Manual.* Palo Alto, CA: Social Ecology Laboratory, Stanford University and Veterans Administration Medical Center.

Moreland, K. L., Fowler, R. D., & Honaker, L. M. (1994). Future directions in the use of psychological assessment for treatment planning and outcome assessment: Prediction and recommendations. In M. E. Maruish (Ed.), *The use of psychological testing for treatment planning* (pp. 581–602). Hillsdale, NJ: Lawrence-Erlbaum.

Morey, L. (1996). *An interpretive guide to the personality assessment inventory (PAI),* Odessa, FL: Psychological Assessment Resources.

Morin, C. M. (1993). *Insomnia: Psychological assesment and management.* New York: Guilford Press.

Morin, C. M., Culbert, J. P., & Schwartz, S. M. (1994). Nonpharmacological intervention for insomnia: A meta-analysis of treatment efficacy. *American Journal of Psychiatry, 151,* 1172–1180.

Morris, R. G., & Morris, L. W. (1991). Cognitive and behavioral approaches with the elderly. *Int. J. Geriatric Psychiat, 6:* 407–413.

Morrison, T. (1990). The site of memory. In R. Ferguson, M. Gever, T. Minh-ha, & C. West (Eds.), *Out There: Marginalization and Contemporary Cultures.* Cambridge, MA: MIT Press.

Morrison, T., Neimeyer, R. A., & Stewart, A. E. (in press). *Trauma, healing, and the narrative emplotment of loss.* University of Memphis.

Mulrow, C., Williams, J., Gerety, M., Rameriz, G., Montel, O., & Kerber, C. (1995). Case-finding instruments for depression in primary care settings. *Annals of Internal Medicine, 122,* 913–921.

Murphy, L. B., & Moriarity, A. E. (1976). *Vulnerability, Coping and Growth.* New Haven: Yale University Press.

Murray, E. J., & Segal, D. L. (1994). Emotional processing in vocal and written expression of feelings about traumatic experiences. *Journal of Traumatic Stress, 7,* 391–405.

Nadler, J., Damis, L., & Richardson, E. (1997). Psychosocial aspects of aging. In P. D. Nussbaum (Ed.). *Handbook of neuropsychology and aging.* New York: Plenum.

Nauta, A., Brooks, J. D., Johnson, J. R., Kahana, E., & Kahana, B. (1996). Egocentric and non-egocentric life events: Effects on the health and subjective well-being of the aged. *Journal of Clinical Geropsychology, 2(1),* 3–21.

Neimeyer, R. A. (1995). Client-generated narratives in psychotherapy. In R. A. Neimeyer & M. J. Mahoney (Eds.), *Constructivism in psychotherapy* (pp. 231–246). Washington, DC: American Psychological Association.

Neimeyer, R. A., & Stewart, A. E. (1996). Trauma, healing, and the narrative emplotment of loss. *Families in Society, 77,* 360-375.

Nemiroff, R. A., & Colarusso, C. A. (1990). In R. A. Nemiroff & C. A. Colarusso (Eds.), *New Dimensions in Adult Development.* New York: Basic Books.

Neugarten, B. L., & Neugarten, D. A. (1994). Policy issues in an aging society. In P. T. Costa, M. Gatz, B. L. Neugarten, T. A. Salthouse, & I. C. Siegler (Eds.), *The adult years: Continuity and change.* Washington: American Psychological Association.

Neugarten, B., Havighurst, R., & Tobin, S. (1961). The measurement of satisfaction. *Journal of Gerontology, 14,* 134–43.

Neugarten, B. L., Crotty, W. J., & Tobin, S. S. (1964). Personality types in an aged population. In Neugarten et al. (Eds.), *Personality in Middle and Later Life.* New York: Atherton Press.

Neugarten, B. L., Havighurst, R., & Tobin, S. S. (1968). Personality and patterns of aging, pp. 173–180. In B. L. Neugarten (Ed.), *Middle age and aging.* New York: Academic Press.

Newman, C. F. (1994). Understanding client resistance: Methods for enhancing motivation to change. *Cognitive and Behavioral Practice, 1,* 47–69.

Nezu, A. M., Nezu, C. M., Friedman, S. H., Faddis, S., & Houts, P. S. (1998). *Helping cancer patients cope.* Washington: American Psychological Association.

Nohler, B. J. (1982). Personal narrative and life course. In P. Baltes & O. G. Grim(Des). *Life span development and behaviour, Vol. 4*. New York: Academic Press.

Norcross, J. C., & Prochaska, J. O. (1988). A study of eclectic (and integrative) views revisited. *Professional Psychology: Research and Practice, 19*, 170–174.

Norman, S. (2000). Training clinical geropsychologists to work in medical settings. *Clinical Geropsychology News, 7*(3), 13.

Norquist, G. S., et al. (1990). Psychiatric disorder in male veterans and nonveterans. *Journal of Nervous and Mental Disease, 178*:328–55.

Norris, F. (1990). Screening for traumatic stress: A scale for use in the general population. *Journal of Applied Social Psychology, 20*, 1704–1718.

Norris, F., & Perilla, J. (1996). Reliability, validity and cross-language stability of the Revised Civilian Mississippi Scale for PTSD. *Journal of Traumatic Stress, 9*, 285–298.

Norris, F. H. (1992). Epidemiology of trauma: Frequency and impact of different potentially traumatic events on different demographic groups. *Journal of Consulting and Clinical Psychology, 60*, 409–418.

Norris, J. T., Gallagher, D., Wilson, A., & Winograd, C. H. (1987). Assessment of depression in geriatric medical outpatients: The validity of two screening measures. *Journal of the American Geriatrics Society, 35*, 989–995.

Ochberg, F. M. (1996). The counting method for ameliorating traumatic memories. *Journal of Traumatic Stress, 9*(4).

O'Donohue, W., & Krasner, L. (1994). *Handbook of psychological skills training*. Needham Heights, MA: Allyn & Bacon.

O'Hanlon, W., & Weiner-Davis, M. (1989). *In search of solutions: A new direction in psychotherapy*. New York: Norton.

Ogilvie, D. M., & Rose, K. M. (1995). Self-with-other representations and a taxonomy of motives: Two approaches to studying persons. *Journal of Personality, 63*, 643–680.

Olio, K. A., & Cornell, W. F. (1993). The therapeutic relationship as the foundation for treatment with adult survivors of sexual abuse. *Psychotherapy, 30*, 512–523.

Omer, H. (1994). *Critical Interventions in Psychotherapy*. New York: W. W. Norton & Company, Inc.

Op den Velde, W., Falger, P. R. J., Hovens, J. E., de Groen, J. H. M., Lasschuit, L. J., Duijn, H. V., & Schouten, E. G. W. (1993). Posttraumatic stress disorder in Dutch resistance veterans from World War II. In J. P. Wilson & B. Raphael (Eds.), *International Handbook of Traumatic Stress Syndromes* (pp. 219–230). New York: Plenum Press.

Owsley, C., & Sloane, M. E. (1990). Vision and aging. In F. Boller & J. Grafman (Eds.), *Handbook of neuropsychology* (vol. 4) (pp. 229–249). Amsterdam: Elsevier.

Packs, D. R. (1989). Quality of life of cardiac patients. A review. *Journal of Cardiovascular Nursing, 3*(2), 1–11.

Page, A. C., & Crino, R. C. (1993). Eye-movement desensitization: A simple treatment for post-traumatic stress disorder. *Australian and New Zealand Journal of Psychiatry, 27*, 288–293.

Pallesen, S., Nordhus, I. H., & Kvale, G. (1998). Nonpharmacological interventions for insomnia in older adults: A meta-analysis of treatment efficacy. *Psychotherapy, 35*(4), 472–482.

Paris, J. (1997). Introduction: Emotion and empiricism: Research on childhood trauma and adult psychopathology. *Journal of Personality Disorders, 11*, 1–4.

Parker, R. G. (1995). Reminiscence: A continuity theory framework. *The Gerontologist, 35*(4), 515–525.

Parkes, C. (1971). Psychosocial transitions. *Social Science and Medicine, 5*, 101–115.

Parkes, K. R. (1984). Locus of control, cognitive appraisal, and coping in stressful episodes. *Journal of Personality and Social Psychology, 46*, 655–668.

Parks, C. M. (1985). *Recovery from bereavement*. New York: Basic Books.

Parks, C. M., & Weiss, R. S. (1983). *Recovery from bereavement*. New York: Basic Books.

Parloff, M. B. (1986). Frank's "common elements" in psychotherapy: Nonspecific factors and placebos. American Journal of Orthopsychiatry, 56, 521–530.

Parmelee, P. A., Katz, I. R., & Lawton, M. P. (1989). Depression among institutionalized aged: Assessment and prevalence estimation. *Journal of Gerontology, 44*, M22–M29.

Pascual-Leone, J. (1987). Organismic processes for neo-Piagetian theories, a dialectical and causal account of cognitive development. *International Journal of Psychology, 33,* 410–421.

Pascual-Leone, J. (1990b). An essay on wisdom: Toward organismic processes that make it possible. In R. J. Sternberg (Ed.), *Wisdom: Its nature, origins and development* (pp. 244–278). New York: Cambridge University Press.

Pascual-Leone, J. (1991). Emotions, development, and psycho-therapy: A dialectical-constructive perspective. In J. D. Safran & L. S. Greenberg (Eds.), *Emotion, psychotherapy, and change* (pp. 302–335). New York: Guilford.

Pascual-Leone, J. (1991a). Reflections on life-span intelligence, consciousness and ego development. In C. N. Alexander & E. Langer (Eds.), *Higher stages of human development* (pp. 258–285). New York: Oxford University Press.

Pearce, S. (1983). A review of cognitive-behavioral methods for the treatment of chronic pain. *Journal of Psychomatic Research, 27*(5), 431–440.

Pearlin, L. I., & Mullan, J. T. (1992). Loss and stress in aging. In M. L. Wykle, E. Kahana, & Jo. Kowal (Eds.), *Stress and health among the elderly* (pp. 117–132). New York: Springer.

Pearlin, L. I., Mullan, J. T., Semple, S. J., & Skaff, M. M. (1990). Caregiving and the stress process: An overview of concepts and their measures. *The Gerontologist, 30,* 583–594.

Pelletier, K. R. (1977). *Mind as healer, mind as slayer.* New York: Delta.

Peniston, E. G. (1986). EMG biofeedback-assisted desensitization treatment for Vietnam combat veterans Posttraumatic Stress Disorder. *Clinical Biofeedback and Health, 9,* 35–41.

Penn, P. (1985). Feed-forward: Future questions, future maps. *Family Process, 24,* 299–310.

Penn, P., & Sheinberg, M. (1991). Stories and conversations. *Journal of Strategic and Systemic Therapies, 10*(3&$), 30–37.

Pennebaker, J. W. (1989). Confession, inhibition, and disease. In L. Berkowitz (Ed.), *Advances in experimental social psychology, Vol. 22.* Orlando, FL: Academic Press.

Pennebacker, J. W. (1997). Writing about emotional experiences as a therapeutic process. *Psychological Science, 8,* 162–166.

Perconte, S. (1988). Stability of positive treatment outcome symptom relapse in post-traumatic stress disorder. *Journal of Traumatic Stress, 2,* 127–135.

Persons, J. (1991). Psychotherapy outcome studies do not accurately represent current models of psychotherapy: A proposed remedy. *American Psychologist, 46,* 99–106.

Persons, J. B., & Tompkins, M. A. (1997). Cognitive-behavioral case formulation. In T. D. Eells (Ed.), *Handbook of psychotherapy case formulation* (pp. 314–339), New York: Guilford.

Perls, F., & Hefferline, R., & Goodman, P. (1951). *Gestalt therapy.* New York: Dell.

Perls, F. S. (1947). *Ego, hunger, and aggression.* London: George Allen & Unwin.

Perry, J. C. (1997). The idiographic conflict formulation method. In T. D. Eells (Ed.), *Handbook of psychotherapy case formulation* (pp. 137–165), New York: Guilford.

Perry, N. W. (1992). How children remember and why they forget. *The Advisor, 5*(3), 1–2, 13–15.

Pervin, L. A. (1983). The stasis and flow of behavior: Toward a theory of goals. In M. M. Page (Ed.), *Personality: Current theory and research* (pp. 1–53). Lincoln, NE: University of Nebraska Press.

Pfeiffer, E., & Busse, E. W. (1973). Mental disorder in later life: Affective disorders; paranoid, neurotic, and situational reactions. In E. W. Busse & E. Pfeiffer (Eds.), *Mental illness in later life* (pp. 107–144). Washington, DC: American Psychiatric Association.

Piaget, J. SEVERAL REFERENCES YEAR FOR THIS ONE UNKNOWN

Pinsof, W. M. (1995). *Integrative Problem-Centered Therapy.* New York: Basic Books.

Piper, W. E., Azrin, H. F. A., McCallum, M., & Joyce, A. S. (1990). Patient suitability and outcome in short-term individuals psychotherapy. *Journal of Consulting and Clinical Psychology, 589,* 475–481.

Pitman, R. Altman, B., Longue, R. E., Poise, R. E., & Lasko, N. B. (1995, May). Eye Movement Desensitization and Reprocessing: Efficacy for Trauma Victims. In S. Lazrove (Chair) presented at the annual meeting of the American Psychiatric Association, Miami, FL.

Pitman, R. K., Orr, S. P., Altman, B., Poise, R. E., Lasko, N. B., & Longue, R. E. (1993, May). A controlled study of eye movement desensitization/reprocessing (EMDR) treatment for posttraumatic stress disorder. Paper presented at the annual meeting of the American Psychiatric Association, Washington, DC.

Pleiffer, E. (1977). Psychotherapy and social pathology, pp. 626–649. In J. E. Birren & K. W. Schaie (Eds.), *Handbook of the Psychology of Aging.* New York: Van Nostrand.

Plutchik, R., & Kellerman, H. (1990). *Emotion, Theory, Research, and Experience.* New York: Academic Press, Inc.

Polkinghorne, D. (1988). *Narrative knowing and the human sciences.* Albany, NY: SUNY Press.

Pollock, G. H. (1987). The mourning-liberation process: Ideas on the inner life of the older adult. In J. Sadavoy & M. Leszcz (Eds.), *Treating the elderly with psychotherapy: The scope for change in later life* (pp. 3–29). Madison, CT: International Universities Press.

Polster, E., & Polster, M. (1973). *Gestalt therapy integrated.* New York: Brunner/Mazel.

Poon, L. L. (1985). Differences in human memory with aging: Nature, causes, and clinical implications. In J. E. Birren & K. W. Schaie (Eds.), *Handbook of the psychology of aging* (2nd ed., pp. 427–462). New York: Van Nostrand Reinhold.

Poon, L. W., & Siegler, I. C. (1991). Psychological aspects of normal aging. In J. Sadavoy, L. W. Lazarus, & L. F. Jarvik (Eds.), *Comprehensive Review of Geriatric Psychiatry.* Washington, DC: American Psychiatric Press.

Price, R. (1994). *A whole new life.* New York: Atheneum.

Prigerson, H. G., & Kasl, S. V. (1995). Complicated grief and bereavement-related depression as distinct disorders: preliminary empirical validation among elderly bereaved spouses. *American Journal of Psychiatry 15*(1), 22–30.

Prigerson, H., Frank, E., Kasl, S., Reynolds, C., Anderson, B., Zubenko, G., Sherman, E. (1991). *Reminiscence and the self in old age.* New York: Springer Publishing Company.

Prioleau, L., Murdock, M., & Brody, N. (1983). An analysis of psychotherapy versus placebo studies. *Behav. Brain Sco., 6,* 275–310.

Puente, A. E., & McCaffrey, R. J. (Eds.). (1992). *Handbook of neuropsychological assessment: A biopsychosocial perspective.* New York: Plenum Press.

Pynoos, R., Sternberg, A., & Goenjian, A. (1996). Traumatic stress in childhood and adolescence: recent developments and current controversies. In B. A. van der Kolk, A. C. McFarlane, & L. Weisaeth (Eds.), *Traumatic Stress: The effects of overwhelming experience on mind, body, and society* (pp. 331–358). New York: The Guilford Press.

Rachman, S. (1980). Emotional processing. *Behaviour Research and Therapy, 18,* 51–60.

Rando, T. Grief in clinical practice. Workshop at University of Medicine and Dentistry of New Jersey, Piscataway, NJ, May 14, 1999.

Rapp, S. R., Parisi, S. I., & Walsh, D. A. (1988). Geriatric depression: Physicians' knowledge, perceptions and diagnostic practices. *The Gerontologist, 29,* 252–257.

Raw, S. D. (1993). Does psychotherapy research teach us anything about psychotherapy? *The Behavior Therapist, March,* 75–76.

Reese, H. W., & Rodenheaver, D. (1985). Problem solving and complex decision making. In J. E. Birren & K. W. Schaie (Eds.), *Handbook of the psychology of aging, 2nd ed.* (pp. 474–499).

Reichard, S., Livson, F., & Peterson, P. G. (1962). *Aging and personality: A study of 87 old men.* New York: John Wiley.

Renfrey, G., & Spates, C. R. (1994). Eye movement desensitization and reprocessing: A partial dismantling procedure. *Journal of Behavior Therapy and Experimental Psychiatry, 25,* 231–239.

Rennie, D. (1994). Storytelling in psychotherapy: The client's subjective experience. *Psychotherapy, 31,* 234–244.

Rennie, D. L. (1994). Storytelling in psychotherapy: The client's subjective experience. *Psychotherapy, 31,* 2.

Resnick, H. S., Falsetti, S. A., Kilpatrick, D. G., & Freedy, J. R. (1996). Asessment of rape and other civilian trauma-related post-traumatic stress disorder: Emphasis on assessment of potentially traumatic events. In T. W. Miller (Ed.), *Stressful life events* (2nd ed.). New York: International Universities Press.

Resnick, H. S., Foy, D. W., Donahoe, C. P., & Miller, E. N. (1989). Antisocial behavior and post-traumatic stress disorder in Vietnam veterans. *Journal of Clinical Psychology, 45,* 861–866.

Resnick, H. S., Kilpatrick, D. G., Dansky, B. S., Saunders. B. E., & Best, C. L. (1993). Prevalence of civilian trauma and posttraumatic stress disorder in a representative national sample of women. *Journal of Consulting and Clinical Psychology, 61*(6), 984–991.

Resick, P. A., & Schnicke, M. K. (1992). Cognitive processing therapy for sexual assault victims. *Journal of Consulting and Clinical Psychology, 60*(5), 748–756.

Resick, P. A., Jordan, C. G., Girelli, S. A., Hutter, C. K., & Marhoefer-Dvorak, S. (1988). A comparative outcome study of behavioral group therapy for sexual assault victims. *Behavior Therapy, 19*, 385–401.

Retzlaff, P. D. (Ed.) (1995). *Tactical psychotherapy of the personality disorders: An MCMI-III-based approach.* Boston: Allyn and Bacon.

Reyna, V. F. (1995). Interference effects in memory and reasoning: A fuzzy-trace theory analysis. In F. N. Dempster & C. J. Brainerd (Eds.), *Interference and inhibition in cognition* (pp. 29–58). San Diego, CA: Academic Press.

Reyna, V. F., & Brainerd, C. J. (1995). Fuzzy-trace theory: An interim synthesis. *Learning and Individual Differences, 7*(1), 1–75.

Reynolds, C. F., 3rd, Frank, E., Dew, M. A., Houck, P. R., Miller, M., Mazumdar, S., Perel, J. M., & Kupfer, D. J. Treatment of 70(+)-year-olds with recurrent major depression. Excellent short-term but brittle long-term response. *American Journal of Geriatric Psychiatry, 7*(1):64–9, 1999 Winter.

Reynolds, C. F., 3rd, Miller, M. D., Pasternak, R. E., Frank, E., Perel, J. M., Cornes, C., Houck, P. R., Mazumdar, S., Dew, M. A., & Kupfer, D. J. Treatment of bereavement-related major depressive episodes in later life: a controlled study of acute and continuation treatment with nortriptyline and interpersonal psychotherapy. *American Journal of Psychiatry, 156*(2):202–8, 1999 Feb.

Rhodewalt, F., Hays, R. B., Chemers, M. M., & Wysocki, J. (1984). Type A behavior, perceived stress, and illness: A person-situation analysis. *Personality and Social Psychology Bulletin, 10*, 149–159.

Rice, L. N., & Greenberg, L. S. (1984). The new research paradigm. In L. N. Rice & L. S. Greenberg (Eds.), *Patterns of change; Intensive analysis of psychotherapy process* (pp. 7–25). New York: Guilford.

Rimm, D. C., & Masters, J. C. (1974). *Behavior therapy: Techniques and empirical findings.* New York: Academic Press.

Roberts, G., & Holmes, J. (1999). *Healing stories: Narrative in psychiatry and psychotherapy.* Oxford: Oxford University Press.

Robins, L. N., Helzer, J. E., Weissman, M. M., Orvaschel, H., Gruenberg, E., Burke, J. D., & Regier, D. A. (1984). Lifetime prevalence of specific psychiatric disorders in three sites. *Archives of General Psychiatry, 41*, 949–958.

Robinson, J. A. (1976). Sampling autobiographical memory. *Cognitive Psychology, 8*, 578–595.

Robinson, L. A., Berman, J. S., & Neimeyer, R. A. (1990). Psychotherapy for the treatment of depression: A comprehensive review of controlled outcome resources. *Psychological Bulletin, 108*, 30–49.

Rockey, L. S. (1997). Memory assessment of the older adult. In P. D. Nussbaum (Ed.). *Handbook of neuropsychology and aging.* New York: Plenum.

Rogers, C. (1951). *Client-centered therapy.* London: Constable.

Rogers, M. L. (1995). Factors influencing recall of childhood sexual abuse. *Journal of Traumatic Stress, 8*(4), 691–716.

Ronis, D. L., Bates, E. W., Garfein, A. J., Buit, B. K., Falcon, S. P., & Liberzon, I. (1996). *Journal of Traumatic Stress, 9*(4).

Rorty, A. O. (1976a). *The identities of persons.* Berkeley: University of California Press.

Rorty, A. Q. (1976). *A Literary Postscript: Characters Persons, Selves, Individuals. The Identity of Persons.* Berkeley: University of California Press.

Rosen, J., Fields, R. B., Hand, A. M., Falsettie, G., & van Kammen, D. P. (1989). Concurrent posttraumatic stress disorder in psychogeriatric patients. *Journal of Geriatric Psychiatry and Neurology, 3*, 65–69.

Rosenheck, R., & Fontana, A. (1994). Long term sequelae of combat in World War II, Korea and Vietnam: A comparative study. In R. J. Ursano, B. G. McCaughey, & C. S. Fullerton (Eds.). *Individual and community responses to trauma and disaster: The structure of human chaos* (pp. 330–359). Cambridge, UK: Cambridge University Press.

Rosow, I. (1974). *Socialization to Old Age.* Berkeley: University of California Press.

Ross, M., & Conway, M. (1986). Remembering one's own past: The construction of personal histories. In R. M. Sorrentino & E. T. Higgins (Eds.), *Handbook of motivation and cognition: Foundations of social behavior* (pp. 122–144). New York: Wiley.

Rothbaum, B. O., & Foa, E. B. (1996). Cognitive-behavioral therapy for posttraumatic stress disorder. In B. A. van der Kolk, A. C. McFarlane, & L. Weisaeth (Eds.), *Traumatic Stress: The effects of overwhelming experience on mind, body, and society* (pp. 491–509). New York: The Guilford Press.

Rotter, J. B. (1966). Generalized expectancies for internal versus external control of reinforcement. *Psychological Monographs, 80,* 1–28.

Rowe, J. W. (1990). Toward successful aging: Limitation of the morbidity associated with normal aging. In W. R. Hazard, R. Andres, E. L. Bierman, & J. P. Blass (Eds.), *Principles of Geriatric Medicine and Gerontology, 2nd ed.* (pp. 331–348). New York: McGraw Hill.

Rowe, J. W., & Kahn, R. L. (1987). Human aging: Usual and successful. *Science, 237:* 143–149.

Rowe, J. W., & Kahn, R. L. (1998). *Successful aging.* New York: Pantheon.

Roy-Byrne, P., Dagadakis, C., Ries, R., Decker, K., Jones, R., Bolte, M. A., Scher, M., Brinkley, J., Gallagher, M., Patrick, D. L., & Mark, H. (1995). A psychiatrist-rated battery of measures for assessing the clinical status of psychiatric inpatients. *Psychiatric Services, 46,* 347–352.

Rubin, D. C. (Ed.) (1986). *Autobiographical memory.* Cambridge, UK: Cambridge University Press.

Rubin, D. C., Wetzler, S. E., & Nebes, R. D. (1986). Autobiographical memory across the life-span. In D. C. Rubin (Ed.), *Autobiographical Memory* (pp. 202–2211). Cambridge: Cambridge Unversity Press.

Ruegg, R., & Frances, A. (1995). New research in personality disorders. *Journal of Personality Disorders, 9*(1), 1–48.

Ruskin, P. E., & Talbott, J. A. (1996). *Aging and posttraumatic stress disorder.* Washington, DC: American Psychiatric Press.

Rutter, M. (1987). Psychosocial resilience and protective mechanisms. *American Journal of Orthopsychiatry, 57*(3), 316–331.

Rutter, M., & Maughan, B. (1997). Psychosocial adversities in childhood and adulthood. *Journal of Personality Disorders, 11,* 4–19.

Rybarczyk, B. (1995). Using reminiscence interviews for stress management in the medical setting. In B. Haight & J. D. Webster (Eds.), *The art and science of reminiscing: Theory, research, methods and applications* (pp. 205–217). Washington, DC: Taylor & Francis.

Rybarczyk, B., & Bellg, A. (1997). *Listening to life stories: A new approach to stress intervention in health care.* New York: Springer.

Ryckman, R. M., Robbins, M. A., Thornton, B., & Cantrell, P. (1982). Development and validation of a physical self-efficacy scale. *Journal of Personality and Social Psychology, 42,* 891–900.

Ryff, C. D. (1984). Personality development from the inside: The subjective experience of change in adulthood and aging, pp 243–279. In P. B. Baltes & O. G. Brim, Jr. (Eds.), *Life Span Development Behavior, vol 6.*

Sadavoy, J. (1994). Integrated psychotherapy for the elderly. *Canadian Journal of Psychiatry, 39(8, Suppl. 1),* 19–26.

Sadavoy, J., & Fogel, B. (1992). Personality disorders in old age. In J. E. Birren, R. Bruce Sloan, & G. D. Cohen (Eds.), *Handbook of Mental Health and Aging, 2nd ed.* (pp. 433–462). New York: Academic Press.

Sadavoy, J. (1987). Character disorders in the elderly: An overview. In J. Sadavoy & M. Leszcz (Eds.), *Treating the elderly with psychotherapy: The scope for change in later life* (pp. 175–229). Madison, CT: International Universities Press.

Safran & Greenberg, L. S. (1991). Emotion, Psychotherapy, & Change. New York: Guilford Press.

Safran & Segal, (1990). *Interpersonal process in cognitive therapy.* New York: Basic Books, Inc.

Safran, J. D., & Greenberg, L. S. (1988). The treatment of anxiety and depression from an affective perspective. In P. C. Kendal & P. Watson (Eds.), *Negative affective condition*. New York: Academic Press.

Salthouse, T. A. (1991). *Theoretical perspectives on cognitive aging*. Hillsdale, NJ: Erlbaum.

Salthouse, T. A. (1994). Age-related changes in basic cognitive processes. In P. T. Costa, M. Gatz, B. L. Neugarten, T. A. Salthouse, & I. C. Siegler (Eds.), *The adult years: Continuity and change*. Washington: American Psychological Association.

Salzman, C., & Lebowitz (1991). *Anxiety in the elderly: Treatment and research*. New York: Springer.

Salzman, C. (1982). A primer on geriatric psychopharmacology. *American Journal of Psychiatry, 139*, 67–74.

Samuel, R. (1975). *Village life and labour*. London: Routledge and Kegan Paul.

Sarason, I. G., Johnson, J. H., & Siegel, J. M. (1978). Assessing the impact of life changes: Development of the life experiences survey. *Journal of Consulting and Clinical Psychology, 46*, 932–946.

Sarbin, T. (Ed.) (1986). *Narrative psychology: The storied nature of human conduct*. New York: Praeger.

Saunders, B., Arata, C., & Kilpatrick, D. (1990). Development of a crime-related post-traumatic stress disorder scale for women within the Symptom Checklist-90-Revised. *J. Traum. Stress, 3*, 439–448.

Schacter, D. L. (1999). The seven sins of memory insights from psychology and cognitive neuroscience. *American Psychologist, 54*(3), 182–203.

Schacter, D. L., Kihlstrom, J. F., Kihlstrom, L. C., & Berren, M. B. (1989). Autobiographical memory in a case of multiple personality disorder. *Journal of Abnormal Psychology, 98*, 508–514.

Schafer, R. (1992). *Retelling a life: Narration and dialogue in psychoanalysis*. New York: Basic Books.

Schaefer, J. A., & Moos, R. H. (1992). Life crises and personal growth. In B. N. Carpenter (Ed.), *Personal coping: Theory, research, and application* (pp. 149–170). Westport, CT: Praeger.

Schaie, K. W., & Geiwitz, J. (1982). *Adult Development and Aging*. Boston: Little, Brown.

Schaie, K. W., & I. A. Parkham (1976). Stability of adult personality traits: Fact or fable. *Journal of Personal & Social Psychology, 34*, 146–158.

Schaie, K. W. (1989). The hazards of cognitive aging. *The Gerontologist, 29*, 484–493.

Scheier, M. F., & Carver, C. S. (1985). Optimism, coping, and health: Assessment and implications of generalized outcome expectancies. *Health Psychology, 4*, 219–247.

Schieber, F. (1992). Aging and the senses. In J. E. Birren, R. B. Sloane, & G. D. Cohen (Eds.), *Handbook of mental health and aging* (pp. 251–306). San Diego, CA: Academic Press.

Schindler, F. E. (1980). Treatment by systematic desensitization of a recurring nightmare of a real life trauma. *Journal of Behaviour Therapy and Experimental Psychiatry, 11*, 53–54.

Schiraldi, G. R. (2000). *The post-traumatic stress disorder sourcebook: A guide to healing, recovery, and growth*. Los Angeles: Lowell House.

Schnurr, P. P. (1996). Trauma, PTSD, and physical health. *PTSD Research Quarterly, 7*(3), 1–3.

Schnurr, P. (September, 1997). "War Trauma of WWII and Korean Veterans." Presentation at the Readjustment Counseling Service Meeting, Nashua, NH.

Schnurr, P. P., & Aldwin, C. M. (1993). Military service: Long-term effects on adult development. In R. Kastenbaum (Ed.), *Encyclopedia of adult development*. Phoenix, AZ: The Onyx Press.

Schnurr, P. P., Aldwin, C. M., Spiro, A., Stukel, T., & Keane, T. M. (unpublished manuscript). A longitudinal study of PTSD symptoms in older veterans. Poster Session for the Symposium on The Future of VA Mental Health Research. Department of Veterans Affairs Office of Research and Development and National Foundation for Brain Research,. Washington, DC.

Schnurr, P. P., Friedman, M. J., & Rosenberg, S. D. (1993). Premilitary MMPI scores as predictors of combat-related PTSD symptoms. *American Journal of Psychiatry, 150*, 479–483.

Schramke, C. (1997). Anxiety disorders (p. 80–97). In P. Nussbaum (Ed.), *Handbook of neuropsychology and aging*. New York: Plenum.

Schulz, R. (1982). Emotionality and aging: A thoretical and empirical analysis. *Journal of Gerontology, 37*, 42–51.

Schulz, R. (1985). Emotion and affect. In J. E. Birren & K. W. Schail (Eds.), *Handbook of the Psychology of Aging, 2nd ed.* (pp. 531–543). New York: Van Nostrand Reinhold.

Scogin, F., & McElreath, L. (1994). Efficacy of psychosocial treatments for geriatric depression: A quantitative review. *Journal of Consulting Clinical Psychology, 62,* 69–74.

Scogin, F., Hamblin, D., & Beutler, L. E. (1987). Bibliotherapy for depressed older adults: A self-help alternative. *The Gerontologist, 27,* 383–387.

Scogin, F., Rickard, H. C., Keith, S., Wilson, J., & McElreath, L. (1992). Progressive and imaginal relaxation training for elderly persons with subjective anxiety. *Psychology and Aging, 7,* 419–424.

Seligman, M. (1975). *On Depression, Development, and Death.* San Francisco, CA: Freeman.

Seligman, M. E. P. (1975). *Helplessness.* San Francisco: Freeman.

Seligman, M. E. P. (1998). *Learned optimism.* New York: Pocket Books.

Sewell, K. (1996). Constructional risk factors for a post-traumatic stress response following a mass murder. *Journal of Constructivist Psychology, 9.*

Shalev, A. Y., Orr, S. P., Peri, T., Schreiber, S., & Pitman, R. K. (1992). Physiologic responses to loud tones in Israeli patients with Posttraumatic Stress Disorder. *Archives of General Psychiatry, 49,* 870–875.

Shalev, A. Y., Peri, T., Caneti, L., & Schreiber, S. (1996). Predictors of PTSD in injured trauma survivors. *American Journal of Psychiatry, 53,* 219–224.

Shanan, J. (1985). Personality types and culture in later adulthood. In: *Contributions to Human Development, vol. 12.* New York: Basic Books.

Shapiro, F. (1989b). Eye movement desensitization: A new treatment for post-traumatic stress disorder. *Journal of Behavior Therapy and Experimental Psychiatry, 20,* 211–217.

Shapiro, F. (1993). *Eye movement desensitization and reprocessing: Level II Manual.* Pacific Grove, CA: EMDR Pub.

Shapiro, F. (1994). Eye movement desensitization and reprocessing new treatment for anxiety and related trauma. In L. Hyer (Ed.), *Trauma victim: Theoretical considerations and practical suggestions.* Muncie, IN: Accelerated Development Press.

Shapiro, F. (1995). *Eye Movement Desensitization and Reprocessing: Basic principles, protocols, and procedures.* New York: Guilford.

Shay, J. (1994). *Achilles in Vietnam: Combat trauma and the undoing of character.* New York: Atheneum.

Shazer de, S. (1988). *Clues.* New York: W. W. Norton & Company.

Shea, M. T., Elkin, I., Imber, S. D., Sotsky, S. M., Watkins, J. T., Collins, J. F., Pilkonis, P. A., Beckham, E., Glass, D. R., Dolan, R. T., & Parloff, M. B. (1992). Course of depressive symptoms over follow-up: Findings from the National Institute of Mental Health Treatment of Depression Collaborative Research Program. *Archives of General Psychiatry, 49,* 782–787.

Sherman, E. (1981). *Counseling the aged: An integrative approach.* New York: Free Press.

Sherman, E. (1991). *Reminiscence and the self in old age.* New York: Springer Publishing Company.

Shore, J. H., Tatum, E. L., & Vollmer, W. M. (1986). Psychiatric reactions to disaster: The Mount St. Helens experience. *American Journal of Psychiatry, 143,* 590–595.

Siegel, D. J. (1995). Memory, trauma, and psychotherapy. *Journal of Psychotherapy of Practice and Research, 4*(2), 93–122.

Siegler, I. C. (1994). Developmental health psychology. In P. T. Costa, M. Gatz, B. L. Neugarten, T. A. Salthouse, & I. C. Siegler (Eds.), *The adult years: Continuity and change.* Washington: American Psychological Association.

Siegler, I. C., George, I. K., & Lkun, M. A. (1979). Cross-sequential analysis of adult personality. *Development Psychology, 15,* 350–351.

Siever, L. J., & Davis, K. L. (1991). A psychobiological perspective on the personality disorders. *American Journal of Psychiatry, 148,* 1647–1658.

Silberschatz, G., Fretter, P. B., & Curtis, J. T. (1986). How do interpretations influence the process of psychotherapy? *Journal of Consulting and Clinical Psychology, 54,* 646–652.

Silver, C. B. (1992). Personality structure and aging style. *Journal of Aging Studies, 6*(4), 333–350.

Silver, R. L., Boon, C., & Stones, M. H. (1983). Searching for meaning in misfortune: Making sense of incest. *Journal of Social Issues, 39,* 81–102.

Singer, J. A., & Salovey, P. (1993). *The Remembered Self: Emotion and Memory in Personality.* New York: The Free Press, MacMillan, Inc.

Sirles, A. T., & Seleck, C. S. (1989). Cardiac disease and the family: Impact, assessment, and implications. *Journal of Cardiovascular Nursing, 3,* 23–32.

Slater, P. E., & Scarr, H. A. (1964). Personality in old age. *Genetic Psychological Monographs, 70,* 229–269.

Sluyter, G. V., & Mukherjee, A. K. (1993). Total quality management for mental health and mental retardation services: A paradigm for the '90's. Annandale, VA: National Association of Private Residential Resources.

Smith, J. C. (1999). *ABC relaxation training: A practical guide for health professionals.* New York: Springer.

Smith, L. (1993). *Necessary knowledge: Piagetian perspectives on constructivism.* Hillsdale, NJ: Erlbaum.

Smith, L. D. (1995). *Clinician's manual for the cognitive-behavioral treatment of post traumatic stress disorder.* RTR Publishing Company: Perry Point, MD.

Smith, M. L., Glass, G. V., & Miller, T. I. (1980). *The benefits of psychotherapy.* Baltimore, MA: Johns Hopkins University Press.

Smith, M., Glass, G. V., & Yunik, S. S. (1982). The psychologist as Geriatric Clinician. In T. Millon, C., & R. Meagher (Eds.), *Handbook of Clinical Health Psychology* (pp. 227–249). New York: Plenum Press.

Smith, M. L., Glass, G. V., & Miller, T. I. (1980). *The benefits of psychotherapy.* Baltimore, MA: Johns Hopkins University Press.

Smyth, L. (1995). *Clinicians's manual for the cognitive-behavioral treatment of post traumatic stress disorder.* Havre de Grace, MD: RTR Publishing Company.

Smyth, L. D. (1994). *Clinician's manual for the cognitive-behavioral treatment of post traumatic stress disorder.* Havre de Grace, Maryland: RTR Publishing Company.

Snow, K. Cognitive behavioral therapy with compromised older adults. Presentation at the 52nd Annual Scientific Meeting of the Gerontological Scociety of America at San Francisco, CA, November, 1999.

Snyder, D. K., Wills, R. M., & Grady-Fletcher, A. (1991). Long-term effectiveness of behavioral versus insight oriented marital therapy: A 4-year follow-up study. *Journal of Counsulting and Clinical Psychology, 59,* 138–141.

Sohnle, S. J. (2000). The Millon Index of Personality Styles and recalled relaxation states for one's preferred relaxation activity. In J. C. Smith (Ed.), *Advances in ABC Relaxation Research.* New York: Springer.

Solomon, K. (1981). Personality disorders and the elderly. In J. R. Lion (Ed.), *Personality disorders, diagnosis and management* (pp. 310–338). Baltimore: Williams & Wilkins.

Solomon, S, Gerrity, E. T., & Muff, A. M. (1992). Efficacy of treatments for posttraumatic stress disorder. *Journal of the American Medical Association, 268,* 633–638.

Solomon, Z., Bleich, A., Koslowsky, M., & Kron, S. (1991). Posttraumatic stress disorder: Issues of co-morbidity. *Journal of Psychiatric Research, 25,* 89–94.

Solomon, Z, Mikulincer, M, & Rivka, A. (1991). Monitoring and blunting: Implications for combat-related post-traumatic stress disorder. *Journal of Traumatic Stress, 4*(2), 209–221.

Solomon, Z., Mikulincer, M., & Hobfoll, S. E. (1987). Objective versus subjective measurement of stress and social support: Combat-related reactions. *Journal of Consulting and Clinical Psychology, 55,* 577–583.

Sonnanburg, K. (Summer 1996). Meaningful measurements in psychotherapy. *Psychotherapy, 33*(2), 160–170.

Southwick, S. M., Yehuda, R., & Giller, E. L. (1991). Characterization of depression in posttraumatic stress disorder. *American Journal of Psychiatry, 148,* 179–183.

Spar, J. E., & LaRue, A. (1990). *Concise guide to geriatric psychiatry.* Washington, DC: American Psychiatric Press.

Sperry, L. (1995). *Handbook of diagnosis and treatment of the DSM-IV personality disorders.* New York: Bruner Mazel.

Spiegel, D. (1993). *Living beyond limits: New hope and healing for facing life-threatening illness.* New York: Times Books.

Spiegel, D., & Classen, C. (1999). *Group therapy for cancer patients: A research-based handbook of psychosocial care*. New York: Basic Books.

Spiro, A., Aldwin, C. M., Levenson, M. R., & Schnurr, P. P. (1993). Combat-related PTSD among older veterans. Poster Session for the Symposium on The Future of VA Mental Health Research and Development and National Foundation for Brain Research, Washington, DC.

Spitzer, R. L., & Williams, J. B. (1985). Structured clinical interview for DSM-III-Revised, SCID. Version prepared for the National Vietnam Veterans Readjustment Study. NY: State Psychiatric Institute, Biometrics Research Dept.

Spitzer, R. L., Williams, J. B. W., Gibbon, M., & First, M. B. (1990). *Structured clinical interview for DSM-III-R personality disorders (SCID-II)*. Washington, DC: American Psychiatric Press Inc.

Spreen, D., & Strauss, E. (1991). *A compendium of neuro-psychological tests*. New York: Oxford University Press.

Starratt, C, & Peterson, L. (1997). Personality and normal aging. In P. D. Nussbaum (Ed.), *Handbook of neuropsychology and aging* (pp. 15–31). New York: Plenum.

Steenbarger, B. N. (1994). Duration and outcome in psychotherapy; An integrative review. *Professional Psychology: Research and Practice, 25*, 111–119.

Steinberg, M. (1997). Assessing posttraumatic dissociation with the structured clinical interview for DSM-IV dissociative disorders. In J. Wilson & T. Keane (Eds.), *Assessing psychological trauma and PTSD* (pp. 160–191). New York: Guilford Press.

Steinmetz Breckenridge, J., Thompson, O. W., Breckenridge, N. J., & Gallagher, D. E. (1985). Behavioral group therapy with the elderly. A psychoeducational approach. In E. Upper & S. M. Ross (Eds.), *Handbook of Behavioral Group Therapy* (pp. 275–299). New York/London: Plenum.

Stephens, J. H., & McHugh, P. R. (1991). Characteristics and long-term follow-up of patients hospitalized for mood disorders in the Phipps Clinic, 1913–1940. *Journal of Nervous and Mental Disease, 179*, 64–713.

Stern, D. N. (1985). *The interpersonal world of the infant: A view from psychoanalysis and developmental psychology*. New York: Basic Books.

Stevens-Long, J. (1990). Adult development: Theories past and future. In R. A. Nemiroff & C. A. Colarusso (Eds.), *New Dimensions in Adult Development* (pp. 125–169). New York: Basic Books.

Stewart, J. (1995). Reconstruction of the self: Life-span-oriented group psychotherapy. *Journal of Constructivist Psychology, 8*, 129–148.

Stiles, W. B. (1994). Producers and consumers of psychotherapy research ideas. *Journal of Psychotherapy Practice and Research, 1*, 305–307.

Stone, (1993) AS ABOVE.

Stone, M. (1993). *Abnormalities of personality: Within and beyond the realm of treatment*. New York: Norton.

Storandt, M. (1983). *Counseling and therapy with older adults*. Boston: Little, Brown and Company.

Storandt, M., & VandenBos, G. R. (Eds.). (1994). *Neuro-psychological assessment of dementia and depression in older adults: A clinician's guide*. Washington, DC: American Psychological Association.

Stricker, G., & Trierweiler, S. J. (December, 1995). The local clinical scientist: A bridge between science and practice. *American Psychologist, 50*, 12, 995–1002.

Strickland, B. R. (1989). Internal-external control expectancies: From contingency to creativity. *American Psychologist, 44*, 1–12.

Strupp, H. H. (1996). The tripartite model and the Consumer Reports study. *American Psychologist, 51*(10), 1017–1024.

Strupp, H. H., & Binder, J. (1984). *Psychotherapy in a new key: A guide to Time-Limited Dynamic Psychotherapy*. New York: Basic Books.

Stutman, S., & Baruch, R. (1992). A model for the process of fostering resilience. In H. Tomes (Chair), The process of fostering resilience: Roles for psychologists and media. Symposium conducted at the annual meeting of the American Psychological Association, Washington, DC.

Suinn, R. M. (1990). Anxiety management training: A behavior therapy. New York: Plenum Press.

Svartbergm, N., & Stiles, T. C. (1991). Comparative effects of short-term psychodynamic psychotherapy: A meta-analysis. *Journal of Consulting and Clinical Psychology, 59*, 704–714.

Suls, J., Marco, C. A., & Tobin, S. (1991). The role of temporal comparison, social comparison, and direct appraisal in the elderly's self evaluations of health. *Journal of Applied Social Psychology, 21*, 1125–1144.

Summers, M., & Hyer, L. (1994). PTSD among the elderly. In L. Hyer (Ed.), *Trauma victim: Theoretical issues and practical suggestions* (pp. 633–671). Accelerated Development, Muncie, IN.

Summers, M. N., Hyer, L., Boyd, S., & Boudewyns, P. A. (1996). Diagnosis of later-life PTSD among elderly combat veterans. *Journal of Clinical Geropsychology, 2*, 103–117.

Sutker, P. B., & Allain, A. N. (1996). Assessment of PTSD and other mental disorders in World War II and Korean conflict POW survivors and combat veterans. *Psychological Assessment, 8*, 18–25.

Sutker, P., Bugg, F., & Allain, A. (1991). Psychometric prediction of PTSD among POW survivors. *Journal of Consulting and Clinical Psychology, 3*, 105–110.

Sutker, P., Wibstead, D., Galina, Z., & Allain, A. (1991). Cognitive deficits and psychopathology among former prisoners of war and combat veterans of Korea. *American Journal of Psychiatry, 148*, 67–72.

Svartbergm N, & Stiles, T. C. (1991). Comparative effects of short-term psychodynamic psychotherapy: A meta-analysis. *Journal of Consulting and Clinical Psychology, 59*, 704–714.

Sweet, A. (1995). A theoretical perspective on the clinical use of EMDR. *The Behavior Therapist. January*, 5–6.

Tait, R., & Silver, R. (1984, August). Recovery: The long term impact of stressful life experience. Paper presented for the 92nd Annual Convention of the American Psychological Association, Toronto.

Tang, T. Z., & DeRubeis, R. J. (1999). Sudden gains and critical sessions in cognitive-behavioral therapy for depression. *Journal of Consulting and Clinical Psychology, 67*(6), 894–904.

Tangney, J. P. (1995). Recent advances in the empirical study of shame and guilt. *American Behavioral Scientist, 38*(8), 1132–1145.

Teasdale, J. D., Segal, Z. V., Williams, J. M. G., Ridgeway, V. A., Soulsby, J. M., & Lau, M. A. (2000). Prevention of relapse/recurrence in major depression by mindfulness-based cognitive therapy. *Journal of Consulting and Clinical Psychology, 68*(4), 615–623.

Tedeschi, R. G., & Calhoun, L. G. (1995). *Trauma and Transformation Growing in the Aftermath of Suffering*. Thousand Oaks, CA: Sage Publications, Inc.

Tedeschi, R. G., Park, C. L., & Calhoun, L. G. (1998). Posttraumatic growth: Conceptual issues. In R. G. Tedeschi, C. L. Park, & L. G. Calhoun (Eds.), *Posttraumatic Growth*. Mahwah, NJ: Lawrence Erlbaum.

Tennant, C. C., Goulston, K., & Dent, O. (1993). Medical and psychiatric consequences of being a prisoner of war of the Japanese: An Australian follow-up study. In J. P. Wilson & B. Raphael (Eds.), *International Handbook of Traumatic Stress Syndromes* (pp. 231–240). New York: Plenum Press.

Teri, L., & Curtis, J. (1991). Cognitive-Behavior therapy with depressed older adults. Paper presented at the National Institutes of Mental Health Consensus Conference on the Diagnosis & Treatment of Depression in Late Life. Washington, DC.

Teri, L., Curtis, J., Gallagher-Thompson, D., & Thompson L. (1994). Cognitive-behavioral therapy with depressed older adults. In L. S. Schneider, C. F. Reynolds, B. D. Lebowitz, & A. J. Friedhoff (Eds.), *Diagnosis and treatment of depression in late life: Results of the NIH consensus development conference* (pp. 279–291). Washington, DC: American Psychiatric Press.

Teri, L., & Uomoto, J. M. (1991). Reducing excess disability in dementia patients: Training caregivers to manage patient depression. *Clinical Gerontologist, 10*(4), 49–63.

Terr, L. (1983). Chowchilla revisited: The effects of psychic trauma four years after a school bus kidnapping. *American Journal of Psychiatry, 140*, 1543–1550.

Terr, L. (1991). Childhood traumas: An outline and overview. *American Journal of Psychiatry, 148*, 10–20.

Terr, L. (1994). *Unchained memories: True stories of traumatic memory loss*, New York: Basic Books.

Terrell, C. J., & Lydon, W. J. (1995). Narrative and psychotherapy. *Journal of Constructivist Psychology, 9*, 27–44.

Thase, M. E. (1990). Relapse and recurrence in unipolar major depression: Short-term and long-term approaches. *Journal of Clinical Psychiatry, 51[6(suppl)]*, 51–57.

The Counseling Psychologist (April 1995). Delayed Memory Debate, 23(2). Division of Counseling Psychology of the American Psychological Association: Sage Periodicals Press.

Thoits, P. A. (1983). Dimensions of life events that influence psychological adistress: An evaluation and synthesis of the literature. In H. B. Kaplan (Ed.), *Psychosocial Stress: Trends in Theory and Research* (pp. 33–103). Orlando, FL: Academic Press.

Thomae, 1976 not in references.

Thomae, H. (1970). Theory of aging and cognitive theory of personality. *Human Development, vol. 3.* Basel: Karger.

Thomae, H. (1992). Emotion and personality. In: *Handbook of Mental Health and Aging* (pp. 355–375). San Diego, CA: Academic Press.

Thompson, I. W., Gallagher, D., & Czirr, R. (1988). Personality disorder and outcome in the treatment of late-life depression. *Journal of Geriatric Psychiatry, 21*, 133–153.

Thompson, L. W., Davies, R., Gallagher, D., & Krantz, S. E. (1986). Cognitive therapy with older adults. *Clinical Gerontologists, 5*(3/4), 245–279.

Thompson, L. W., & Gallagher, D. (1984). Efficacy of psychotherapy in the treatment of late-life depression. *Advances in Behavior Research and Therapy, 6*, 127–139.

Thompson, L. W., Gallagher, D., & Breckenridge, J. S. (1987). Comparative effectiveness of psychotherapies for depressed elders. *Journal of Consulting and Clinical Psychology, 55*, 385–390.

Thompson, L. W., Gallagher, D., & Czirr, R. (1988). Personality disorder and outcome in the treatment of late-life depression. *Journal of Geriatric Psychiatry, 21*, 133–146.

Thompson, L. W., Gallagher, D., & Breckenridge, J. S. (1987). Comparative effectiveness of psychotherapies for depressed elders. *Journals of Consulting and Clinical Psychology, 55*, 385–390.

Thompson, L. W., Gantz, F., Florsheim, M., Del Maestro, S., Rodman, J., Gallagher-Thompson, D., & Bryan, H. (1991). Cognitive/behavioral therapy for affective disorders in the elderly. In W. Myers (Ed.), *New techniques in the psychotherapy of older patients* (pp. 3–19). Washington, DC: American Psychiatric Press.

Thompson, P. (1988). *The voice of the Past: Oral history, 2nd ed.* Oxford: Oxford University Press.

Thomson, L. W., Gallagher, D., Hanser, S., Gantz, F., & Steffen, A. (1991, November). Comparison of desipramine and cognitive/behavioral therapy in the treatment of late-life depression. Paper presented at the meeting of Gerontological Society of America, San Francisco.

Thygesen, P. Hermann, K., & Willnger, R. (1970). Concentration camp survivors in Denmark: Persecution, disease, disability, and compensation. *Danish Medical Bulletin, 17*, 65–105.

Timiras, P. (1972). *Developmental physiology and aging.* New York: MacMillan.

Tomkins, S. S. (1987). Script theory. In J. Aronoff, A. I. Rabin, & R. A. Zucker (Eds.), *The emergence of personality.* New York: Springer.

Tomm, K. (1989). Externalizing the problem and internalizing personal agency. *Journal of Strategic and Systemic Therapy, 8*(1), 54–59.

Tomm, K. (1993). The courage to protest: A commentary on Michael White's work. In S. Gilligan & R. Price (Eds.), *Therapeutic Conversations* (pp. 62–80). New York: Norton.

Tornstam, L. (1996). Gerotranscendence—A theory about maturing into old age. *Journal of Aging and Identity, 1*(1), 37–50.

Tornstam, L. (1997). Gerotranscendence in a broad cross-sectional perspective. *Journal of Aging and Identity, 2*(1), 17–36.

Tracey, T. J., & Ray, P. B. (1984). The stages of successful time-limited counseling: An interactional examination. *Journal of Counseling Psychology, 31*, 13–27.

Tromp, S., Koss, M. P., Figueredo, A. J., & Tharan, M. (1995). Are rape memories different?: A comparison of rape, other unpleasant and pleasant memories among employed women. *Journal of Traumatic Stress, 8*(4), 607–627.

Trower, P., & Dryden, W. (1989). "Resistance" in a process approach to social skills training: The role of cognitive blocks and how these can be overcome. In W. Dryden & P. Trower (Eds.), *Cognitive psychotherapy: Stasis and change* (pp. 123–138.) New York: Springer.

Tuokko, H., & Hadjistavropoulos, T. (1998). *An assessment guide to geriatric neuropsychology.* Mahwah, NJ: Lawrence Erlbaum Associates.

Turkat, I. D. (1990). *The personality disorders: A psychological approach to clinical management.* New York: Pergamon.

Turner, S. W., McFarlane, A. C., & van der Kolk, B. A. (1996). The therapeutic environment and new explorations in the treatment of posttraumatic stress disorder. In B. A. van der Kolk, A. C. McFarlane, & L. Weisaeth (Eds.), *Traumatic Stress: The effects of overwhelming experience on mind, body, and society* (pp. 537–558). New York: The Guilford Press.

Uddo, M., Vasterling, J., Brailey, K., & Sutker, P. (1993). Memory and attention in posttraumatic stress disorder. *Journal of Psychopathology and Behavioral Assessment, 15,* 43–52.

Ullman, S. E., & Siegel, J. M. (1996). Traumatic events and physical health in a community sample. *Journal of Traumatic Stress, 9*(4).

Valent, P. (1999). *Trauma and fulfillment therapy.* Philadelphia: Brunner/Mazel.

Valliant, G. E., & Perry, J. C. (1990). Personality disorders. In H. I. Kaplan & B. J. Sadock (Eds.), *Comprehensive textbook of psychiatry, 5th ed., Vol. 2* (pp. 1352–1387). Baltimore: Williams & Wilkins.

Van den Dale, L. (1975). Ego development and preferential judgment in life-span perspective. In N. Datan & L. Ginsberg, (Eds.), *Life-Span developmental psychology: Normative life crises.* New York: Academic Press.

van der Hart, O., Brown, P., & Turco, R. N. (1990). Hypnotherapy for traumatic grief: Janetian and modern approaches integrated. *American Journal of Clinical Hypnosis, 32,* 263–271.

van der Kolk (1999). *Complex post traumatic stress disorder (DESNOS).* Invited address, Mount Sainai Medical Center, New York, NY.

van der Kolk. B. A. (1988). The trauma spectrum: The interaction of biological and social events in the genesis of the trauma response. *Journal of Traumatic Stress, 1,* 273–290.

van der Kolk, B. A., & Fisler, R. (1995). Dissociation and the fragmentary nature of traumatic memories: Overview and exploratory study. *Journal of Traumatic Stress, 8*(4), 505–525.

van der Kolk, B. A. (1996). The complexity of adaptation to trauma: Self-regulation, stimulus discrimination, and characterological development. In B. A. van der Kolk, A. C. McFarlane, & L. Weisaeth (Eds.), *Traumatic Stress: The effects of overwhelming experience on mind, body, and society* (pp. 3–23). New York: The Guilford Press.

van der Kolk, B. A., & Fisler, R. (1995). Dissociation the fragmentary nature of traumatic memories: Overview and exploratory study. *Journal of Traumatic Stress, 8*(4), 505–525.

van der Kolk, B. A., & Greenberg, M. S. (1987) The psychobiology of the trauma response: Hyperarousal, constriction, and addiction to traumatic reexposure. In B. A. van der Kolk (Ed.), *Psychological trauma* (pp. 63–87). Washington, DC: American Psychiatric Press.

van der Kolk, B. A., McFarlane, A. C., & van der Hart, O. (1996). A general approach to treatment of posttraumatic stress disorder. In B. A. van der Kolk, A. C. McFarlane, & L. Weisaeth (Eds.), *Traumatic Stress: The effects of overwhelming experience on mind, body, and society* (pp. 3–23). New York: The Guilford Press.

van der Kolk, B. A., & Saporta, J. (1991). The biological response to psychic trauma: Mechanisms and treatment of intrusion and numbing. *Anxiety Research, 4,* 199–212.

van der Kolk, B. A. (1988). The trauma spectrum: The interaction of biological and social events in the genesis of the trauma response. *Journal of Traumatic Stress, 1,* 273–290.

van der Kolk, B. A., & Fisler, R. (1995). Dissociation and the fragmentary nature of traumatic memories: Overview and exploratory study. *Journal of Traumatic Stress, 8*(4), 505–525.

van der Kolk, B. A., & McFarlane, A. C. (1996). The black hole of trauma. In B. A. van der Kolk, A. C. McFarlane, & L. Weisaeth (Eds.), *Traumatic Stress: The effects of overwhelming experience on mind, body, and society* (pp. 3–23). New York: The Guilford Press.

van der Kolk, B. A., Mandel, R., Pelcovitz, D., & Roth, S. (1992a, June). Update of 'DES NOS' data analysis. Presentation at the meeting of the International Society for Traumatic Stress Studies World Conference, Amsterdam, The Netherlands.

van der Kolk, B. A., van der Hart, O., & Marmar, C. R. (1995). Dissociation and information processing in posttraumatic stress disorder. In B. A. van der Kolk, A. C. McFarlane, & L. Weisaeth (Eds.), *Traumatic Stress: The effects of overwhelming experience on mind, body, and society* (pp. 3–23). New York: The Guilford Press.

van der Kolk, B. A., Weisaeth, L., & van der Hart, O. (1996). History of trauma in psychiatry. In B. A. van der Kolk, A. C. McFarlane, & L. Weisaeth (Eds.), *Traumatic Stress: The effects of overwhelming experience on mind, body, and society* (pp. 3–23). New York: The Guilford Press.

Varela, F. J., Rosch, E., & Thompson, E. (1991). *The embodied mind: Cognitive science and human experience.* Cambridge, MA: MIT Press.

Vasterling, J. J., Sementilli, M. E., & Burish, T. G. (1988). The role of aerobic exercise in reducing stress. *Diabetes Educator, 14*(13), 197–201.

Vaughan, K., Armstrong, M. F., Gold, R., O'Connor, N., Jenneke, W., & Tarrier, N. (1994). A trial of eye movement desensitization compared to image habituation training and applied muscle relaxation in post-traumatic stress disorder. *Journal of Behavior Therapy and Experimental Psychiatry, 25,* 283–291.

Velicer, W. F., Hughes, S. L., Fava, J. L., Prochaska, J. O., & Diclemente, C. C. (1995). An empirical typology of subjects within stage of change. *Addictive Behaviors, 20,* 299–320.

Verwoerdt, A. (1976). *Clinical Geropsychiatry.* Baltimore, MD: Williams & Wilkins.

Verwoerdt, A. (1988). *Clinical geropsychiatry.* Baltimore, MD: Williams and Wilkins.

Verwoerdt, A. (1988). Towards a political economy of ageing. *Ageing and Society, 1,* 73–94.

Viederman, M., & Perry, S. (1980). Use of the psychodynamic life narrative in the treatment of depression in the medically ill. *General Hospital Psychiatry, 2,* 77–85.

Villereal, G. (1991). An application of the Veterans Diagnostic Scale as a rapid assessment instrument. Unpublished doctoral dissertation, University of Pittsburg.

Viney, L. L. (1987). A sociophenomenological approach to lifespan development complementing Erikson's psychodynamic approach. *Human Development, 30,* 125–136.

Viney, L. L., Benjamin, Y. N., & Preston, C. (1990). Personal construct therapy for the elderly. *Journal of Cognitive Psychotherapy, 4,* 211–224.

Vinokur, A., & Selzer, M. L. (1975). Desirable versus undesirable life events: Their relationship to stress and mental distress. *Journal of Personality and Social Psychology, 32,* 329–337.

Wagner, B. M. (1990). Major and daily stress and psychopathology: On the adequacy of the definitions and methods. *Stress Medicine, 6,* 217–226.

Wagner, B. M., Compas, B. E., & Howell, D. C. (1988). Daily and major life events: The PERI Life Events Scale. *Journal of Health and Social Behavior, 19,* 205–229.

Wallston, K. A., Smith, R. A., King, J. E., Smith, M. S., Rye, E., & Burish, T. G. (1991). Desire for control and choice of antiemetic treatment of cancer chemotherapy. *Western Journal of Nursing Research, 13*(1), 12–29.

Wallsten, S. M. (1997). Elderly caregivers and care receivers: Facts and gaps in the literature. In P. D. Nussbaum (Ed.), *Handbook of neuropsychology and aging* (pp. 467–482). New York: Plenum.

Walter, J. L., & Peller, J. E. (Eds.) (1992). *Becoming solution-focused in brief therapy.* New York: Brunner/Mazel.

Wang, S., Wilson, J. P., & Mason, J. (1996). Stages of decompensation in combat-related posttraumatic stress disorder: a new conceptual model. *Integrative Physiological and Behavioral Science, 31,* 237–253.

Wasylenki, D. A. (1989). Psychodynamics and aging. In D. A. Wasylenki, B. A. Martin, D. F. Clark, E. A. Lennox, L. A. Perry, & M. K. Harrison (Eds.), *Psychogeriatrics: A Practical Handbook.* London: Jessica Kingsley.

Waters, E. B., & Goodman, J. (1990). *Empowering older adults: Practical strategies for counselors.* San Francisco: Jossey-Bass.

Watkins, C. E. (1991). What have surveys taught us about the teaching and practice of psychological assessment? *Journal of Personality Assessment, 56,* 426–437.

Watson, C. G., Juba, M. P., Manifold, V., Kucala, T., & Anderson, P. E. D. (1991). The PTSD Interview: Rationale, description, reliability, and concurrent validity of a DSM-III-based technique. *Journal of Clinical Psychology, 47,* 179–188.

Watson, D., & Clark, L. A. (1984). Negative affectivity: The disposition to experience aversive emotional states. *Psychological Bulletin, 96,* 465–490.

Watson, D., & Pennebaker, J. W. (1989). Health complaints, stress, and distress: Exploring the central role of negative affectivity. *Psychological Review, 96,* 233–253.

Watzlawick, P. (1990). Therapy is what you say it is. In J. K. Zeig & S. G. Gilligan (Eds.), *Brief therapy: Myths, methods and metaphors* (pp. 55–61). New York: Brunner/Mazel.

Waxman, H. M., & Carner, E. A. (1984). Physicians' recognition, diagnosis, and treatment of mental disorders in elderly medical patients. *The Gerontologist, 24,* 593–597.

Weathers, F. W., & Litz, B. T. (Spring, 1994). Psychometric properties of the clinician-administered PTSD scale, CAPS-1. *PTSD Research Quarterly, 5*(2), 6–8.

Weinberger, M., Darnell, J. C., & Martz, B. L. (1986). The effect of positive and negative life changes on the self-reported health status of elderly adults. *Journal of Gerontology, 41,* 114–119.

Weingarten, K. (1992). A consideration of intimate and non-intimate interactions in therapy. *Family Process, 31,* 45–59.

Weisaeth, L. (1984). Stress reactions in an industrial accident. Unpublished doctoral dissertation. Oslo, Norway.

Weiss, D. S., Marmar, C. R., Schlenger, W. E., Fairbank, J. A., Jordan, B. K., Hough, R. L., & Kulka, R. A. (1992). The prevalence of lifetime and partial PTSD in Vietnam theater veterans. *J. Traum. Stress, 5,* 365–376.

Webster, J. (1997). The reminiscence functions scale: A replication. *International Journal of Aging and Human Development, 44*(2), 137–148.

Wells, G., & Loftus, E. F. (1984). *Eyewitness testimony,* New York: Cambridge University Press.

Wells, K. B., Burnam, M. A., Rogers, W., Hays, R., & Camp, P. (1992). The course of depression in adult outpatients: Results from the Medical Outcomes Study. *Archives of General Psychiatry, 49,* 788–794.

Werner, H. (1948). *Comparative psychology of mental development* (rev. ed.). Madison, CT: International Universities Press.

Westen, D. (1998). Case formulation and personality diagnosis: Two processes or one? In B. J. Washington (Ed.), *Making diagnosis meaningful* (pp. 111–138). Washington, DC: American Psychological Association.

Wheeler, E., & Knight, B. (1981). Morrie: A case study. *Gerontologist, 21,* 323–328.

Whitbourne, S. K. (1985). The psychological construction of the life span. In J. E. Birren & K. W. Shaie (Eds.), *Handbook of psychology and aging* (pp. 594–618). New York: Van Nostrand Reinhold.

Whitbourne, S. K. (1987). Personality development in adulthood and old age: Relationships among identity style, health, and well-being, pp. 189–216. In K. W. Schaie & C. Eisdoorfer (Eds.), *Annual Review of Gerontology and Geriatrics, Volume 7.* New York: Springer.

White, H. (1980). The value of narrativity in the representation of reality. *Critical Inquiry, 7,* 5–28.

White, J. (1980). *Rothschild Bildings: Life in an east end tenement block 1887–1920.* London: Routledge and Kegan Paul.

White, M. (1986a). Family escape from trouble. *Case Studies, 1,* 1.

White, M. (1986b). Negative explanation, restraint and double description: A template for family therapy. *Family Process, 25,* 169–184.

White, M. (1987). Family therapy and schizophrenia: Addressing the "in-the-corner" lifestyle. *Culwich Centre Newsletter,* 7–11.

White, M. (1988/9). The externalizing of the problem and the re-authoring of lives and relationships. *Dulwich Centre Newsletter,* 3–20.

White, M. (1988a). The process of quesitonint: A therapy of literary merit? *Dulwich Centre Newsletter,* 8–14.

White, M. (1989). Selected papers. Adelaide, Australia: Duwich Centre Newsletter, 3, 21–40.

White, M., & Epston, D. (1990). *Narrative means to therapeutic ends.* New York: Norton.

Widdison, H., & Salisbury, H. (1990). The delayed stress syndrome: A pathological grief reaction? *Omega, 20*(4), 293–305.

Widner, S. (1994). Self-Complexity as a Stress Buffer in an Elderly Population. Unpublished Dissertation. Ann Arbor, MI.

Williams, L. M. (1995). Recovered memories of abuse in women with documented child sexual victimization histories. *Journal of Traumatic Stress, 8*(4), 649–673.

Wilson, J. P. (1988). Understanding the Vietnam veteran. In F. Ochberg (Ed.), *Posttraumatic therapy and victims of violence.* New York: Brunner/Mazel.

Wilson, J., & Keane, T. (1997). *Assessing psychological trauma and PTSD.* New York: Guilford Press.

Wilson, J. P., & Zigelbaum, S. D. (1983). The Vietnam veteran on trial: The relation of posttraumatic stress disorder to criminal behavior. *Behavioral Sciences and the Law Journal, 1,* 25–50.

Wilson, S. A., Tinker, R. H., & Becker, L. A. (1994, August). Eye Movement Desensitization and Reprocessing Method in the Treatment of Traumatic Memories. Paper presented at the 102nd Convention of the American Psychological Association, Los Angeles, CA.

Wolfe, B. E. (1995). Self pathology and psychotherapy integration. *Journal of Psychotherapy Integration, 5*(4), 293–312.

Wong, P. T., & Watt, L. M. (1991). What types of reminiscence are associated with successful aging? *Psychology and Aging, 6,* 272–9.

Worden, J. W. (1982). *Grief counseling and grief therapy: A handbook for the mental health practitioner.* New York: Springer Company.

Worden, J. W. (1991). *Grief counseling and grief therapy: A handbook for the mental health practitioner* (2nd ed.). New York: Springer.

Wright, M. (1986). Priming the past. *Oral history, 14*(1), 60–65.

Yehuda, R., Kahana, B., Schmeidler, J., Southwick, S. M., Wilson, S., & Giller, E. L. (1995). Impact of cumulative lifetime trauma and recent stress on current posttraumatic stress disorder symptoms in Holocaust survivors. *American Journal of Psychiatry, 152,* 1815–1818.

Yost, E., Beutler, L. E., Corbishley, M. A., & Allender, J. R. (1986). *Group cognitive therapy: A treatment approach for depressed older adults.* New York: Pergamon.

Young, J. E. (1990). *Cognitive therapy for personality disorders: A schema-focused approach.* Sarasota, FL: Professional Resource Press.

Yule, W., & Williams, R. M. (1990). Post-traumatic stress reactions in children. *Journal of Traumatic Stress, 3,* 279–295.

Yullie, J. C. (1993). We must study forensic eyewitnesses to know about them. *American Psychologist, 48,* 572–573.

Zalewsi, C., Thompson, W., & Gottesman, I. (1994). Comparison of neuropsychological test performance in PTSD, generalized anxiety disorder, and control Vietnam Veterans. *Assessment, 1,* 133–142.

Zarit, S. (1996). Interventions with family caregivers. In S. H. Zarit & B. G. Knight (Eds.), *A guide to psychotherapy and aging* (pp. 163–220). Washington, DC: American Psychological Association.

Zarit, S., Eiler, J., & Hassinger, M. (1985). Clinical assessment. In J. Burren & K. Schaie (Eds.), *Handbook of the psychology of aging* (pp. 725–754). New York: Van Nostrand Reinhold.

Zarit, S. H., & Knight, B. G. (1986). *A guide to psychotherapy and aging.* Washington, DC: American Psychological Association.

Zeiss, A. M., & Lewinsohn, P. M. (1986). Adapting behavioral treatment for depression to meet the needs of the elderly. *The Clinical Psychologist, 39,* 98–100.

Zeiss, R. A., & Dickman, H. R. (1989). PTSD 40 years later: Incidence and person-situation correlates in former POWs. *Journal of Clinical Psychology, 45,* 80–87.

Zeiss, R. A., Delomonico, R. L, Zeiss, A. M., & Dornbrand, L. (1991). Psychological disorder and sexual dysfunction in elders. In L. K. Dial (Ed.), *Clinics in geriatric medicine: Sexuality and the elderly* (pp. 133–151). Philadelphia: W. B. Saunders.

Zivian, M. T., Gekoski, W., Knox, V. J., Larsen, W., & Hatachette, V. (Fall/1994). Psychotherapy for the elderly: Public Opinion. *Psychotherapy, 31*(3).

Zonderman, A. B., Leu, V. L., & Costa, P. T., Jr. (1986). Effects of age, hypertension history, and neuroticism on health perceptions. *Experimental Gerontology, 21,* 449–458.

Zeiss, R. A., & Steffen, A. M. (in press). Interdisciplinary health care teams: The basic unit of geriatric care. In L. L. Carstensen, B. A. Edelstein, & L. Dornbrand (Eds.), *The handbook of clinical gerontology.* Newbury Park, CA: Sage.

Zung, W. W. K. (1971). The differentiation of anxiety and depressive disorders: A biometrics approach. *Psychosomatics, 12,* 380–384.

Zweig, R. A., & Hillman, J. (1996). Personality disorders in adults: A review. In E. Rosowsky, R. C. Abrams, & R. A. Zweig, *Personality disorders in older adults: Emerging issues in diagnosis and treatment* (pp. 31–53). Mahwah, NJ: Lawrence Erlbaum Associates.

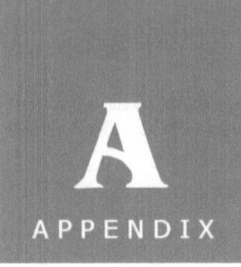

APPENDIX

Cognitive Behavioral Therapy: Application

We describe our method of CBT. We often use a 10–20 session standard CBT trial on everyday problems, usually as they relate to PTSD. If the client is depressed, we address this first, using our method. Often this therapy is sufficient for change. Yes, often the treatment of depression is sufficient to change of many PTSD symptoms.

CBT is a structured therapy (Box A-1). CBT also does not aim to change the client per se—rather, its purpose is to teach clients techniques for changing thought and behavior patterns that they can generalize to other aspects of their lives. A heavy emphasis is on the role of thinking: Thoughts are the central person elements that influence symptoms, emotions, and behavior patterns. In fact, CBT is really a model of coping that is person-oriented, educative, and collaborative. Additionally, CBT attempts to define complaints as solvable problems.

If you reduce CBT to its essentials, it consists of a series of questions that address cognitions. First, there is the Socratically arrived at data that is called *socialization*. Then, the Colombo-style advances on logic: (a) What is the evidence? (b) What are alternative explanations? (c) Are there poor attributions? and (d) Why are the perceived outcomes so terrible? If these do not bear fruit, then the cognitive schema, the silent assumptions of living, comes under attack. The DTR (Dysfunctional Thought Record) is used liberally, as well as other cognitive or behavioral methods. In the wings are ever-present interventions of activity, graded task assignments, and mastery/reward experiments.

The key to CBT is the ability to get the patient onboard. With older people it is often helpful to label the problem as medical. As part of this we take pains to foster one other point: that the person can control thoughts and behaviors and that these are as effective as any medication and leave a better legacy (learned skills for continued change). Then the therapist must frame the problem as "external," as an adversary to defeat. The discussion of goals and personal efficacy arrives in an easier form at this point. The work that follows is made less effortful by this formulation.

Box A-1
Cognitive Therapy: Rationale

1. The content of a person's thinking affects mood and leads to a specific emotional response.
2. The person's interpretation of data determines the emotional response.
3. The person sees awareness as a continuum rather than as a dichotomy separating conscious from unconscious experience.
4. The patient and therapist are in partnership.
5. The problem is owned by the patient.
6. Making incorrect judgments becomes a deep habit. To break the habit requires consciousness (awareness). Recognition of thoughts perpetuating habit. Substitution of accurate for inaccurate judgments; feedback.
7. Automatic thoughts are without logical sequence of steps, such as in goal-oriented thinking or problem solving. They happen as if by reflex.
8. Automatic thoughts are plausible to the one thinking them. They are often idiosyncratic; more prone to reflect distortion of reality than other thoughts.
9. Individuals may have a deficit of self-monitoring of thoughts and impulses.
10. The meaning of a person's experiences is very much determined by his/her expectations of their immediate and ultimate consequences.
11. Irrationality can be understood in terms of inadequacies in organizing and interpreting data that are present (vs. unconscious).
12. The most observable events (behaviors) are preceded by a thought process.
13. There is a conscious thought between an external event and a particular emotional response.
14. People are practical scientists: They make observations, set up hypotheses, check their validity, and eventually form generalizations that will later serve as a guide for making rapid judgments of situations.
15. Intuitive knowledge is important.
16. To understand . . . we need to get inside the conceptual system and see the world through that person's eyes.
17. Rules are programs by which one deciphers and evaluates experience and regulates behavior.
18. Rules are one of the umbrellas under which behavior is attempted to be understood.

☐ Socialization (1–3 Sessions)

Socialization is critical. This is both friendly persuasion and education (Box A-1). To explain the process of PTSD, we emphasize the role played by the trauma, by loss, by the sense of helplessness, and by the negative attributions of self, other, and future. We often use a downward spiral scheme, as well as outlines of the person's own cycle of thinking, behaving, physiology, and emoting. We of course emphasize the power of thinking. We use the DTR. At this beginning phase, a judicious therapeutic

---

Box A-2
Adaptations with Older Adults

- Adaptations to sensory deficits (large print, etc).
- Adaptations to cognitive deficits (memory aids—tapes, written assignments, notebooks).
- Emphasis on qualities representing relative strengths of older adults.
- Slower pacing of material.
- Multimodal training (say it, show it, do it).
- Strategies for staying on track in session.
- Plans for generalization of training.
- Right to be respected.
- Reinforce patient's knowledge of personal strengths.
- Use experience of handling past problems.
- Constant focus on commitment (What might get in the way of . . .).

---

attempt is made to address automatic thoughts and to assure the client that these influence behavior. With many patients we identify potential self-defeating patterns (personality). We clarify the role of the patient and the role of the therapist, and the need for a working partnership. With the elderly, often negative beliefs center around self-management and control of symptoms.

Data are obtained at each session. Baseline measures are obtained at the start of treatment and a brief self-report measure is taken before each session. At intake, clients complete the Beck Depression Inventory (BDI; Gallagher, 1986) and the Impact of Events Scale (IES), and perhaps the Beck Anxiety Inventory. It is completed prior to each therapy session. Homework is emphasized, especially the DTR (see below).

Also, special needs of older folks are attended to (Box A-2). Cognitive slowing or sensory deficits may be a problem. The therapist uses different sensory modalities. This includes repeating themes or concepts both verbally and visually (e.g., using a blackboard), as well as have the patient take notes. Also it is helpful to provide a tape recording of the session for review between sessions, particularly for those patients exhibiting more severe sensory and/or cognitive impairment. Handouts and written feedback also are necessary. Summarizations are used, requesting the client to reiterate themes at the end of the session. They also assist many patients in the "deep processing" of the material.

Socialization means that the client becomes immersed in the processes of therapy at the beginning. We also want the person to know that "small wins are good wins." In all this, we solicit commitment.

☐ Skills of CBT

The skills of CBT are addressed in several areas. These are thinking (the flagship of CBT), mood, the influence of mood on thinking and behavior especially (especially activity scheduling and mastery/pleasure of acts), and, finally, relaxation.

Dysfunctional Thought Record and Thinking Techniques (Sessions 4–13)

The therapeutic phrase "What were you just thinking then?" is iterated again and again, starting in just about every session. From the beginning, therefore, the elicitation of automatic thoughts is practiced. In the PTSD caring process, there is curative power in thinking, the elicitation of the sensitive construals that represent/subserve/infect the trauma complexity. Automatic thoughts are staples in CBT therapy: They are the gateway to beliefs and schemas and the most accessible form of client interaction. It is this datum that is to be challenged, to be tested for evidence, to be probed for alternative explanations, and to be changed. In this effort too the therapist is sensitive to any shift during the session, any problematic situation, and is always ready to role play and use imagery.

The main focus of the therapy is to teach the client a variety of cognitive and behavioral skills that are applicable to the stated goals. In Sessions 3 or 4, the three-column DTR, the most used cognitive tool of CBT (Beck et al., 1979), is explained. They include the event, the cognitive distortions (actual thoughts), and emotions. Skills include the repetitive (daily) use of both the three and later the five-column DTRs (adding the challenges and the later reformulation of thoughts as well as ratings) to (a) identify cognitive distortions, (b) examine the evidence to support or dispute particular beliefs, and (c) teach the client specific skills for challenging unhelpful thoughts and developing alternative views.

This technique is so simple as to be abused because its value is taken for granted. In the five-column DTR the task is to identify one or more situations that have been recent problems. Emotions are identified and rated. The client is then told to look at what "you told yourself": "Do you see any distortions in your thinking (like the ones we discussed last week)?" The evidence is evaluated. The client is then asked if those thoughts are helpful. "Could you have said something different to yourself?" The next task is to generate alternative thoughts. The client is taught errors of thinking especially those most apt at older age. Eventually a reformulation is developed. Ratings of beliefs and emotions are also provided. The vertical arrow technique is also used: "What does it mean about you as a person?" The "vertical arrow" works backward along the client's chain of reasoning until arriving at his or her erroneous premise.

Other techniques are used also. Often the client can see a tension between head and heart. A rational emotive role play may assist in the separation of these two (What does your brain say? What does your heart say?) The person is not their feelings and can be greater than these. Feelings do not make truth. Often the client benefits from a discussion of the advantages/disadvantages of their beliefs, from developing a yardstick to better assess their situation, and from acting "as if" things were different. (See Box A-3.)

Often too the older client benefits from an attack on core reasons for lack of change—"I cannot change," "Small change is meaningless," "Change won't make me feel better." The therapist should always consider asking how likely the client is to carry out a task. Reasons to the contrary are important and rich with therapeutic material. Always such techniques are used in the context of "It is understandable that you would believe. . . ."

Mood and Behavior

Daily mood monitoring or a Pleasant Events Schedule (PES), or preferably both (Gallagher-Thompson, 1980), are used. Clients track their mood between sessions,

---

Box A-3
Cognitive Therapy Generic Model

1. Get example (write it down).
    (a) Get situation (a).
    (b) Get feelings or behavior (c).
    (c) Get thoughts (b)—write them down.
2. Restate thoughts in clear way or as a fear statement.
3. Rate belief and fear.
4. Intervene.
    (a) Is it true? Ever not true? (Reality testing)
    (b) How else could you view it? (Alternative explanation)
    (c) Is it as bad as it seems? (Lower importance)
    (d) Is it all your fault? (Reattribution)
    (e) How likely is it to happen? (Decatastrophize)
    (f) Is my standard too high? (Criteria testing)
5. Rerate belief and fear.
6. Teach thinking errors, especially overgeneralization, awfulizing, excessive demands on self or others, mind reading and "should" statements.
7. Use vertical arrow technique: What does this say about you as a person?: Is that important? Does it matter?
8. Homework assignment: Test belief and fear.
    (a) Get feedback to check perceptions.
    (b) Act differently and observe.
    (c) Look for contrary evidence.
    (d) Practice alternative thoughts.
    (e) Assure homework compliance.

---

rate the level of depression, and give one or two reasons why they think they felt the way they did or mention daily events. At some point they fill out the PES and identify several events for application in their life. These are then performed over time and the mood ratings continue. The results are plotted. Often the mood scales are elevated as a result of the pleasant events.

Journal writing (self-monitoring) can be used too, as trauma/depressed elders under- or overestimate the frequency of key events. In this way, skill deficits are identified, and training, like assertive behavior, can be applied.

Relaxation

DTR

Content of 3-column Technique

| Situation | Emotion | Cognitive |

Content of 6-column Technique

| Situation | Emotion Rate | Cognition Authentic Thought |
| Evidence | Balanced Thought | Mood Rate |

☐ Post Script

Termination is never far away. It is also elusory. It has been our experience that the continuance of therapy is a good thing. This involves an open door policy, including booster sessions, continued phone contact, and periodic mailings. Each client receives a "Maintenance Guide" that is a summary document of their sessions, strengths and weaknesses, as well as a focus on issues of potential relapse. Clients are schooled to watch for triggers, cope with problems, and apply an armamentarium of techniques. For this, booster sessions are encouraged.

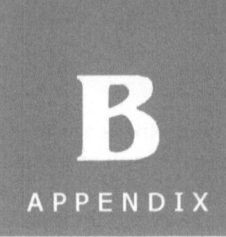

Treatment Rules for Personality Disorders

☐ Overall Rx for PDs

Therapy is not defined by techniques but by conceptualization. It is a model of care that has rules. In clients with PDs, their "head" changes before their gut. This points to what is necessary for the treatment of a PD; the person must experience the "sensation of the PD" and "know" that this is a problem state before change takes place. As a general rule, the clinician attacks the overall rigidity in the PD (the built-in constraints), to increase flexibility and decrease self-defeating patterns.

In addition, a key feature of this therapy is the "connection" between mood changes and interpersonal problems. The patient knows that they cause problems. Problems re-occur most in disputes, grief, role transitions, and as a function of skill deficits. In fact, a linking of the mood and event is most helpful. An understanding of setbacks is critical – What did you want in that situation? What options did you have to achieve what you wanted? What could you have done? What can you do next time? The patient needs to know what it is that they want and how they can get this. This is best with a review of the important relationships in the person's life. It is best done in the here and now, and done honestly.

Initial Questions of "Do I?"

What is involved with this patient with Axis II?
How do I interface with the treatment of Axis I?
The conceptualization of a PD person may alter over time
Think double—Axis I and Axis II
Think modules and stages
What about medications?
Who to bring in? Who's in charge?
Take time to Dx

If You Decide to Treat Axis II, Then Know That …

PD work is hard and boring
Therapist must be active and in charge
Therapist must define roles (therapist and patient)
Therapist must educate/negotiate
Therapist must prepare for the long haul
Therapist must prepare for resistance (No pain/no gain)
Therapist must be explicit with PDs. Tell the patient. Can't be done in inpatient setting: Too tough to do all the time in Rx.
Therapist must get commitment

Overall Goals: Do the Vision Thing

Symptoms count most at the gate: Attend to them.
Axis II integrative therapy
   Polarities
   Domains

Particulars

1. Goal Thinking around Personality

The therapist is doing therapy. This starts with the formulation of goals.

What do you want from therapy?
How would you be different?
How do you get in your way?
Imagine a year form now …

Typical PD statements

Either you are X or you have a belief that you are so.
Although self-defeating, it is who I am.
What does your brain say?; What does the gut say?
Imagine life 10 years form now with this belief?
Perhaps you are not yet ready for this form of therapy

2. Cognition First

Remember that all PDs have automatic thoughts. These are fed by beliefs. These of course could be images. But cognitive distortions bind anxiety and other psychopathologies by constructing a secondary reality that reduces the dissonance between the inner and outer world. Secondary realities are fostered further by the many cognitive distortions. At its root, thinking is generally causing the problem. It fosters a kind of mind reading and faulty prediction. Additionally, feelings or sensations may disrupt the proceedings. If so, the feeling requires a full investigation, labeling, unearthing, and desensitizing (below). Finally, problems could arise due to the fear of the future. Here the strategy is to normalize; to reach the edge of the unknown is a problem for everyman.

In general the therapist is tightening or loosening cognitions. Tightening would involve questions such as: "Tell me more about that." Loosening would involve queries like: "When were you not that way?" The therapist needs to be therapeutically practical. This involves the constant deconstructing of negative or self-defeating thoughts by reframing, challenge self-limiting constructions, and so forth.

As part of the case formulation, the issue of core beliefs are central to the plan. These evolve to automatic thoughts (ATs). In fact, a Beck model of this process is:

Core Beliefs⟶Intermediate Beliefs⟶Automatic Thoughts
Attitude
Assumptions
Rules

Core beliefs then are the "core cognitions" of the person's PD. They are subserved by intermediate beliefs and ATs. It is through the examination of ATs that common themes emerge. Several techniques are used to expose the core belief:

Downward arrow
Core belief worksheet
Early Learning
Education

Several techniques are used to address the core belief:

Advantages/Disadvantages of belief
Cognitive continuum
Behavioral experiments
Act "as if"
Role play, emotional side and rational side
Monitoring core beliefs
Restructure early memories.
Coping cards
Imagery and rehearsal
SUDS (subjective units of distress)
Disputation and rational reaction
Debriefing
Capsule summaries used frequently.

3. Get Small in Therapy

Above all, the therapist needs to set the agenda (agenda setting) (Burns, 1999). That is, he/she needs to be molecular and get the individual problem situation. Several methods apply.

Role play; use Anxiety Management Training methods
Get a molecular representation of the problem. Be data centered.
Special techniques—Cognitive restructuring
   Identify automatic triggers
   Label them
   Dispute with challenges (probability/severity)
   Develop coping strategies
   Challenge schema
   Exposure to negative beliefs
   Experiments (expect to pass or use coping card)
   Breathing and self rewards

4. Emotion

People with a PD are addicted to the "comfort" of the emotion. The therapist needs to respect affect: Affect recruits cognitions. The therapist needs to identify emotions and help the person to tolerate previously unacceptable emotions. This may involve an attention to the imagery in emotions. The use of experiential, "now" techniques is most helpful here.

5. Be an Interpersonal Therapist

The therapist needs to point out "now events." Statements apply such as:

> "You seem to want me to . . ."
> "Are you aware that . . ."
> "Has it ever happened that you . . ."
> Be Reflexive and nonreflexive.

The therapist can maintain a present focus with genuine inner contact. He/she can bring the person into the present by attending to current feeling, sensations, and thoughts. Remember that memory is present consciousness.

6. Be Developmental

The therapist can assure that the life span is respected. Actually in this case this involves a focus on the naturalness of early learnings: "How could you be otherwise." Statements apply such as:

> If you have a screen or filter around you, then you will see things in a certain way.
> What if this way of processing has been in existence since childhood?
> What would be the effect of continually seeing things in this way?
> Can you see how your core belief feels true and yet is false?

The clinician can make vivid the notion that: "This really was you!" The clinician can attend to issues of the past and enable a sense of agency in the context of the past. Now, the person canm change.

7. Use a Core Conflict Model

The clinician can ground problems in selected systems. This is a systematic evocative unfolding. The sequence is:

> This was you.
> > You expected . . .
> > Your job was . . .
> > You could only see . . .
> Anchor past times when similar: See how data could be only interpreted this way; identify themes in your life
> Identify the price paid (pain)
> Wonder if patient wants to change

This sequence can be performed on any "puzzling" issue. The therapist can then get back to the issues of PD in light of the particulars of the situation.

8. Identify and Highlight Core Personality Issues

Schizoid:
  Obvious⟶
    I am okay except for ...
    Social skills and reduce craziness
    Give feedback on Pt's responses
  Subtle⟶
    Get interpersonal involvement and go after wherever the emotion is
Avoidant:
  Obvious⟶
    I may get hurt ...
    Evaluation anxiety
    Going blank
    Mind reading
  Subtle⟶
    Microanalysis of event
    Childhood repetition experiences
Depressive:
  Obvious⟶
    I am not good enough
    Use CBT especially helplessness
    Pt accepts pain
    Use BDI
  Subtle⟶
    Be proactive
Dependent:
  Obvious⟶
    I need other people ...
    Continuum
    Dichotomous thinking
  Subtle⟶
    Decision making problem
    Who they are as people
Histrionic:
  Obvious⟶
    I must be loved ...
    Controlling or reactive
    Be specific
  Subtle⟶
    Explore relationships in detail
    Fear loss of exciting life
    What do they want?
Narcissist:
  Obvious⟶
    I am special
    Do they want something or are they depressed?
    Stroke (reward) and spit (challenge)
  Subtle⟶
    Unmet expectation
    Be psychodynamic/existential

Antisocial:
  Obvious⟶
    If I do not act, they will . . .
    What does he/she want (clarify your role)
    Anger management
    Choice review
  Subtle⟶
    Feelings are teachable moments
Sadistic:
  Obvious⟶
    I am right, you are not . . .
    Be behavioral and contractual
  Subtle⟶
    Be genuine and reality based
Compulsive:
  Obvious⟶
    I must avoid mistakes . . .
    Perfection and inflexibility
    Get to feel
  Subtle⟶
    Get to be happy
    Get molecular (get decisive action/stabilize self other conflict)
Negativistic:
  Obvious⟶
    I want help but . . .
    Contain, contain, contain
    Watch hostility
    Predict next problem and relapse prevent
  Subtle⟶
    Get two columns of cognitions
Self Defeating:
  Obvious⟶
    Life is unfair and I will prove it . . .
    Teach about the personality
  Subtle⟶
    Abused as a child
    Feeling are unspecified and unclear
    What is success?

Schizotypal/Paranoid/Borderline Personalities are structurally deficient (mini-psychotic breaks, social withdrawal, severe rigidity, and severe disconnection with thoughts and reality).

9. Use Monitors and Know When to Back Off

The therapist needs to have the patient monitor cognitions, emotions, and behaviors on a regular basis. This implies the use of many CBT methods. They should also support effort, not results.

In the pursuit of a goal too the client will get frustrated and the therapist needs to back up and re-build alliance and then re-state goals and progress. One technique that is helpful is advantages/disadvantages (Burns, 1999). The therapist should also employ paradox (You may not be ready for this). The following is a list of PD resistance issues.

Personality-Based Resistance Issues/Questions

1. Use labels for resistance as in "the alone personality" to heighten and objectify the problem.
2. Pay special attention to details of patient, session to session
3. Acknowledge that therapy is difficult and that change requires some anxiety
4. Speak in client' language and avoid judgments
5. Gently confront unpleasantness in the therapeutic relationship
6. Don't skip uncomfortable issues
7. Be careful with compliments, giving credit for work done
8. Ask for feedback
9. Use paradox→"You may not be ready for this. . ."
10. Assess skill levels→"What skills does the client lack that might make it practically difficult or impossible at this point for him or her to actively collaborate with treatment?"
11. Respect past→"When and under what circumstances has the client been similarly disinclined to try to change or accept help in the past?"
    —"What other relationships in the client's past and present are called to mind by the current conflict between the client and therapist?";
    —"How is the current scenario in therapy similar to and distinct from previous situations in the client's life when he or she resisted change or direction?"
12. Think cognitive→What was going through your mind just then?
    —"And what did that mean to you?"
13. Think for secondary gains→"What would occur if you were to change?"
14. Think environment→Does the client have a spouse who is actively sabotaging the client's progress?
15. Monitor self→Is the therapist acting in a disengaged manner?

10. Relapse Prevention

The therapist needs to apply the techniques of relapse prevention. They constitute an idea of the person with a PD is in a "new" deficit -stresses of life and PD overlearned patterns are more persuasive than the skills of the person. People with PDs must be educated here. One method is the use of the "map of US." Relapse works like a map of the bottom of the US: There are dips in performance as with Texas, then successes, then dips again (Florida). Naturally booster sessions are needed.

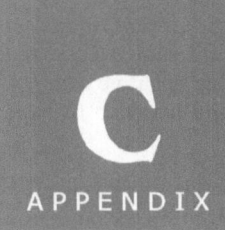

APPENDIX

EMDR Relaxation Procedure

The eight-step exercise (modified from Shapiro, 1995) is as follows:

Step 1: *Image*. The clinician and client identify an image of a safe place that the client can easily evoke and that creates a personal feeling of calm and safety.

Step 2: *Emotions and sensations*. The clinician asks the client to focus on the image, feel the emotion, and identify the location of the pleasing physical sensations.

Step 3: *Enhancement*. The clinician may use soothing hypnotic tones to enhance the imagery and affect. He should take care to convey a sense of safety and security for the client, who is asked to report when she feels the emotions.

Step 4: *Eye movements*. The positive response is further expanded by including a series of eye movements. The clinician should use the direction and speed of movement that the client has identified as most comfortable and should say, "Bring up the image of a place that feels safe and calm. Concentrate on where you feel the pleasant sensations in your body and allow yourself to enjoy them. Now concentrate on those sensations and follow my fingers with your eyes." At the end of the set the clinician asks the client, "How do you feel now?" If the client feels better, the clinician should do four to six more sets. If the client's positive emotions have not increased, the clinician should try alternative directions of eye movements until the client reports improvement.

Step 5: *Cue word*. The client is then asked to identify a single word that fits the picture (e.g., "relax," "beach," "mountain," "trees") and to rehearse it mentally as pleasant sensations and a sense of emotional security are noticed and enhanced by the clinician's directions. This procedure is repeated four to six times, along with additional eye movements.

Step 6: *Self-cueing*. The client is then instructed to repeat the procedure on her own, bringing up the image and the word and experiencing the positive feelings (both emotions and physical sensations), without any eye movements. When the client has successfully repeated the exercise independently, the clinician points out how the client can use it to relax during times of stress.

Step 7: *Cueing with disturbance.* To emphasize the preceding point, the clinician asks the client to bring up a minor annoyance and notice the accompanying negative feelings. The clinician then guides the client through the exercise until the negative feelings dissipate.

Step 8: *Self-cueing with disturbance.* The clinician then asks the client to bring up a disturbing thought once again and to follow the exercise, this time without the clinician's assistance, to its relaxing conclusion.

Once this exercise has been completed, the clinician should instruct the client to practice it at home every day by calling up the positive feelings and the associated word and image while she uses a relaxation tape.

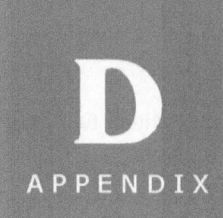

APPENDIX

Relaxation

We provide two components. There is the 12-8-4-4-0 muscle tension program, followed by the relaxation log. We use these together. The log, however, is suitable for use with any relaxation method.

MUSCLE RELAXATION PLUS IMAGERY

This relaxation method is set forth in five steps. It is best to try each step at least **twice per day,** 10–15 minutes at a time, **for a week.**

GOAL: To be able to tell yourself to relax, and then feel yourself begin to feel calm all over.

> *Note:* *It will be necessary to reach this level of skill, so that later you can test yourself in situations in which you are angry.*

Step 1.
Keeping a record: Find the worksheet labeled "Daily Log."

In the far left column, record the date.

Next to the date, write down how calm or upset you feel now, from 0–10, with ten being the most upset you can imagine (see scale at top).

After you practice your relaxation, write down how calm you were able to get during the practice session.

Use this record before and after each practice session. It will help you to keep track of your progress.

Muscle Relaxation: Sit in a comfortable position. Move through the twelve muscle groups in the chart on the next page. With each muscle group, **tense that area for about ten seconds, then relax for about twenty seconds.** Note that for the arms and legs, the exercise is performed first with one, then the other, then both. As you do the exercise, **let your mind focus on the difference** between the tension and the relaxation. Notice the relaxation settling in, as the tension in that area drifts away. After you complete the sequence of twelve muscle groups, sit quietly for a couple of minutes. Let your mind focus on a personal image, as described below.

Imagery: Bring to mind a scene that you have experienced in person, a real memory that is calm and peaceful. Let it become as clear as possible, with all of the senses. *What do you see, hear, feel (touch, temperature), smell?*

12 MUSCLE GROUPS

Lower arm: left, right, both together	Make fist, palm down, and pull wrist up toward upper arm.
Upper arm: left, right, both together	Tense biceps. With arms by side, pull upper arm back and toward the side without touching. (Try not to tense lower arm while doing this; let lower arm hang loosely.)
Lower leg and foot: left, right, both together	Extend leg so it is straight. Point toe upward toward knees.
Thighs	Pull knees together until upper legs feel tense.
Abdomen	Pull in stomach toward back.
Chest and breathing	Take a deep breath and hold it about ten seconds, then release.
Shoulders and lower neck	Shrug shoulders, then bring shoulders up until they touch the ears.
Back of neck	Put head back and press against back of chair.
Lips	Press lips together; don't clench teeth or jaw.
Eyes	Close eyes tightly, but not too hard (be careful if you wear contact lenses).
Lower forehead	Pull eyebrows toward each other and down.
Upper forehead	Raise eyebrows, wrinkling the top of your forehead.

8 MUSCLE GROUPS

Both arms
Both lower legs
Abdomen
Chest
Shoulders
Back of neck
Eyes
Forehead

Both arms: Hold both arms in front of you, bending at the elbow. Tense the biceps and pull the wrist back.

Step 2: Move through a sequence of tense-release exercises with eight muscle groups.

For the **eyes** and the **back of neck,** tense and relax as usual. Then repeat, tensing only **half as strongly** as the time before, then relax. Finally, tense half as much as the time before (one quarter of the original strength).

At the end, bring to mind your personal image, as before, for one or two minutes.

Do this exercise twice daily for at least one week.

4 MUSCLE GROUPS

Both arms
Chest
Shoulders/neck
Face

Slightly hunch shoulders while drawing the neck in and back.

Close eyes tightly while drawing up the rest of the face.

Step 3: Move through a sequence of four muscle groups. For neck/shoulders and face, repeat at **half strength,** then repeat again at **one quarter strength.**

Sit quietly for one or two minutes, using personal image as before.

Repeat exercise twice daily for at least one week.

Step 4: Try to feel the feeling of relaxation in each of the four areas, without going through the tense-release exercises. If necessary, perform the tense-release sequence. Sit quietly, using the image as before. Repeat twice daily.

Step 5: Take a deep breath. Think the word, "Relax." Notice the relaxation in each area. Let the relaxation settle in and the tension drift away.

DAILY LOG

NAME	LAST 4

Rate from 0 to 10 how tense or upset you felt **before and after** each relaxation practice. Write the number in the appropriate boxes below.

0	1	2	3	4	5	6	7	8	9	10
NONE		SLIGHT		MODERATE			ALOT		AS MUCH AS YOU CAN IMAGINE	

DATE	BEFORE RELAXATION	AFTER RELAXATION	DATE	BEFORE RELAXATION	AFTER RELAXATION

INDEX

ABOUT THE AUTHORS

Leon Albert Hyer, Ph.D., is a professor of Psychiatry and Director of Geropsychological Services at the University of Medicine and Dentistry of New Jersey. Prior to 1998, Dr. Hyer held the posisiton of co-Director of the Augusta War Trauma Project at the VA Medical Center, was a professor at the University of Georgia, and maintained a part-time private practice over his years in Georgia. He has received the Veterans Administration Superior Performance Award ten times since 1983. Dr. Hyer's concentration in gerontology and traumatology is clear through his varied appointments and programs over nearly 25 years.

Steven James Sohnle, Psy.D., holds a postdoctoral fellowship in geropsychology at University of Medicine and Dentistry of New Jersey/University Behavioral Health Care in Edison, New Jersey. Doctor Sohnle's current work includes individual and group psychotherapy with older adults, neuropsychological testing and report writing for dementia and Huntington's Disease diagnostic and management clinics, and cognitive and personality testing with adults.